D1716244

Methods in Biotechnology and Bioengineering

(For Pharmacy and Other Biosciences)

Methods in Biotechnology and Bioengineering

(For Pharmacy and Other Biosciences)

S.P. Vyas
M.Pharm., Ph.D.
Post doc. (University of London, UK)
Professor (Pharm. Biotechnology), Deptt. of Pharmaceutical Sciences
Dean, Faculty of Technology
Dr. H. S. Gour University, Sagar (M.P.)

D.V. Kohli
M.Pharm., Ph.D.
Reader, Department of Pharmaceutical Sciences
Dr. H. S. Gour University, Sagar (M.P.)

[redacted]

CBS

CBS PUBLISHERS & DISTRIBUTORS
4596/1-A, 11 Darya Ganj, New Delhi - 110 002 (India)

ISBN : 81-239-0800-8

[redacted]

First Edition : 2002
Reprint : 2003

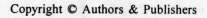

Copyright © Authors & Publishers

All rights reserved. No part of this book may be reproduced or transmitted in any form or by any means, electronic or mechanical, including photocopying, recording, or any information storage and retrieval system without permission, in writing, from the authors and publishers.

Published by :
Satish Kumar Jain for CBS Publishers & Distributors,
4596/1-A, 11 Darya Ganj, New Delhi - 110 002 (India)

Printed at :
India Binding House, Delhi - 110 032

660.6
V99m

Preface

With the invention of recombinant DNA technology and advancement in the knowledge relating to nucleic acid biochemistry, molecular biology and other biotechnologies, we have entered in an era marked by dramatic and discernible changes in the methodologies and altered perceptions about the living systems. Like many others, pharmaceutical biotechnology is one of the disciplines, which emerged very strongly with applied potentials and promises. It has been realized that virtually the health sector would selectively be benefited by pharmaceutical biotechnology and biotechnologicals. With the invention of recombinant technology and its ensuing effects, one can realize that future of pharmaceuticals shall be underwritten by miniaturized molecular drug delivery systems. The applications will cover immunodiagnostics, gene cloning, recombinant protein synthesis, novel pharmaceuticals, gene therapy, molecular vaccines, etc.

Looking back we do feel that venturing into writing a book on Pharmaceutical Biotechnology, probably the first of its kind, was a stupendous task driven by enthusiasm. Nevertheless, it is heartening to admit that it gained widespread appreciation and could define a subject emphatically in an exquisite and vivid manner. Ever since we have been continuously inspired and asked by our colleagues from all over the country, scientists from the laboratory and instructors from institutions that there is a need of workable concise experimental protocols in biotechnology and bioengineering. This is to train the budding pharmacists and biologists in biotechnological and cell biological processes. This would not only fulfil the requirements of regular practical classes but also instil the component of confidence in students in order to make them mature biotechnologists of future. Here resides the ray of hope, which prompted us to present the comprehensive compilation of well-tested protocols from cell biology and biotechnology laboratories. Hope teachers and students shall appreciate this effort.

We are thankful to our families for sparing us of responsibilities, continual encouragement and support during the preparation of the manuscript of the book. We acknowledge the sources of protocols. We are thankful to our scientists Mr. Amit Rawat, Mr. Vivek Mishra, Ms. Preeti Venugopalan, Mr. Praveen Dubey, Mr. Paramjit Singh, Mr. Sanyog Jain, Mr. Prabhakaran D., Mr. Vaibhav Sihorkar, Mr. Sunil Mahor and Mr. Rajendra Pratap Singh for their help in the preparation of manuscript and secretarial assistance. We also express our sincere gratitude to CBS Publishers, New Delhi for their expert assistance in quality publication of this book. We welcome suggestions and comments from teachers, students and other readers, which will help in improving the contents.

S. P. Vyas
D. V. Kohli

Contents

CHAPTER 1

Cell Culture Techniques

- Animal cell culture
- Chronology of cell culture development
- Cell culture laboratory
- Lymph node cell culture
- Mouse macrophage culture
- Bone marrow culture
- Spleen cell culture
- Live cell culture
- Propagation of cell lines
- Mycoplasma testing of cell lines
- Suspension cultures
- Plant cell culture
- Callus cultures
- Organ culture
- Meristem culture
- Micropropagation
- Cloned cauliflower

ANIMAL CELL CULTURE

Growing cells of embryonic, adult tissue of animal or plant origin *in vitro* is called cell culturing. The cells are made free from tissue by mechanical, enzymatic or chemical means. The dispersed cells are resuspended in an appropriate nutrient medium at optimum conditions. These cells are inoculated into culture vessels and then incubated in a stationary position. After settling out, the cells adhere to and stretch out on the surface of vessel and transform into morphology very close to that *in vivo*. These cells multiply until a confluent sheet layer is formed. The primary objective in cell culture procedures is to disrupt/digest intercellular material that binds cells together. The deaggregation of cells of some organ can be achieved by perfusion of organ with an enzyme (e.g. trypsin, collagenase) or a chemical. However, some organs are not easily perfused and therefore the procedure adopts mincing the tissue into small fragments with sharp scissors, scalpels, razor blades or cataract knives. Mechanical dispersion involves pressure homogenization and passage through a nylon or stainless steel mesh is applicable when soft tissues especially those from young embryo are employed.

Animal cell culture techniques are having vast applications in the field of pharmaceutical biotechnology. Cell culture models are used for examining intestinal absorption of drugs, drugs or peptide absorption across blood brain barrier (BBB), hepatic absorption of drugs and for *in vitro* experimentation etc.

CHRONOLOGY OF CELL CULTURE DEVELOPMENT

Primary Cell Culture

These cells are derived from the tissues and organs of animals, which possess a diploid caryotype. These cells when cultured *in vitro*, have the tendency to attach on the surface of the vessel and after a definite time they attain the similar morphology as *in vivo*. Such cells divide mitotically and remain identical to their progenitors. These cells retain the ability to recognize each other when they come in contact. This is attributed to their identical surface components. This is well established that genetically identical cells show a ruffling movement towards each other. When they come in contact, ruffling stops which is termed as contact inhibition of movement.

This phenomenon explains the formation of confluent monolayer on the cultured vessels. After confluent monolayer formation, cells continue to divide mitotically, however at one point the cells growth/ division stops because of overcrowding of cells. This phenomenon is termed as density dependent inhibition of mitosis. After density dependent inhibition, the chances of transformation of normal cells to malignant cells arise and therefore culture should be split into two or more. A chronological pattern of growth of human cells cultured *in vitro* is shown in Figure 1.1, in which, phase I terminates with the formation of the first confluent culture. Phase II shows the continuous subdivision of cells while phase III represents the degeneration of cell culture.

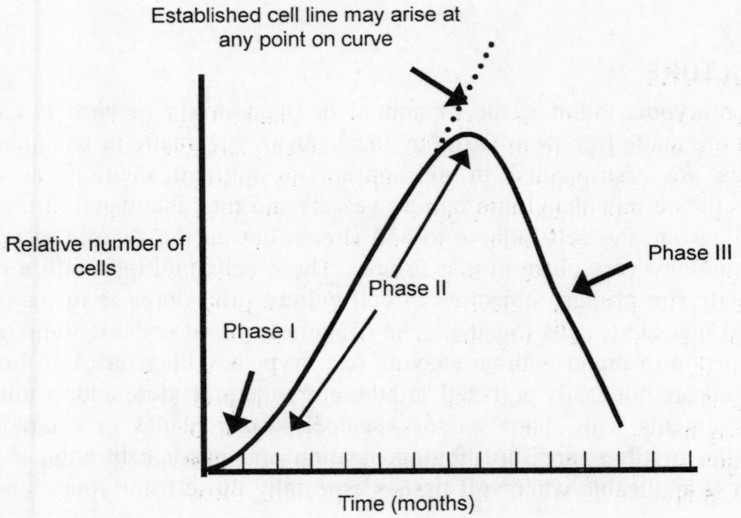

Fig. 1.1. Graphical representation of growth of animal cell culture

Established Cell Lines

Established cell lines are like tumour cells. Such cell lines are generated spontaneously as a rare occurrence in diploid cells. This process is called as transformation. Transformation can be induced in cell culture by three ways

- A cell is diploid culture transformed by some spontaneous event,
- A haploid cell can be transformed by adding a carcinogen to the culture and
- Transformation in haploid cells can be induced by virus.

Cell cultures can be grown in two ways viz. monolayer cultures and suspension cultures.

Monolayer Cultures

When cultures are grown on a supporting surface, they are called monolayer cultures, e.g. cultures grown in glass or plastic bottles, flasks, tubes, Petri dishes, microtitre plates, etc. After dispensing the cells in these vessels, they are incubated in a stationary condition so that the cells form a confluent monolayer.

Suspension Cultures

When the cells are grown in suspension and are not allowed to attach to any support surface, such cultures are called suspension cultures. For this purpose cell suspension is agitated continuously so that the cells remain suspended in suspension.

CELL CULTURE LABORATORY

Cell culture is specifically conducted in a well-defined laboratory premise where by all means near absolute sterility is maintained and modes are available to avoid any possible cross contamination. A well self-contained laboratory (Fig. 1.2) for the purpose houses a range of generally used equipments. Some important equipments with their principles and uses, are discussed as follows.

- Laminar flow cabinets
- Liquid nitrogen containers
- Deep freezers
- Refrigerators
- Balances
- Distillation apparatus
- pH meter
- Incubator
- Water bath
- Centrifuge
- Roller cell culture apparatus
- Surgical kit

Instruments

Centrifuges

The centrifuges used in cell culture laboratory range from bench models for sedimenting cells to ultracentrifuges are also capable of sedimenting small viruses. The performance of the centrifuge is rated as the relative centrifugal force (RCF) expressed in terms of G, which is calculated from the following formula:

$$RCF(G) = 1.118 \times 10^{-5} \times R \times N^2 \quad \text{------------------------------------[1.1]}$$

Where, R= Distance in centimeters from the centre of the centrifuge shaft to the extended tip of the centrifuge tube, N= Revolutions of the centrifuge head per minute (rpm).

It is obvious from the above formula that although the speed of the centrifuge (rpm) is the most important factor, the radius (R) of the centrifuge head also influences the rate of sedimentation. Therefore, it is advisable to state the speed of the centrifuge in G rather than in rpm to avoid errors in techniques caused by using centrifuges of different sizes.

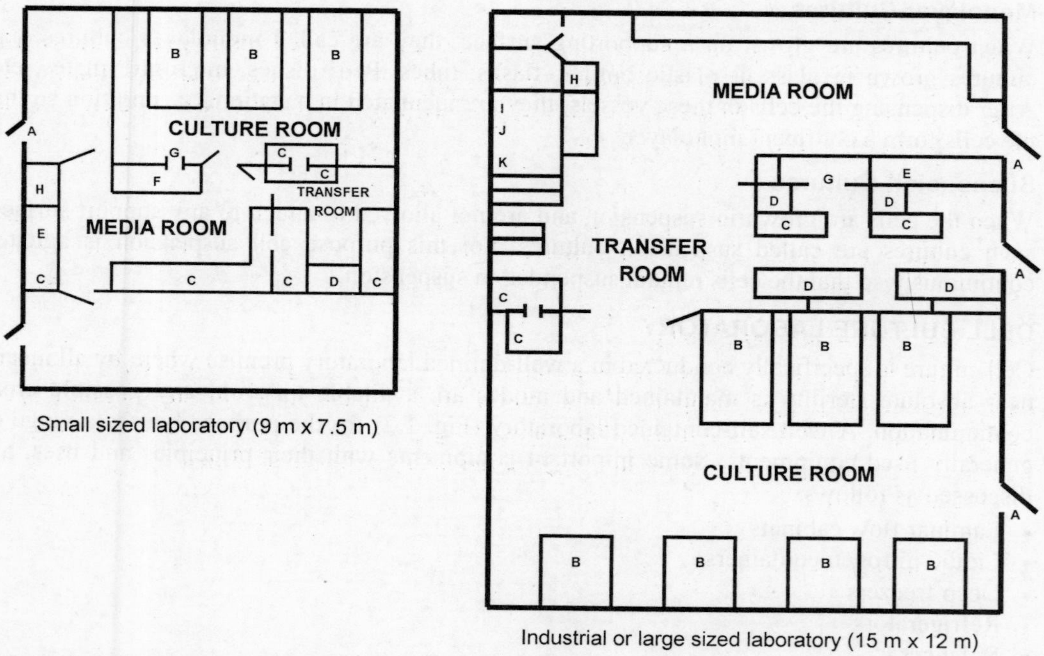

Fig. 1.2. Designs of small and large sized laboratory (A) entrance (B) shelves (C) counter (D) laminar air-flow cabinet (E) sink (F) gas outlet/burner (G) window (H) refrigerator and deep freezer (I) store (J) conference room (K) library

Laminar flow cabinets

These provide a sterile clean area to work and are highly satisfactory for cell culture and virus work. There are different types of laminar flow cabinets such as horizontal model, vertical model (Fig. 1.3) etc. A special model is available for working with dangerous pathogens such as viruses.

Filters

A variety of filters are available, but the most commonly used in the laboratory are the seitz filters with EKS grade, seitz filter pads for sterilization by filtration of reagents and media and the millipore filters. The millipore filters consist of millipore filter holder and filter pads with varying pore diameter. They are suitable for the sterilization by filtration of the reagents and media as well as for removing the microbial contamination in viral samples and also determining the size of virus particles in a viral sample.

Washing of New Glassware

New glassware contain toxic products derived from manufacturing process and packing and hence they should be carefully washed, as suggested below:

- Autoclave at 15 lb/inch^2 pressure for 30 minutes to 1 hour.
- Wash several times with tap water.
- Immerse in a 4% solution of hydrochloric acid in water overnight.
- Rinse in tap water.
- Immerse in detergent solution overnight. Scrub mechanically.
- Rinse in tap water several times to remove the detergent solution.
- Rinse once in double distilled water.
- Put immediately for drying in hot air cabinet at 63-70°C.

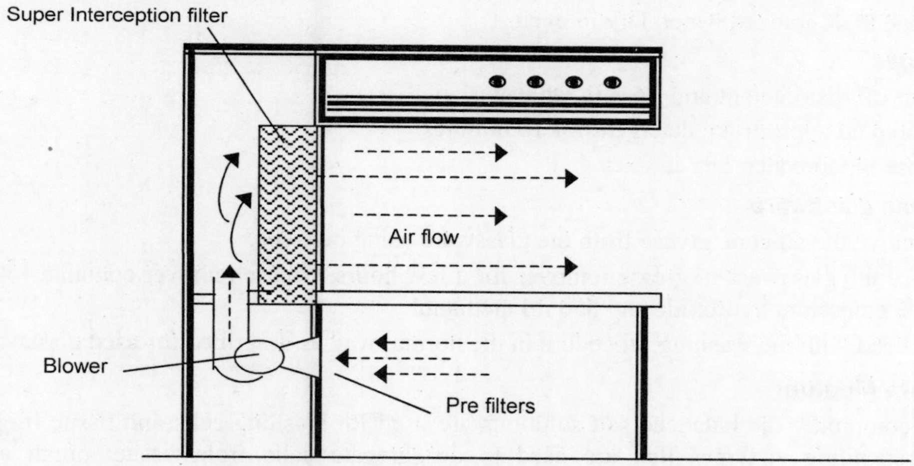

Fig. 1.3. Diagrammatic representation of horizontal laminar flow cabinet

Washing of used glassware

- Scrub the glassware with 10% soap solution.
- Wash with tap water thoroughly.
- Rinse in 0.05% HCl solution to neutralize the alkalinity of the detergent and tap water.
- Thoroughly wash with tap water.
- Rinse several times with triple glass distilled water.
- Put for drying in a hot air cabinet at 63-70°C.

Washing of rubber bungs

The above mentioned procedure is followed for rubber bungs, which are in use. New rubber bungs are subjected to the following treatment after autoclaving at 15 lb/inch^2 pressure for 30 minutes.

- Rinse in hot tap water.
- Boil in 20% sodium hydroxide solution for 20 minutes.
- Rinse in hot tap water.
- Boil in 20% hydrochloric acid solution for 20 minutes.
- Rinse in hot tap water. Rinse thoroughly in glass distilled water.

Sintered glass filters

- Sintered glass filters should be cleaned with strong acids after use. Concentrated sulphuric acid with a few crystals of sodium nitrate and sodium chlorate is passed through the filter.
- After this the filter should be rinsed with a large volume of glass distilled water.

Pipettes

- Wash in tap water.
- Boil in appropriate detergent solution for 10 minutes.
- Wash in continuous flow pipette washer for 4 hours.
- Rinse in de-ionized water. Dry in oven.

Syringes

- Pour off disinfectant and rinse in tap water.
- Boil in an appropriate detergent for 10 minutes.
- Rinse in tap water. Dry in oven.

Silicone glassware

- Remove the silicone grease from the glassware using benzene.
- Place the glassware in grease remover for a few hours. Grease remover contains 150 ml of 50% potassium hydroxide and 850 ml methanol.
- Proceed with the washing procedure in the normal way as described for used glassware.

Culture Medium

Most commonly the balanced salt solutions are used for washing cells and tissue fragments, for suspending enzymes that are used to deaggregate cells from tissue/ organ and for separation of cells from glass and plastic surfaces and as a basic unit in formulating cell culture media. Some commonly used media used in animal cell culture are given in Table 1.1.

Enzymes Used for Organ and Tissue Deaggregation

Trypsin

Trypsin (EC 3.4.4.4) is a pancreatic digestive enzyme found in the intestine, which is optimally active at pH 8.2. Trypsin preferentially catalyses hydrolysis of peptide bond between the carboxylic group of arginine and lysine and the amino acid next in sequence in the polypeptide chain. Enzyme also acts as an amidase and an esterase. Highly purified trypsin is available in 10 ml vials containing 125,000 NF units and in 25 ml vial containing 250,000 NF units.

Note

NF unit is used to define the potency of the enzyme for hydrolyzing N-benzoyl-L-arginine ethylester hydrochloride at 25°C. One unit is defined as that quantity of enzyme that causes a change in absorption at 253 nm of 0.003 unit/minute.

Table 1.1. Composition of various mediums used in animal cell culture

Component	Mol. wt.	Quantity in mg/l					
		Ringer's	Earle's	Hank's	Dulbecco's	Eagle's MEM	CMF -PBS
NaCl	58.44	6500	6800	8000	8000	6800	8000
KCl	74.56	140	400	400	200	400	300
$CaCl_2.2H_2O$	146.99		265	186			
$MgSO_4.7H_2O$	110.99	120	200	140	100		
$MgCl_2.6H_2O$	246.50		200	200			
Na_2HPO_4	203.31					200	
$Na_2HPO_4.7H_2O$	141.96				1150		730
$NaH_2PO_4.7H_2O$	267.96			90			
$NaH_2PO_4.H_2O$	138.0		140	60		1400	
KH_2PO_4	136.09		2200	350	200		200
$NaHCO_3$	84.01	200		1000		2000	
Glucose	180.16			10		1000	2000
Phenol red						10	

Preparation of trypsin

The following procedure is used for the preparation of trypsin solution

- Take 2.5 g of trypsin powder and place into a 1000 ml beaker. Add 5 ml of calcium and magnesium free physiological balanced salt (CMF-PBS).
- Stir it to make smooth paste.
- With continuous stirring add 900 ml of CMF-PBS to dissolve paste. Make the quantity sufficient to 1000 ml.
- Filter it to remove any residual material. Adjust the pH to 7.8 using 0.1N NaOH.
- Sterilize the solution by filtration. Dispense in bottles and store at –20°C.

Procedure for Typsinization

Tissue fragments are washed several times with BSS and transferred to a 500 ml trypsinization vessel (Fig. 1.4). Cover it to a level of 150 ml with the 0.25% of trypsin in CMF-PBS warmed to 37°C. Keep the flask on the rotary shaker for 1 hour. Collect the cells.

Another apparatus is also used to obtain the continuous dispersion of cells from tissue fragments. Tissue fragments are placed into a specially constructed flask (Fig. 1.5) and the flow of trypsin from a reservoir is controlled by a pinchcock. The fragments are agitated with a magnetic stirrer bar. A sump containing numerous holes is annealed into the bottom of the flask. This sump allows the suspended cell passage through it and by a receiving hole suspended cells are collected.

Collagenase

Collagenase (EC 3.4.4.19) acts specifically on native collagen at near physiological pH. The enzyme hydrolyzes polypeptides containing protein. It requires Ca^{++} for its activity. This enzyme is not used in phosphate as its potency diminishes in the presence of phosphate ions. This enzyme is useful for the deaggregation of cells from organs rich in connective tissue. In cell culture procedure a concentration of 0.01 to 0.05% is used.

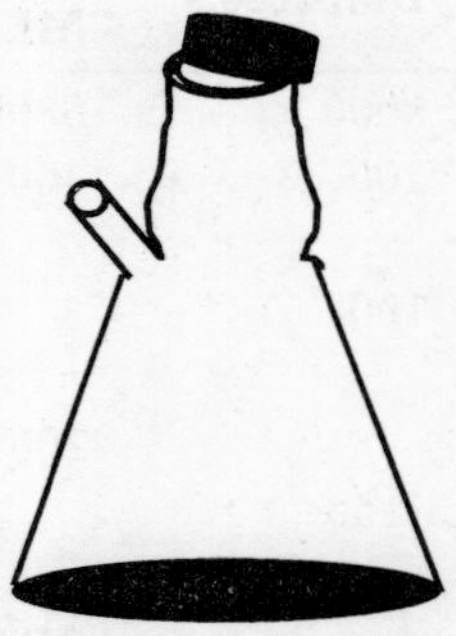

Fig. 1.4. Trypsinization flask

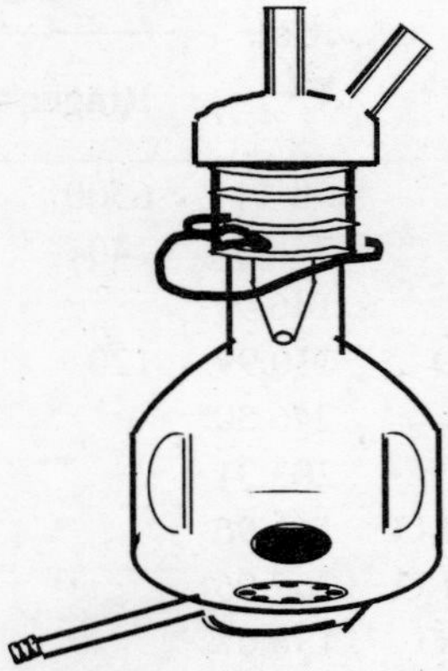

Fig. 1.5. Continuous trypsinization flask

Papain

Papain (EC 3.4.4.10) is a protease that hydrolyzes peptides and ester bonds. This enzyme is activated by cysteine and is useful in the dispersion of adult skeletal muscles with 0.01% cysteine in CMF-BSS at a concentration of 0.05%. Papain is less stable at room temperature and therefore a short but repeated treatment of tissue is preferable.

Elastase

Elastase (EC 3.4.4.7) is a pancreatic enzyme, which can digest a number of proteins. It can digest the fibrous protein, elastin, which is an integral part of connective tissues. Crystalline elastase is used at 0.05% for deaggregation purposes.

Chemical Compounds Used for Organ / Tissue Deaggregation

Chelating agent

The divalent cations Ca^{++} and Mg^{++} play an important role in maintaining integrity of the surface of animal cells. Omission of these cations weakens the integrity of cells. Ethylene diamine tetraacetic acid (EDTA) and Ethyleneglycol-bis-(β-aminoethylether)-N,N,N',N'-tetraacetic acid (EGTA) are used for the omission of divalent cation as they form stable complex with them.

EDTA is available in three forms

- Disodium hydrogen ethylene diamine tetraacetic acid.H_2O (Mol. Wt. 372.24)
- Tetrasodium methylene diamine tetraacetic acid.$2H_2O$ (Mol. Wt. 416.21)
- Tetrasodium methylene diamine tetraacetic acid. $3H_2O$ (common name Versene, Mol. Wt. 434.22)

Concentration in between 0.01 to 0.11 M is usually used for deaggregation of cells. For improved dispersion with trypsin, Versene is combined with trypsin.

EGTA (Mol. Wt. 380.25) chelates Ca^{++} but not Mg^{++} and is used for removing cells from a glass or plastic substrate at a concentration of 0.5 mM in combination with 0.05% trypsin.

Potassium complexing agent

Deaggregation with potassium complexing agent e.g. tetraphenylboron is based on the assumption that K^+ rather than Ca^{++} is predominantly involved in intercellular adhesion. Tetraphenyl boron is used at a concentration of 5 mM.

Cell Counting Procedures in Cell Culture

Counting using haemocytometer

Cell in suspension can be counted using haemocytometer. Haemocytometer is divided into 5 big squares each of, which is further, divided into 16 small squares (Fig. 1.6). Number of cells in the total 80 small square is counted.

Total cell count in $1mm^3$ volume is calculated using the following formula:

$$\text{Total cell count per mm}^3 = \frac{\text{Total number of cells x Dilution x 4000}}{\text{Total number of squares counted}} \quad \text{------------- [1.2]}$$

Procedure

- Dilute the cell suspension by approximation to bring the total number of cell count in between 100 to 1000.
- Set up haemocytometer by putting a precision ground cover slip on the raised support arm so that the two ruled areas in the upper and lower portions of slides are covered.
- Stir the diluted cell suspension with a capillary pipette and place a drop at the opening between haemocytometer and the coverslip in both the upper and lower chambers. The drop flows under the coverslip by capillary action and fills the chambers.
- Place haemocytometer onto stage of a microscope and locate the ruled area.
- When C1 is centred count all the cells in the 16 squares. (Cells that are counted include those touching the inner lines on the right and top but those touching the left and bottom lines are omitted). Move the focus to areas C2, C3, C4 and C5 and count all the cells.

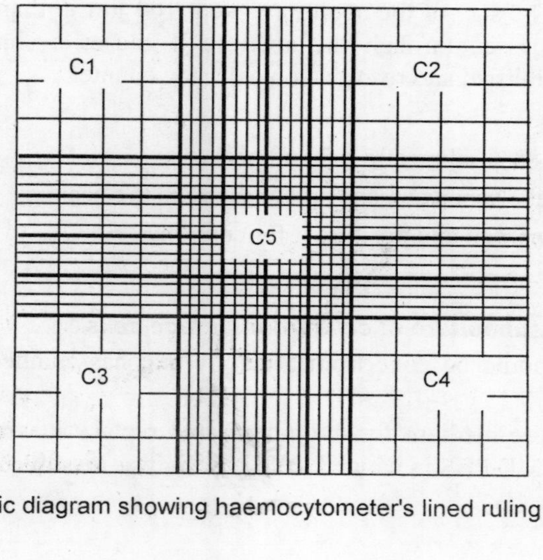

Fig. 1.6. Schematic diagram showing haemocytometer's lined ruling of one chamber

Viability Determination

To estimate the total viable cell population erythrosin B and trypan blue dyes are used. These dyes have negatively charged chromophore, which interacts with the damaged cell only.

Stock solutions

Erythrosin B

A 10X stock solution is prepared by dissolving 0.4 g of the dye in 100 ml Hanks' BSS.

Trypan Blue

A 10X stock solution is prepared by dissolving 0.2 g of the dye in100 ml of Hanks' BSS.

Procedure

- Mix a 0.5 ml cell suspension with 4.5 ml of dye. Dilute the cell suspension.
- Count both total and viable cell populations with haemocytometer as described previously.

Nuclear Count

To count cells attached to glass surface, nuclear count method is applied. In this method, citric acid destroys the cell membrane and crystal violet stains the nucleus.

Reagent

Dissolve 21.01 g of citric acid and 0.1 g crystal violet in 1 litre of distilled water. Add 100 mg of trypan blue and dissolve. Autoclave it for 10 minutes at 121°C.

Procedure

Mix 1 ml of cell suspension with 4 ml of citric acid-crystal violet reagent for 15 minutes. Count the nuclei in haemocytometer.

Electronic Cell Counting

Cells are poor conductor of electrical current compared to a saline solution and on this principle cells can be counted in a suspension by drawing through a small aperture through which current is continuously being conducted. An assembly of electronic cell counter is shown in Figure 1.7. Two large surface platinum electrodes are immersed in an electrolyte solution of 0.85% NaCl. A mercury manometer with electrical leads for metering sample volume is also placed. The size of the aperture is kept 100 μm in diameter, which is 75 μm long. When a cell is passed through the aperture it causes a sharp drop in electrical conductivity which is amplified and recorded on a decade counter.

Procedure

- Measure 24.5 ml of 0.85% saline into a 50 ml beaker.
- Withdraw 0.5 ml of cell suspension and add to saline in the beaker.
- Mix the cell suspension well and position it for counting.

Monolayer Culture

General procedure for subculture of cells from surface cells

- Subculture of cells should be done from a culture that has attained a form of confluent sheet.
- Decant the used culture medium for the culture and replace it with an equal volume of lukewarm media of CMF-PBS in which 0.25% trypsin was dissolved.

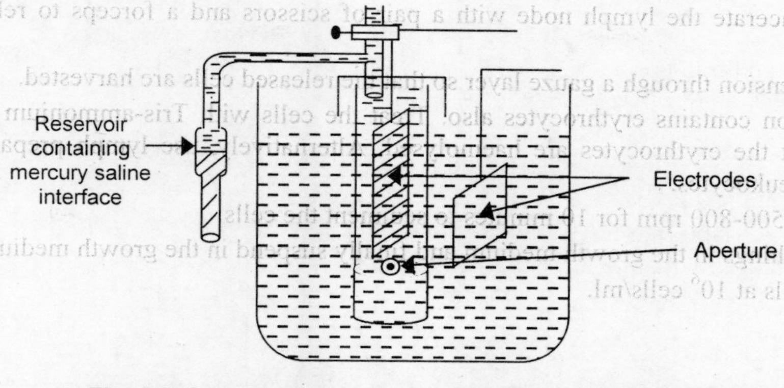

Fig. 1.7. Schematic diagram showing electronic cell counter

- Maintain the pH around 7.8 and incubate at 37°C for 5 to 10 minutes. The enzyme action dislodges the cells from inert surface.
- Gently triturate the suspension to disperse the cells.
- Add 1/10 volume of foetal calf serum of total volume suspension. This will stop the future activity of enzyme.
- Transfer the cell suspension to a conical flask and centrifuge at 200g for 5 minutes. This will pelletize the cells.
- Decant the trypsin solution and disperse the pellet in the same volume of complete growth medium.
- Count the cells and add the addition media so as to produce 2-3 x10^5 cells/ml.
- Inoculate the suspended cells in to clean sterilized culture vessel and keep the vessels in an incubator maintained at 37°C.

PROTOCOL 1.1

LYMPH NODE CELL CULTURE

Materials and Equipment

Lymph node, BSS medium, Tris-ammonium chloride buffer, Centrifuge, Haemocytometer, CO_2 incubator

Procedure

- Collect a lymph node from a young animal from which culture is desired, e.g., bovine, swine, ovine, etc. For this purpose, collect a precapsular lymph node or a mesenteric lymph node without any damage to it.
- Transfer the lymph node to a Petri dish containing BSS. Remove the fibrous tissues, fat and other connective tissues attached. Then remove the capsule.
- Transfer the lymph node to a fresh Petri dish and wash it.

- Tease and macerate the lymph node with a pair of scissors and a forceps to release the cells.
- Pass the suspension through a gauze layer so that the released cells are harvested.
- The suspension contains erythrocytes also. Treat the cells with Tris-ammonium chloride buffer so that the erythrocytes are haemolysed. Alternatively, use lymph preparation to separate the leukocytes.
- Centrifuge at 500-800 rpm for 10 minutes to sediment the cells.
- Give two washings in the growth medium and finally suspend in the growth medium.
- Adjust the cells at 10^6 cells/ml.

PROTOCOL 1.2

MOUSE MACROPHAGE CULTURE

Materials and Equipment

BSS medium, Heparin, Ethanol, Surgical kit, Centrifuge, CO_2 incubator, Haemocytometer.

Procedure

- Keep the culture medium and the glassware to be used in the refrigerator to prevent the macrophage from sticking to the glass surface. Give preference to siliconized glassware.
- Select a 1-2 month old mouse and sacrifice it by cervical dislocation.
- Pin the mouse to the post-mortem board keeping the abdominal portion upward and wash it with 70% ethanol.
- Lift the skin from the abdominal wall with the help of a forceps, cut a median longitudinal line, and separate the outer skin to expose the abdominal wall. If the abdominal perforation occurs at this stage, discard the mouse.
- Inject 2.5 ml of culture medium along the mid anterior line avoiding puncturing the gut, after which the abdominal wall is ballooned up.
- With the help of fingertips, gently massage the abdominal wall to release the macrophages from the cell walls.
- Take preservative-free heparin in a syringe (2 IU/ml) and insert the needle into the flank and slowly aspirate the fluid.
- Transfer the fluid into a sterile chilled centrifuge tube.
- Centrifuge at 800 rpm for 10 minutes and resuspend the cells in 10 ml growth medium.
- Suspend cells in the growth medium and count the cells. Adjust the cell density at 2×10^6 cells/ml.
- Distribute them in cell culture vessels and incubate in humidified atmosphere containing 5% CO_2 at 37°C.

PROTOCOL 1.3

BONE-MARROW CULTURE

Materials and Equipment

CMF-BSS medium, Heparin, Tris-ammonium buffer, RPM-1640, Surgical kit, Centrifuge, CO_2 incubator, Isopaque-Ficoll column.

Procedure

- Select a healthy animal preferably below one month of age and sacrifice it.
- Take out the long bones of the legs, preferably femur.
- Remove the skin under aseptic conditions.
- Cut the bone from one end and collect the loosely associated tissue from the bone in a beaker containing CMF-PBS and heparin (20 IU/ml, preservative free). Disperse the cells by pipetting.
- Remove the red blood cells by gradient centrifugation on Isopaque-Ficoll or tris-ammonium chloride buffer.
- Adjust the cell population at 1-3 x 10^6 nucleated marrow or blood cells per ml. Use RPM-1640 growth medium containing 20% foetal bovine calf serum and antibiotics.
- Incubate the cells dispensed in various cell culture vessels at 37°C in a humidifier incubator with 5% CO_2 and 95% air.
- Transfer the non-adherent cells to the next vessel when there is an increase in number. For this purpose, harvest the medium containing cells, centrifuge, and resuspend in a fresh growth medium.
- Dispense it in a fresh culture vessel and incubate.

PROTOCOL 1.4

SPLEEN CELL CULTURE

Materials and Equipment

BSS medium, Centrifuge, CO_2 incubator, Isopaque-Ficoll column, Tris-ammonium buffer.

Procedure

- Collect a spleen from a young animal of the desired species in a Petri dish containing BSS.
- Remove the adherent fat and wash the spleen several times.
- Mince the spleen with the help of a pair of scissors so as to release the cells.
- Pass the suspension through muslin cloth layer.
- As the cell suspension would contain erythrocytes also, to remove them, treat with Tris-ammonium buffer or separate by using Isopaque-Ficoll.

- Adjust the cell density at 2×10^6 cell/ml and dispense in suitable culture vessels and incubate at 37°C in 5% CO_2 atmosphere.

PROTOCOL 1.5

LIVER CELL CULTURE

Materials and Equipment

BSS medium, chicken serum, Centrifuge, CO_2 incubator, CMF-Hank's BSS, CMG-BSS, Trypsin, Collaginase.

Procedure

- Collect a liver tissue from the foetal or a newborn animal. In the case of human liver cell culture, collect a liver from an infant or embryo at autopsy or hysterectomy or such surgical procedures.
- Place the liver tissue immediately into a chilled culture medium and transport it on ice bath to the laboratory.
- Wash the liver fragments several times with CMF-Hank's BSS containing 1% chicken serum.
- Mince the liver tissue into 1-2 mm^2 fragments using a pair of curved scissors.
- Transfer the tissue fragments to a 50 ml or 100 ml Erlenmeyer flask and wash them several times with CMF-BSS.
- Add cell dissociation medium (0.1% trypsin and 0.1% collagenase in CMG-BSS) to the flask and shake it gently in a shaker bath at 37°C for 20 minutes.
- Shake it in such a way that the fragments are not settled and are always in motion.
- Take out the flask from the shaker bath, allow the fragments to settle, and then collect the supernatant solution containing the dispersed cells and transfer it to a chilled centrifuge tube.
- Add equal volume of chilled Cuorure medium and put the tube in the refrigerator.
- Make several collections of the dispersed cells, if necessary, as described above.
- Centrifuge the cells at 600g for 10 minutes and then give two washings in the culture medium.
- Finally suspend the cells in modified Ham's F12K culture medium containing 15% foetal calf serum.
- Count the cells by haemocytometer and adjust the cell density at $1\text{-}2 \times 10^5$ cells/ml.
- Dispense in Petri dishes and incubate at 37°C in a humidified incubator with CO_2.
- Replace the medium 2-3 times a week.

PROTOCOL 1.6

PROPAGATION OF CELL LINES

The definition of cell line has already been given along with its distinction from the primary cell culture. The greatest advantage in using a cell line is that it gives an unlimited amount of cells by continued passages. The cell lines always grow uniformly and can be grown on glass or plastic surfaces as monolayers as well as in suspension. The subculturing of cell lines is done in the similar way as for secondary cultures. The established cell lines, their media requirement and virus sensitivity are given in Table 1.2.

Equipment

A flow hood, An incubator with temperature, humidity and CO_2 control, An inverted microscope, Refrigerator, Deep Freezer, Liquid nitrogen freezer, Tissue culture plates, T-flasks, Multiwell plates, Roller bottles.

Propagation of Cell Lines

Adherent cells preparation

- To remove any traces of serum, briefly rinse the provided cell monolayers with trypsin-EDTA.
- 1 ml Trypsin-EDTA is added to a 100 mm dish and incubated for 1-4 minutes.
- Trypsin is inactivated by the addition of 9.0 ml of complete medium (DAEM high glucose, 5-10% serum, penicillin streptomycin solution, L-glutamine as required). Cells are pipetted out up and down several times to ensure complete removal of the cells from the dish.
- By using haemacytometer cells are counted and a dilution of cells is seeded which allows for future growth but is not too low to retain viability of the culture by cross feedings. New culture vessel is to be used for this.

Suspension cells

To prepare suspension, cells are counted and diluted into fresh medium. Dilution of cells is seeded that allows cell growth but is not too low to retain viability of the culture by cross feeding (See suspension cell culture generation, protocol 1.8).

PROTOCOL 1.7

MYCOPLASMA TESTING OF CELL LINES

Mycoplasmas are present as an impurity in the cell culture. A simple and reliable method for the detection of mycoplasma concentration is generally used, in which mycoplasma binds with fluorescent dye and upon examination with a fluorescent microscope, produces what appeared to be a fluorescent cytoplasm.

Procedure

- In 35 mm or 60 mm Petri dishes the test cultures are seeded at the regular intervals.

Table 1.2. Established cell lines, their media requirement and virus sensitivity

Species	Cell lines	Derivation	Growth medium	Split ratio	Morph-ology	Viral susceptibility
Cattle	MDBK	Bovine kidney	MEM, 10% Foetal bovine serum (FBS), 2 mM glutamine	1:10	Fib.	BVD, IBR, VSV
	IMR-31	Buffalo lung	Mc-Coy's 5A, 20% FBS, 2mM Glutamine	1:2	Fib.	HSV, Vaccinia, Pseudo-Rabies, Bovine entero-virus
Hamster	BHK21/CI 13	Pooled kidneys from 1 day old syrian hamsters	Eagle's MEM glasgow modified, 10% FBS, 2 mM Glutamine, 10% Tryptose phosphate broth	1:30	Fib.	FMDV, rabies, Pseudorabies, Adenovirus, VSV, Reovirus, Polyoma
Human	Hela	Cervical carcinoma	MEM, 10% FBS, 2mM Glutamine	1:40	Epith.	Poliovirus, Adenovirus
	HEp2	Carcinoma of larynx	Eagle's basal medium 15% FBS, 2mM Glutamine	1:20	Epith.	Poliovirus, Adenovirus, VSV
	KB	Oral epidermoid carcinoma	MEM, 5% FBS, 2mM Glutamine	1:20	Epith.	Poliovirus, Adenovirus
Monkey	BSC-1	African green	MEM, 10% FBS, 2mM Glutamine	1:2	Epith.	Polio, VSV, SV40
	Vero	monkey kidney	Medium 199, 5% FBS, 2 mM glutamine	1:15	Fib.	Semliki forest virus, Tacaribe, herpes simplex
Mouse	Clone M3	Melanoma cloudman S91	Ham's F10, 2.5% FBS, 15% Horse serum, 3 mM Glutamine	1:2	Epith.	HSV, Vaccinia, VSV, Pseudorabies
	NCTC clone	C3H/An mouse areolar and adipose tissue	Ham's F10, 2.5% FBS, 15% Horse serum, 2 mM Glutamine	1:4	Neur-oblast	HSV, Vaccinia, VSV
	L 929	Swiss mouse embryos	Eagle's medium, Dulbecco's modified, 10% FBS, 2mM Glutamine	1:20	Fib.	Polyoma, HSV, Vaccinia
Pig	PK15	Clone of pig kidney PK-29	MEM 5% FBS, 2mM Glutamine	1:20	Epith	Hog cholera, African swine fever, FMDV
Rabbit	RK13	Rabbit kidney	MEM, 10% FBS, 2mM Glutamine	1:15	Epith	Rubella, HSV, Herpes B

Fib : Fibroblast-like; Epith. : Epithelial-like; FBS : Foetal bovine serum; HSV : Herpes simplex virus; RS : respiratory syncytial
VSV : Vesicular stomatitis virus; IBR : Infectious bovine rhinotracheitis; FMDV : Foot & mouth disease virus

- Cultures are incubated until they reach between 20-50% confluence. (Complete confluence may hinder the mycoplasma visualization).
- Then media is removed and cells are rinsed with PBS twice.
- Again cells are rinsed with a solution of one part of PBS and one part of acetic acid/ methanol.
- Cells are then rinsed with pure acetic acid/ methanol.
- Cold acetic acid / methanol is added to the cells and then incubated in -20°C freezer for 10 minutes.
- Then acetic acid / methanol are removed and cells are rinsed with deinonized water.
- Then Hoechst 33258 dye solution (50 ng/ml in PBS) is added to the cells and incubated at room temperature for 10 minutes.
- Stain is removed by rinsing cells twice with deionized water.
- Coverslip is mounted using one drop of mounting solution (50% glycerol, 44 mM citrate, 111 mM sodium phosphate, pH 5.5) and blot off surplus from the coverslip with a Kimwipe. Seal the edges with clear fingernail polish.
- Slide is examined by epifluorescence. Mycoplasma will produce bright particulate or filamentous extracellular fluorescence over the cytoplasm and some times in intercellular spaces. If the contamination is low, all of the cells will not show extranuclear fluorescence so scan the entire culture before declaring a culture negative.

Cell Freezing

- A cell suspension is prepared and centrifuged to get the cells in the form of pellet.
- Cells are resuspended in freezing medium at a concentration of 10^6-10^7 cells/ml.
- One ml of suspension is dispensed into each freezing vial.
- Vials are placed in the polystyrene box and box is placed into a –70°C freezer and freeze overnight.
- Store vials under liquid nitrogen.

Thawing frozen cells

- Stored vials are removed from the liquid nitrogen freezer and thawed in a 37°C water bath.
- Cells are transferred to a T-75 flask containing 35 ml of media. Incubate the culture at 37°C. After 8-10 hours, culture medium is replaced with fresh medium.

PROTOCOL 1.8

SUSPENSION CULTURES

When a larger yield of cells is required, the suspension culture is the best method. The cells are grown in suspension without allowing them to attach on the surface of the vessel and this is achieved by constant stirring of the vessel contents. The O_2, CO_2, pH and other environmental conditions are provided to suit the requirements of the cells. For cultivating cells on a moderate scale a suitable vessel with a plastic enclosed magnet is available, and after adding the cell suspension the vessel is placed on a magnetic stirrer so that the cells are maintained continuously in suspension. For suspension culture on a large scale, larger size fermenter vessels of several hundred litre capacity are employed with electronic controls for maintaining all the required optimum conditions. Suspension cultures are mainly employed for the production of viruses on a large scale for the manufacture of vaccine.

Procedure for suspension cell culture generation

- Initial culture to set a suspension culture should be of 5×10^4 to 5×10^5 cells/ml.
- Inoculate 150 ml of cell suspension in a 500 ml Erlenmeyer flask.
- Cap the flask tightly and place it on a rotary shaker with a speed of 110 rpm in a 35°C incubator. For this purpose spinner flasks are used (Fig. 1.8).
- Add 0.12% methylcellulose (15cps) to the complete medium. This will stabilize the suspension.
- If culture medium is without serum, add a drop of 0.025% trypsin two three times in a week to maintain dispersed population of cells. When serum is used in culture, add 1 ml of 0.025% trypsin solution daily.

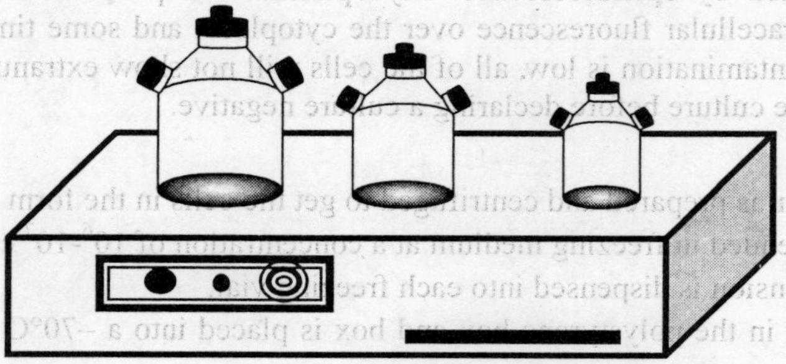

Fig. 1.8. Diagram of spinner flask

PLANT TISSUE CULTURE

The term plant tissue culture implies for the maintenance and propagation of plant cells, tissues and organs in an artificial prepared medium. The basic principle of the plant tissue culture is that a cell is totipotent that is having the capacity and ability to develop into whole organism. Plant cell culture is used to cultivate cells in quantity, or as clones from the single cell, to grow whole plant from isolated meristems and to induce callus or even single cell to develop into whole plant either by organogenesis or directly by embryogenesis *in vitro*. The production of haploid cells through tissue culture from anthers or isolated microspores and of protoplasts from higher plant cells, serve the basic tools for genetic engineering and somatic hybridization.

Preparing Media

One of the most complete media is Murashige and Skoog's shoot multiplication medium B (MSMB). At the appropriate time, order a pretransplant medium (Murashige syngonium stage III pretransplant medium with sucrose). A gelling agent, preferably a blend of agar and agar substitute, such as Agar gel is also needed.

- Add the powdered medium to the distilled water and stir. Adjust the pH to pH 5.7 using 1N NaOH or 1N HCl and pH indicator paper (3.5 - 6.8), or a pH meter.
- Thereafter add the agar. Use about 5 g per litre of medium. Heat and stir until the medium is clear (clarity indicates that agar has melted).
- Dispense the media into test tubes.

Sterilizing the Media

- Pour about one and a half inches of water into the autoclave.
- Place the tubes upright in the autoclave. To hold them upright place them in a wide mouth jar and make a wire or wooden rack, or tie them with string in bundles of ten. Process at 15 lb for 15 minutes.

Preparing Explant

- An explant is the part of a plant that is in culture. Select a young runner where the bud on the end has not yet opened. Cut it off from the plant one inch or so from the end. Transport the tips in a plastic bag with a wet, but not dripping wet, paper towel. If the runner tips are not going to be processed immediately, keep them in a refrigerator for a day or two.
- Fill a pint jar half full of sterile water (boiled, pressure cooked tap water or the store-bought bottled distilled water). Add 2 or 3 drops of liquid dish washing detergent (or Tween 20, a wetting agent).
- Place the runner tips in the jar and replace the screw-on lid. Vigorously shake the jar by hand for one minute.
- Pour off the water, rinse two or three times with fresh sterile water. Repeat this operation (or dip in 70% alcohol for a few seconds and rinse).
- In another container add 30 ml of household bleach to 270 ml of sterile water (10% bleach). To this add 2 drops of detergent. Add the explants and shake intermittently for 10 minutes.
- Quickly drain and add sterile water, cover and shake. The explants are now ready and can be taken to the transfer chamber.

Starting the Explants

The transfer chamber should be ready with the walls and workspace wiped or sprayed with 10% bleach/sterile water solution or 70% isopropyl alcohol (not if using a Bunsen burner). There should be a container of 10% bleach/sterile water and a container of 1% bleach/sterile water to sterilize and rinse the instruments and gloved hands of the operator.

- Immerse the forceps and knife for 30 seconds or more in the 10% bleach then rinse in the 1% bleach and rest them on a sterile holder or paper towel to dry for a few seconds.
- With the forceps place a sterile paper towel on the workspace. With the forceps place a runner tip on the towel. Place the forceps in the other hand to hold the tip while the first hand uses the knife or scalpel to cut off 1 cm of the stem.
- Place the knife in the 1/10 bleach, move the forceps to that hand. Grab a sterile test tube of medium with the other hand, hold it by the base. With the little finger of the hand holding the forceps, remove the cap and cradle it there while use the forceps to firmly lay the bud on the medium.
- Recap the test tube and seal with a piece of Scotch tape (or Parafilm).

Growing

- Place the test tubes in the planter tray (or other appropriate holder) and place the tray on a shelf under fluorescent light, which is 8-10 inches above the top of the tubes. Room temperature and continuous light is acceptable, but 16 hours light/ 8 hours darkness is standard. Check daily for contaminants. If any are found, sterilize the tube and contents before discarding the contents.
- Transfer the explant every two weeks or so until it is actively growing. In one to two months the culture can be divided into two pieces, each of which is about 0.5 cm in diameter. Continue to divide and transfer until enough plantlets are obtained. The plantlets should be singulated as they are transferred to prerooting medium, which has no hormones (or only IAA).

Transplanting

- When the plantlets begin to root, perhaps two to four weeks, transplant them to a light artificial soil mix, such as peat/ pearlite, in a seedling tray.
- Cover with clear plastic and place on a lighted shelf or in a shaded greenhouse. After two or three weeks begin leaving the plastic off for a period of time each day. The time the plantlets are left uncovered should get longer each day, until after about a week, the cover can be left off completely.

Types of Plant Tissue Cultures

Plant tissue cultures are broadly divided into three categories.

- Callus culture
- Organ culture
- Meristem culture

PROTOCOL 1.9

CALLUS CULTURE

In vivo, callus is frequently formed as a result of wounding at the cut edge of a root or stem, following invasion by microorganisms or damage resulting from insect feeding. Endogenous auxin and cytokinin control its formation. By incorporation of these plant growth regulators into a growth medium, callus can be induced to form *in vitro* on explants of parent tissue. The initiation of callus material from angiosperms, gymnosperms, ferns, mosses and liverworts can be achieved in this way.

Materials

The medium components are enlisted in Table 1.3.

Plant growth regulator stock solutions (1 mg/ml).

Naphthalene acetic acid, indole acetic acid and 2,4-dichlorophenoxyacetic acid present in the solution should be titrated with NaOH. Kinetin, gelatin and benzylaminopurine can be dissolved in dilute NaOH or 95% aqueous ethanol. Store at 4°C.

Plant Material

A wide range of plant organs and specialized tissues are used to initiate callus formation.

0.1M NaOH

Agar

Incubator (temperature controlled 25±2°C with additional light control facility).

Murashige and Skoog's medium (Table 1.4).

Table 1.3. Components of media for preparation of callus culture

Code no.	Compound	Concentration in medium (mg/l)	Amount in stock solution*	Stock volume (ml)
1.	NH_4NO_3	1650	8.25 g	400 ml
2.	KNO_3	1900	9.50 g	400 ml
3.	$MgSO_4.7H_2O$	370	1.85 g	400 ml
4.	KH_2PO_4	170	0.85 g	400 ml
5.	KI	0.83	4.18 mg	400 ml
6.	H_3BO_3	6.20	31.00 mg	400 ml
7.	$MnSO_4.7H_2O$	22.30	111.50 mg	400 ml
8.	$ZnSO_4.7H_2O$	8.6	43.00 mg	400 ml
9.	Myo-inositol	100.00	0.50 g	400 ml
10.	$CaCl_2.2H_2O$	440.00	2.20 g	400 ml
11.	$FeSO_4.7H_2O$	27.8	139.25 mg	100 ml
12.	$Na_2EDTA.2H_2O$	37.3	186.25 mg	100 ml
13.	$CuSO_4.5H_2O$	0.025	12.50 mg	100 ml
14.	$Na_2MoO_4.2H_2O$	0.25	12.50 mg	10 ml
15.	$CoCl_2.6H_2O$	0.025	12.50 mg	100 ml
16.	Nicotinic acid	0.50	25.0 mg	10 ml
17.	Pyridoxine-HCl	0.50	25.0 mg	10 ml
18.	Thiamine-HCl	0.10	5.0 mg	10 ml
19.	Glycine	2.00	100.0 mg	10 ml
20.	Sucrose	30.0 g/l		

**All solutions should be stored at -20°C.*

Procedure

Medium preparation

- Dissolve compounds 1-10 in 250 ml double-distilled water. Add 1 ml each of solutions of 13, 14 and 15 and make up the volume to 400 ml. Label it as stock solution A.
- Dissolve 11 and 12 in 50 ml double-distilled water and make up the volume to 100 ml. Label it as stock solution B.
- Dissolve sucrose (30 g) in 600 ml double distilled water.
- Add solution A (80 ml) and solution B (20 ml).
- Stir well and dilute to 700 ml.
- Add 0.2 ml each of solutions of 16, 17, 18 and 19. Adjust the pH of the solution to 5.5 with 0.1M NaOH and dilute to 1 litre.

- Add the chosen plant growth regulators to the appropriate concentration. It is advisable to prepare several batches of media containing a variety of combinations and concentrations of auxin and cytokinin for initiation of a new callus line.

The following supplements to Murashige and Skoog's medium (MS medium) have proven useful to initiate callus in a number of species:

Benzylaminopurine (5 mg/l) and naphthalene acetic acid (1 mg/l)
Kinetin (1 mg/l) and naphthalene acetic acid (1 mg/l)
Kinetin (0.2 mg/l) and 2,4-dichlorophenoxyacetic acid (1 mg/l)
Kinetin (0.2 mg/l) and naphthalene acetic acid (1 mg/l)
Add agar (1%)

If the medium is to be used in Erlenmeyer flasks, then the agar should be premelted in a water bath and the medium dispensed into the culture vessels. The flasks, after stoppering, should be sterilized in an autoclave at 120°C for 15 minutes (1.06 kg/cm^2).

The medium should be autoclaved and cooled to 40°C, if it is to be used in presterilized containers.

Table 1.4. Composition of Murashige and Skoog's medium

Material	Quantity (mg/l)	Material	Quantity (mg/l)
KNO_3	1900	$FeSO_4.7H_2O$	11.1
$CaCl_2$	880	H_3BO_3	12.4
NH_4NO_3	825	$MnSO_4.H_2O$	33.6
$MgSO_4.7H_2O$	370	$ZnSO_4.7H_2O$	21.0
KCl	350	KI	1.66
KH_2PO_4	170	$Na_2MoO_4.2H_2O$	0.5
Na_2EDTA	14.9	$CoCl_2.6H_2O$	0.05

Sterilization of seed material

- Place seeds in ethanol for 30 seconds, remove and place in any proprietary bleach for 30 minutes (shaking occasionally) and remove.
- Wash the seeds 4 to 5 times with sterile double distilled water and place them on appropriate media so that they are not in contact with each other.
- Incubate in the dark for one week and then transfer to the desired incubation conditions and observe daily for callus formation.

Sterilization of stem explants

- Remove non woody stem from the plant and cut into 5 cm length and wash with double-distilled water and remove the leaves and axillary buds.
- Place the explants in appropriate bleach for 5 minutes, remove and wash 4 to 5 times with fresh, sterile double distilled water.
- Trim away the end 2-3 mm of the explant and cut the remaining tissue into 2 cm length.
- Cut these in half lengthwise and place the cut side down on the agar.
- Incubate the explants and water daily for callus formation.

- Once sufficient callus growth has taken place, remove it from the explant and transfer to fresh medium. The callus line can be maintained by subculture at regular intervals (every 2-4 weeks). The callus should be divided and transferred onto fresh medium.

Notes

Heat labile components in some media (like kinetin) should be filter sterilized using a 0.22 μ membrane filter.

The method of sterilization of any one medium component should remain consistent as its final concentration in the medium depends on its method of sterilization.

The media should be stored at 4°C and then returned to room temperature prior to use, to prevent media desiccation.

It is preferable to initiate and maintain callus lines in either continuous light or continuous dark so that the effect of photo period can be easily investigated.

PROTOCOL 1.10

ORGAN CULTURE

Each cell may be capable of developing into an entire plant when provided with the correct environmental stimuli. Organogenesis is the development of adventitious organs or primordia (embryoid) from undifferentiated cell mass (callus) in tissue culture. Research has demonstrated that successful organogenesis in callus cultures can be achieved by the correct choice of medium components, selection of a suitable inoculum and control of the physical environment. The manipulation of plant growth regulator concentration is probably the most widely used technique for the induction of organogenesis and this methodology has formed the basis of the propagation of commercially important plants via tissue culture in recent years. Organogenesis is controlled mostly by a balance between cytokinin and auxin. A relatively high ratio of auxin : cytokinin induces root formation in callus tissues whereas, a low ratio induces shoot formation. Caulogenesis is a type of organogenesis by which only adventitious shoot bud initiation takes place in callus tissue. When it is applicable for root, it is known as rhizogenesis. Anomalous structures developed during organogenesis are called organoids.

The localized meristematic cells on a callus which give rise to shoots and/or roots is termed as meristemoids.

Materials

Medium

The formula defined for the maintenance of callus tissue as a reference (as already described) can be used to prepare a number of media varying in both the concentration and ratio of plant growth regulators. The plant growth regulator supplements, benzylaminopurine (from 0.05 mg/l to 5.00 mg/l) and naphthalene acetic acid (from 0.05 mg/l to 1.00 mg/l) to MS medium can be used to investigate the control of organogenesis in callus tissue.

Culture vessels

Wide neck 100 ml Erlenmeyer flasks containing 30 ml of medium and closed with cotton wool bungs covered with a single layer of aluminum foil are ideal for this purpose.

Callus material

Callus material, which has been initiated and maintained on a defined growth medium, incubated (temperature should be controlled 25±2°C) with additional control of light intensity.

Procedure

- Subculture the maintenance callus under sterile conditions onto the newly prepared media containing different concentrations of plant growth regulators. Incubate in continuous light and observe daily for organogenesis.
- Subculture after the usual interval, taking care to transplant any tissue showing a morphogenic response.
- Study the effect of high levels of the auxin naphthalene acetic acid and the cytokinin, benzyl aminopurine (in excess of 1.00 mg/l) on the production of callus and the effect of low level of benzylaminopurine (below 1 mg/l) on the shoot formation.
- Isolate both roots and shoots initiated from the callus material and maintain on an appropriate medium independently.

Notes

The use of 2,4-dichlorophenoxy acetic acid in plant tissue culture may be responsible for the loss of the ability of some callus cultures to undergo organogenesis. Therefore, the callus material, which has been maintained on a medium containing 2,4-dichlorophenoxyacetic acid is avoided.

Induction of Embryogenesis in Suspension Culture

The embryos that arise from the vegetative cells of the plant are called somatic embryos. This asexual reproduction is an alternative to sexual reproduction. These structures were termed embryoids, initially but now they are named as somatic embryos because of their similarity to zygotic embryos. The origin of somatic embryos is different from zygotic embryos which result from the fusion of gametes. This phenomenon is also called adventive or asexual embryogenesis. In contrast to buds, somatic embryos have a bipolar axis with an apical meristem and a root, and as they have no vascular connection with the mother callus, they are easily detached by the swirling action of the agitated medium.

Culture preparation in a liquid medium is strenuous. When the tissue is inoculated, it sinks and rapidly dies because of lack of oxygen. To prevent asphyxia, the liquid must be agitated to dissolve air in the medium. The culture of somatic embryos in a liquid medium, however, has numerous advantages. The swirling medium naturally separates the embryo, which are then easily observed. Thus, the embryos can be fractionated according to their stages. They can be obtained in great quantity and used as a basis for a large-scale micropropagation.

To induce somatic embryogenesis in suspension, three types of medium are required. The first medium contains agar and auxin; this differentiates the somatic tissue and provokes initiation of embryogenic cells (primary culture). The second medium is liquid and also contains auxin, ensures the multiplication of these cells. The third medium is also liquid but does not contain auxin and allows the cells to express embryogenic potential.

Temperature and light in the culture rooms are regulated. Temperature has to be regulated at approximately 25°C. Continuous light ($1W/m^2$) can be supplied by ordinary fluorescent tubes placed over the rotary shaker.

Culture medium

Callus tissue require all those substances which the plant tissue normally obtained from their phloem and xylem. Most culture media contain necessary minerals, an energy source, one or few vitamins and hormones. The mineral solution of Murashige and Skoog's can be used for culture of somatic embryos. Generally stock solutions are prepared in advance at 100X concentration.

- 2 ml of a stock solution containing 5.57 g of $FeSO_4.7H_2O$ and 7.45 g of Na_2EDTA per litre. In addition, the following items must be put into the medium sucrose 30 g/l, glutamic acid 400 mg/l, vitamin B_1 1 mg/l, 2,4-dichlorophenoxy acetic acid 1 mg/l and agar 1 g/l. Adjust the pH to 5.5.
- For mature embryo growth, use half-strength M S medium containing 5 g/l sucrose.
- Sieves (1mm grid) made of stainless screens (tea sieves) to fraction suspension culture and transfer only the smaller embryos in the new flask.
- Subsequent plantlet development requires filter paper bridge apparatus and small pots containing soil mixture.

Procedure

The method to get embryogenic suspension culture involves three steps. First, embryogenic tissue is initiated by culture on an agar medium with auxin, it is then transferred to liquid medium with auxin and then transferred into a liquid medium without auxin.

Initiation of embryogenic tissue

The solidified medium containing 2,4-dichlorophenoxy acetic acid is most effective for growth initiation. When the callus has developed potentiality for embryogenesis, i.e. 5 weeks at least after explant isolation, it is transferred to a liquid medium.

Establishment of embryogenic suspension culture

- Remove the callus from the culture tube with the help of sterile forceps and transfer to a Petri dish containing filter paper.
- Discard brownish parts of the callus and inoculate a fragment (about 2 g) in a 250 ml Erlenmeyer flask containing 50 ml of medium.
- Place the flasks on an orbital shaker and agitate at 100-150 rpm.
- When the plant material is placed in the medium, there is an initial lag period prior to cell division, followed by an exponential rise in cell number. Finally, the cells enter a stationary stage.
- To maintain the viability of the culture, the cells should be subcultured at the beginning of the stationary phase. It is reached in 2-3 weeks, and the suspension has to be transferred to a fresh medium at regular intervals within this period. A minimum density must be achieved when cells are transferred to fresh medium to maintain embryogenic potential.

- To subculture embryogenic suspension, let the cells settle at the bottom and decant almost all the medium. Suspend the suspension again by gently rotating the flask and transfer one fourth of the entire population to a fresh medium.
- Carry out all these operations using a micropipette. When the cells have settled, pipette out almost all the supernatant above the cells. Then, aspirate one-fourth of the cell population and transfer it into a new medium.
- A population of cells shows a wide range of proembryonic stages (under the dissecting microscopy). It is a mixture of single cells, proembryonic cell clusters and new embryogenic centres and elder embryos.
- Sieve the inoculum during transfer of the suspension to get uniformity.
- Pass the suspension through a 200 μm sieve and then a 100 μm sieve. The proembryonic cells pass through the second sieve while differentiated embryos from the late globular stage are retained and may be examined. Let the suspension settle which has passed the sieves and decant most of the medium to get a suspension with a high density of cells.

Proembryonic cluster

- Embryogenic cell division in the liquid medium and constitution of proembryonic clusters and formation of globular embryos
- A heterogenous population of somatic embryos during maturation without filtration.

PROTOCOL 1.11

MERISTEM CULTURE

When a meristem is cultivated *in vitro*, it produces a small plant within a few weeks bearing 5 to 6 leaves. Then the stem is cut into 5-6 micro cuttings, which under favourable conditions, become fully grown plants.

Materials

Culture vessels

Murashige and Skoog's medium (the medium generally contains 0.8-1% w/v agar. Liquid media may be used in conjunction with paper bridges or fibre supports in the culture vessel).

Ethanol solution (90% v/v)

Sodium hypochlorite (0.5-10% v/v)

Tween 80 (1% v/v)

Growth room provided with a temperature control of 25 ±1°C.

Procedure

- Excise from a suitable donor plant a terminal portion of stem and/or stem segments containing at least one node.
- Cut the donor segments to an appropriate size after exposing the terminal and axillary buds.
- Presterilize it by immersing in 90% v/v ethanol or methylated spirit for 10-30 seconds.

- Sterilize the donor tissue by immersing in a sodium hypochlorite solution. A 0.5-10.0 v/v solution and 15 minutes immersion of the tissue would represent the typical protocol range. When the tissue surfaces are waxy, addition of few drops of Tween 80 to the hypochlorite solution improves wetting of the tissues.
- Then rinse the donor tissues in sterile distilled water.
- Mount the tissue on the stage of a dissection microscope (magnification of 15X). The tissue should be held in place and for this, use a piece of expanded polystyrene covered in white plastic film. The tissue can then be held in place by dissection pins.
- Use the tips of the hypodermic needles to dissect away progressively smaller, developing leaves to expose the apical meristem of the bud. Excise the tissue, which should comprise the apical dome and the required number of the youngest leaf primordia.
- Then transfer it directly on to the selected growth medium.
- Seal the Petri dishes with parafilm tape.
- Transfer the complete meristem-tip culture to a suitable growth room at, typically, 25±1°C and illumination from warm white/cool white fluorescent lamps. A 12-16 hours photoperiod of intensities up to (4000 lux) would be typical of the optimal conditions reported for a wide range of species.
- If the explant is viable, then enlargement, the development of chlorophyll and some elongation should be visible within 7-14 days.
- Maintain the developing plantlet *in vitro* until the internodes are sufficiently elongated so as to allow dissection into nodal explants.
- Remove the plantlets from their culture vessel, under sterile conditions and separate into nodal segments.
- Transfer each of these on to fresh growth medium to allow axillary bud growth. Extension of this bud should be evident within 7-10 days of culture initiation.

Notes

- For sterilization by immersing the donor tissues in sterilant solutions, the concentration and immersion times depend upon the size and nature of the donor tissues.
- Donor tissues should be taken from young, preferably actively growing regions of the plant to ensure success.
- Hypodermic needles used as dissecting tools are sometimes discarded after 2-3 meristem excisions and the presence of leaf primordia is essential for successful culture growth.

PROTOCOL 1.12

MICROPROPAGATION

The most important use of micropropagation technique has been the production of plants. For effective micropropagation, the plant must be in an active and healthy state. The micropropagation technique provides a method whereby viral and bacterial pathogens can be eliminated from infected varieties.

The most appropriate technique of micropropagation is axillary bud multiplication. The advantages of this technique are that large number of uniform, genetically stable plants are produced under sterile conditions. Major steps involved in the micropropagation are shown in the Figure 1.9.

Materials

For selection and sterilization of elite plants

- Elite stock plants free from any sign of disease, stress or surface blemishes. This material should be grown in an environmentally controlled growth cabinet or clean glass house and should be tested for the presence of specific viruses using ELISA technique.
- 70% ethanol containing four drops of surfactant Manoxol/100 ml solution at room temperature
- 2% chloros containing four drops of surfactant Manoxol/100 ml solution at room temperature

For establishment of axillary buds in culture

- Sterile Petri dishes (50 mm diameter) containing approximately 10 ml of medium 1 (Table 1.5) or sterile Petri dishes (85 mm diameter) containing 25 ml of medium 1.
- Incubator or environmentally controlled growth chamber allowing environmental conditions of 20-24°C (depending on variety or species), a 16 hours photoperiod and a light intensity of 4000-6000 lux.

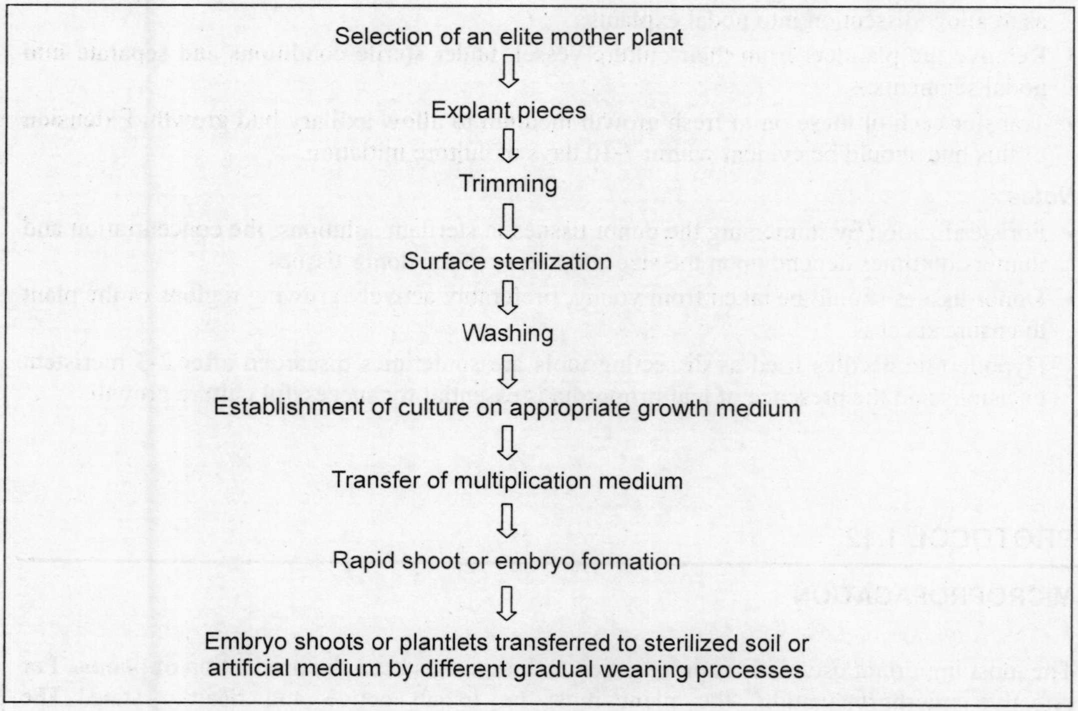

Fig. 1.9. Major steps involved in micropropagation

For multiplication in culture

Sterile jars (250 ml) containing approximately 30 ml of medium 2 or medium 3 (Table 1.5). Environmental conditions as were in establishment of axillary buds.

Table 1.5. Quantity of chemicals (g/l or mg/l) in media used in axillary bud culture of *Solanum* species based on either Murashige and Skoog's medium or Gambourg B5 Medium.

	Medium 1 (MS)	**Medium 2 (MS)**	**Medium 3 (B5)**	**Medium 4 (MS)**
NH_4NO_3	1.65 g	1.65 g	-	1.65 g
KNO_3	1.9 g	1.9 g	2.5 g	1.9 g
$CaCl_2.2H_2O$	0.44 g	0.44 g	0.15 g	0.44 g
$MgSO_4.7H_2O$	0.37 g	0.37 g	0.25 g	0.37 g
KH_2PO_4	0.17 g	0.17 g	-	0.17 g
$(NH_4)_2SO_4$	-	-	13.4 g	-
$NaH_2PO_4.H_2O$	-	-	0.15 g	
FeNaEDTA	36.7 mg	36.7 mg	40.0 mg	36.7 mg
H_3BO_3	6.2 mg	6.2 mg	3.0 mg	6.2 mg
$MnSO_4.4H_2O$	22.3 mg	22.3 mg	10.0 mg	22.3 mg
$ZnSO_4.7H_2O$	8.6 mg	8.6 mg	2.0 mg	8.6 mg
KI	0.83 mg	0.83 mg	0.75 mg	0.83 mg
$Na_2MoO_4.2H_2O$	0.25 mg	0.25 mg	0.25 mg	0.25 mg
$CuSO_4.5H_2O$	0.025 mg	0.025 mg	0.025 mg	0.025 mg
$CoCl_2.6H_2O$	0.025 mg	0.025 mg	0.025 mg	0.025 mg
Nicotinic acid	0.50 mg	0.50 mg	1.0 mg	0.50 mg
Thiamine HCl	0.10 mg	0.10 mg	10 mg	0.10 mg
Pyridoxine HCl	0.50 mg	0.50 mg	1.0 mg	0.50 mg
Glycine	2.0 mg	2.0 mg	-	2.0 mg
Sucrose	20.0 g	20.0 g	20.0 g	20.0 g
Inositol	0.1 g	0.1 g	0.1 g	0.1g
Glutamine	0.1 g	0.1 g	0.1 g	-
BAP(6-benzylamino purine)*	0.25 mg	0.25 mg	0.25 mg	0.05 mg
GA_3 (Gibberellic acid)*	0.1 mg	0.1 mg	-	5.64
NAA(1-naphthalene acetic acid)	-	-	-	8.0 g
pH**	5.64	5.64	5.64	5.64
Agar***	8.0 g	8.0 g	8.0 g	8.0 g

** Varying the hormones allows the above media to be used for axillary bud culture of a wide range of species.*

*** pH adjusted using 0.1M HCl and 0.1M KOH before adding agar and prior to autoclaving.*

**** The amount of agar needed varies depending on the brand used.*

For rooting of in vitro plants and transfers to compost

Sterile jars (250 ml) containing approximately 50 ml of medium 4 (Table 1.6).

Propagation trays, plastic bags, or seed trays covered with glass sheets or a misting or fogging system.

Pots (50 mm diameter) containing compost (3:2, peat:sand) supplemented with nutrients. For potato (*Solanum tuberosum)*, these are :

Osmocote	57 g
Sulphated potash	21 g
Epsom salts	28 g
Frit 252 A	14 g
Lime	170 g
Phosphate	85 g

3:2 peat and sand mix.

Procedure

Selection and sterilization of elite plants

- Excise carefully axillary buds of the desired variety and store in distilled water until enough buds have been obtained.
- Put a maximum of 20 buds into a sterile test tube (use Laminar flow bench).
- Fill to the brim with ethanol solution and leave for 1-1.5 minutes. Decant the ethanol.
- Fill to the brim with chloros solution, replace the top, and agitate at 120 strokes per minute for 12 minutes either manually or with a shaker.
- Decant the chloros solution and refill with sterile distilled water. Rinse in sterile water 3-4 times.
- Store in sterile distilled water until ready to continue (not longer than 2 hours).

Establishment of axillary buds in culture

- Transfer the water and axillary buds into an empty sterile Petri dish.
- Place upto 4 buds in a 50 mm sterile Petri dish or 10 buds in 85 mm sterile Petri dish containing medium 1.
- The base of the bud should stick firmly in the medium but should not be buried.
- Seal the Petri dish with laboratory sealing film, ensuring adequate gaseous exchange by puncturing with a fine sterile needle (at 2-4 times).
- Transfer to incubator or grow at room temperature and leave for 1 week to 2 months depending on the variety.

Multiplication in culture

- When shoot extends, cut internodes, and transfer apical cutting and internodal cuttings to sterile jars containing medium 2 or 3.
- Make sure that the basal portion of the stem is firmly pressed into the medium without burying the explant.

Rooting of in vitro plants and transfer to compost

- Cut off the top 5 mm of *in vitro* plant (apex plus 2 or 3 notes) and transfer to medium 4 (12 plants/150 ml jar).

- Leave for 3-5 days until 3 or 4 small, study roots approximately 5 mm long are visible.
- Remove each plantlet carefully from the jar.
- Remove as much agar as possible without harming the root structure and transfer to damp compost in 5 mm pots.
- Keep in high humidity conditions for 12-24 hours (propagator, plastic bag or misting).
- Transfer to the glass house, preferably placing on top of capillary matting. Shade from direct sunlight.
- Transfer the plants (when approximately) 70 mm high and have begun to loose their juvenile characteristics to large pots or to the field.

Notes

The test for infections by known viruses should be done before initiating the culture, viral pathogens, once in culture are rapidly spread by axillary bud cultures.

PROTOCOL 1.13

CLONED CAULIFLOWER

Various steps involved in the procedure are shown in figure 1.6.

Material

White part of Cauliflower
Sterile distilled water, 100 ml
70% Ethanol, 50 ml
20% Domestos solution (Chlorate solution with added detergent)
Test tubes, containing 2-3 ml of plant tissue growth medium
Sterile Petri dish
Metal forceps and scalpel
Non-adsorbent cotton wool and aluminium foil

Preparation of Plant Tissue Growth Medium (1 litre)

Granulated sugar, 20 g
Agar, 10 g
Murashige and Skoog's (M S) medium, 4.7 g
Kinetin stock solution, 25 ml

- Prepare the kinetin stock solution using 0.1 g kinetin in 1 litre of distilled water. As kinetin is not readily soluble in water, add one or two pellets of sodium hydroxide to solubilize it. Store the stock solution at 4°C.
- In order to prepare the growth medium, dissolve the sugar, MS medium and agar in 725 ml distilled water.
- Mix kinetin in the stock solution, then dispense into test tubes and take 2-3 ml per tube. Plug the tubes with non-absorbent cotton wool and cap them with aluminum foil.

- Autoclave at 121°C for 15 minutes in an autoclave. When cool, the tubes may be refrigerated until they are needed.

Procedure

- Swab the working area with 70% ethanol. Cut out a small piece of cauliflower curd roughly the size of a cherry. Divide the curd into three.
- Sterilize the surface of the tissue by keeping it in a bleach solution e.g. Domestos for nearly 10 minutes. Rinse the explants in three successive beakers of sterile distilled water. Use flamed, cooled forceps for this purpose.
- Leave the explants in a beaker of sterile water (covered with a Petri dish lid) until required.
- From the first tube of growth medium, withdraw the cotton wool plug, then briefly flame the neck. Use flamed, cooled forceps to pick up an explant and quickly drop it into the tube. Return the forceps to the ethanol beaker. Flame the neck of the tube once more. Then replace the plug.
- Similarly transfer the two remaining explants in two fresh tubes of growth medium. Keep the tubes in a warm, light place. Growth should be visible within 10 days.

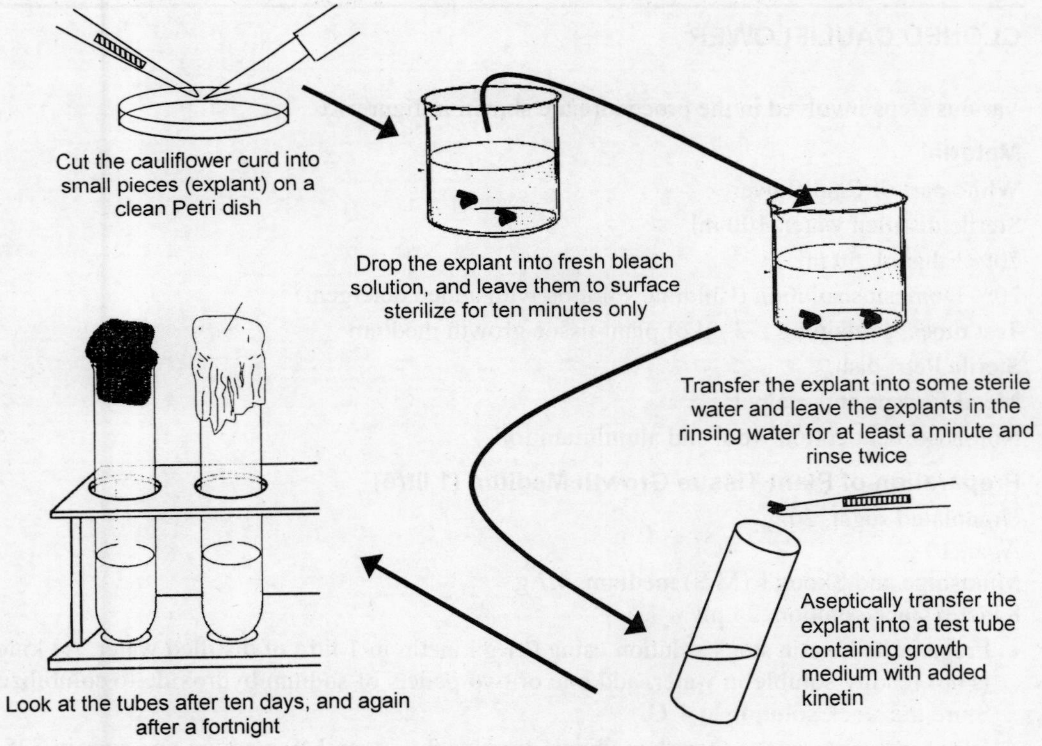

Fig. 1.6. Schematic diagram showing cloning technique of cauliflower

SUGGESTED READINGS

Driessen, F. M., Ubbels, J. and Stadhoudin, J., *Biotech. Bioeng.*, Vol. 19, 821, 1977.

Kuchler, R. J., Biochemical Methods in Cell Culture and Virology, Dowden, Huchinson and Ross, Inc., Strausberg, USA, 1977.

Laboratory Experiments in Biotechnology and Related Areas, Vol. 3, 1988.

Rhinehart, H. and Winston, S., Biology: Visualizing Life, 1994.

Sadasivam, S. and Manickem, A., Biochemical Methods, 2nd Edition, New Age International Publishers, New Delhi, India, 1997.

Stephan, L. C. and Polking, G. F., Public Education Program in Biotechnology, 1995.

Storr, T., Plant Tissue Culture, ISBN, 1985.

Tamine, A. Y. and Deeth, H. C., *J. Food Protection*, 43, 939, 1980.

The Bionet Booklet, Vol. 3, 1995.

Trehan, K., Biotechnology, Wiley Eastern Limited, New Delhi, India, 1991.

Vyas, S. P. and Dixit, V. K, Pharmaceutical Biotechnology, CBS Publishers, New Delhi, India, 1998.

Wagner, M., Bradley, R. and Mennes, M., Homemade Yogurt, Sour Cream and Butter Milk, 1994.

CHAPTER 2

Electrophoresis

- Electrophoresis
- Apparatus for electrophoresis
- Agarose gel electrophoresis for DNA separation
- One dimensional agarose gel elecrophoresis
- Two dimensional agarose gel electrophoresis of DNA replication intermediates
- Electrophoretic separation of proteins
- SDS-polyacrylamide gel electrophoresis
- Southern analysis
- Immunoblot (western blotting)
- Anti-phosphotyrosine western blotting

ELECTROPHORESIS

Electrophoresis may be considered as one of the main techniques for molecular separation in modern cell biology laboratory. Because it is such a powerful technique, and yet reasonably easy and inexpensive, it has become common place. In spite of the many physical arrangements for the apparatus, and regardless of the medium through which molecules are allowed to migrate, all electrophoretic separations depend upon the charge distribution of the molecules being separated. Electrophoresis can be one-dimensional (i.e. one plane of separation) or two-dimensional. One-dimensional electrophoresis is used for most routine protein and nucleic acid separations. Two-dimensional separation of proteins is used for finger printing, and when properly constructed can be extremely accurate in resolving all of the proteins present within a cell (greater than 1500 kD).

The support medium for electrophoresis can be formed into a gel within a tube or it can be layered into flat sheets. The tubes are used for easy one-dimensional separations, while the sheets have a larger surface area and are better for two dimensional separations. When the detergent SDS (sodium dodecyl sulphate) is used with proteins, all of the proteins become negatively charged by their attachment to the SDS anions. When separated on a polyacrylamide gel, the procedure is abbreviated as SDS-PAGE (Sodium Dodecyl Sulphate Polyacrylamide Gel Electrophoresis). The technique has become a standard means for molecular weight determination. Polyacrylamide gels are formed from the polymerization of two compounds, acrylamide and N,N methylene- bis-acrylamide (Bis). Bis is a cross-linking agent for the gels. The polymerization is initiated by the addition of ammonium persulphate along with either β-dimethyl amino-propionitrile (DMAP) or N,N,N,N,-tetramethyl-ethylenediamine (TEMED). The gels are neutral, hydrophilic, three-dimensional networks of long hydrocarbons cross-linked by methylene groups.

The separation of molecules within a gel is determined by the relative size of the pores formed within the gel. The pore size of a gel is determined by two factors, the total amount of acrylamide present (designated as %T) and the amount of cross-linker (%C). As the total amount of acrylamide increases, the pore size decreases. With cross- linking, 5% C gives the smallest pore size. Any increase or decrease in %C increases the pore size. Gels are designated as percent solutions and will have two necessary parameters. The total acrylamide is given as a % (w/v) of the acrylamide plus the bis-acrylamide. Thus, a 7.5%T would indicate that there is a total of 7.5 g of acrylamide and bis per 100 ml of gel. A gel designated as 7.5%T : 5%C would have a total of 7.5 % w/v acrylamide plus bis, and the bis would be 5% of the total (with pure acrylamide composing the remaining 2.5%). Proteins with molecular weight ranging from 10,000 to 1,000,000 may be separated with 7.5% acrylamide gels, while proteins with higher molecular weight require lower acrylamide gel concentrations. Conversely, gels up to 30% have been used to separate small polypeptides. The higher the gel concentration, the smaller the pore size of the gel and the better it will be able to separate smaller molecules. The percent gel to be used depends on the molecular weight of the protein to be separated. Use 5% gels for proteins ranging from 60,000 to 200,000 daltons, 10% gels for a range of 16,000 to 70,000 daltons and 15% gels for a range of 12,000 to 45,000 daltons is generally recommended.

Cationic versus Anionic Systems

In electrophoresis, proteins are separated on the basis of charge, and the charge of a protein can be either +ve or –ve, depending upon the pH of the buffer. In normal operation, a column of gel is partitioned into three sections, known as the Separating or Running Gel, the Stacking Gel and the Sample Gel. The sample gel may be eliminated and the sample introduced via a dense non-convective medium such as sucrose. Electrodes are attached to the ends of the column and an electric current passed through the partitioned gels. If the electrodes are arranged in such a way that the upper bath is –ve (cathode), while the lower bath is +ve (anode), and anions are allowed to flow towards the anode, the system is known as an anionic system. Flow in the opposite direction, with cations flowing towards the cathode is referred to as cationic system.

Tube versus Slab System

Two basic approaches have been used in the design of electrophoresis protocols. One, column electrophoresis, uses tubular gels formed in glass tubes, while the other, slab gel electrophoresis, uses flat gels formed between two plates of glass. Tube gels have an advantage in that the movement of molecules through the gels is less prone to lateral movement and thus there is a slightly improved resolution of the bands, particularly for proteins. It is also more economical, since it is relatively easy to construct home made systems from materials on hand. However, slab gels have the advantage of allowing for two-dimensional analysis, and of running multiple samples simultaneously in the same gel.

Slab gels are designed with multiple lanes set up such that samples run in parallel. The size and number of the lanes can be varied and, since the samples run in the same medium, there is less likelihood of sample variation due to minor changes in the gel structure. Slab gels are the techniques of choice for any blot analysis and for autoradiographic analysis. Consequently, for laboratories performing routine nucleic acid analysis, and those employing antigenic controls, slab gels have become standard. The availability of reasonably low priced commercial slab gel units has increased the use of slab gel systems, and the use of tube gels is becoming rare. The theory and operation of slab gel electrophoresis is identical to tube gel electrophoresis. The choice for system is, however dependent more on the experience of the investigator than on any other factor, and the availability of equipment. While acrylamide gels have become the standard for protein analysis, they are less suitable for extremely high molecular weight nucleic acids (above 200,000 daltons). In order to properly separate these large molecules, the acrylamide concentration needs to be reduced to a level where it remains liquid. The gels can be formed, however, by the addition of agarose, a naturally linear polysaccharide, to the low concentration of acrylamide. With the addition of agarose, acrylamide concentrations of 0.5% can be used and molecular weights of up to 3.5×10^5 daltons can be separated. This is particularly useful for the separation of large sequences of DNA. Consequently, agarose-acrylamide gels are used extensively in genetic laboratories for the determination of gene maps.

APPARATUS FOR ELECTROPHORESIS

Commercially two types of apparatus fitted with a source of variable DC supply are available vertical (Fig. 2.1) and horizontal (Fig. 2.2). Horizontal arrangement is simple to handle and thus frequently used for electrophoresis of proteins and enzymes in starch and agarose gels. Nevertheless, vertical arrangement allows the separation in lesser time in comparison with horizontal. Some of the parts of electrophoresis apparatus are as follows.

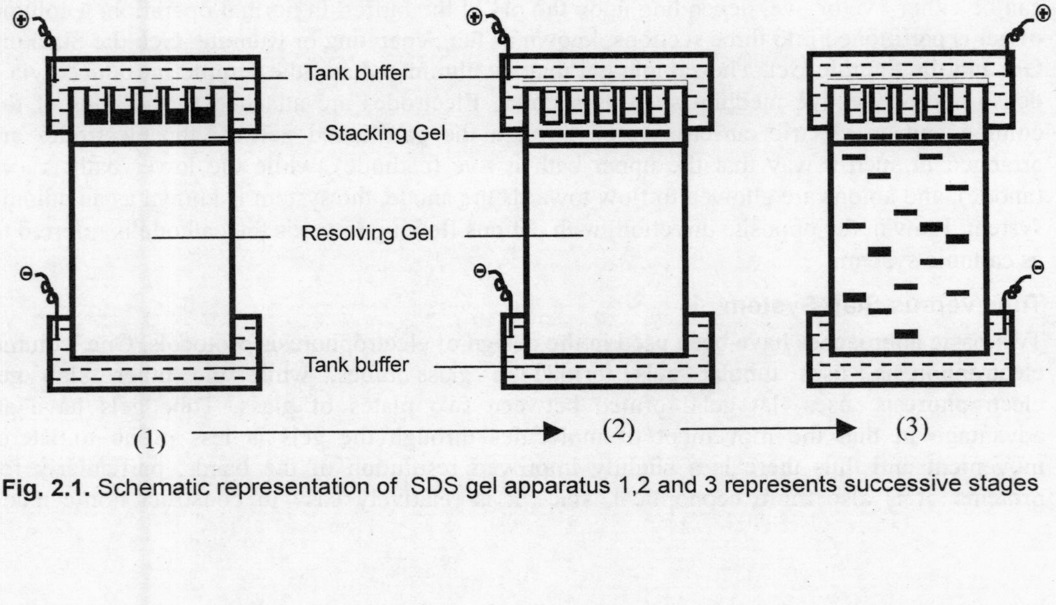

Fig. 2.1. Schematic representation of SDS gel apparatus 1,2 and 3 represents successive stages

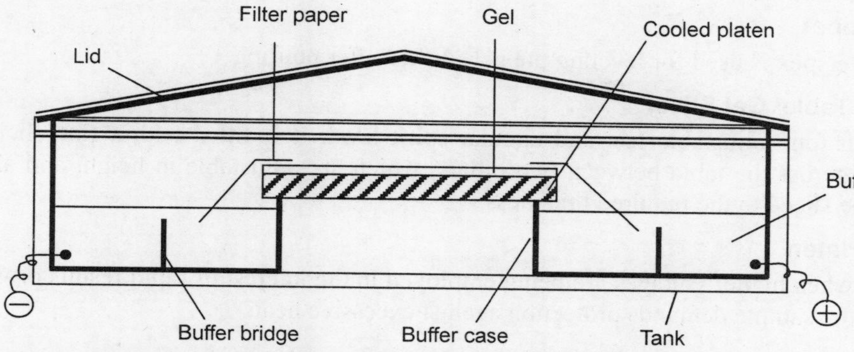

Fig. 2.2. Diagrammatic representation of horizontal electrophoresis apparatus

Gel Trays

Made of Perspex of glass and fitted with removable bezels or glass side pieces 1 cm wide and 0.5 cm depth. Size of the gel trays varies from 5 cm, 10 cm, 15 cm, 18 cm in width and 18 cm to 21 cm in length (Fig. 2.3).

Slot Makers (Comb)

Generally made of plastic and available in 36 or 10 slots each 10 mm wide. For the vertical apparatus the mould is constructed so that wedges of gel are casted at the two ends to provide buttress support when it is finally erected in the vertical position; a slot former for the sample inserts is also included as part of the mould (Fig. 2.4).

Single Sample Applicator

It is an aid for placing of small reproducible quantities at required origin of electrophoresis like pipetting samples on the cellulose acetate strips. The edge of the tool carries a small precision machined between 7 and 15 mm width with delivery volumes of between 0.5 and 5 µl. In use the applicator is dipped into a shallow pool of sample solution pipetted onto a flat surface such as a glass plate, it is then applied lightly to the cellulose acetate in the desired position (Fig. 2.5).

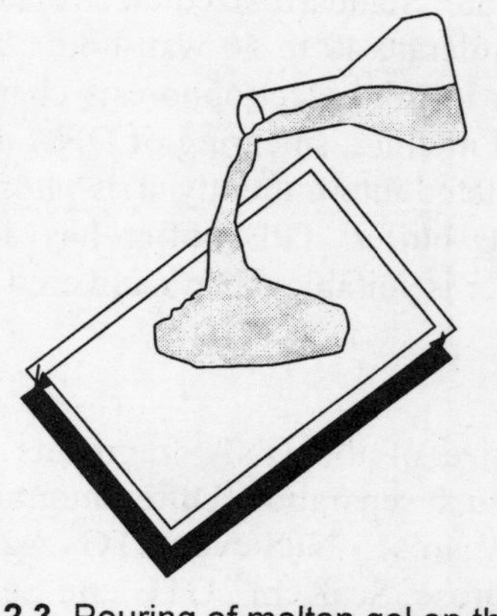

Fig. 2.3. Pouring of molten gel on the plate

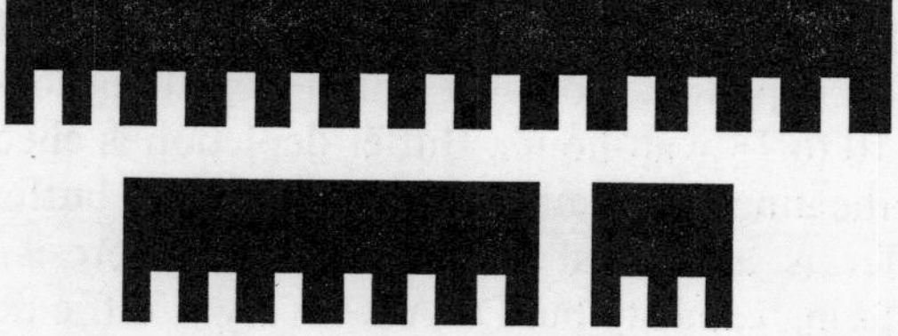

Fig. 2.4. Slot makers with different number of slots

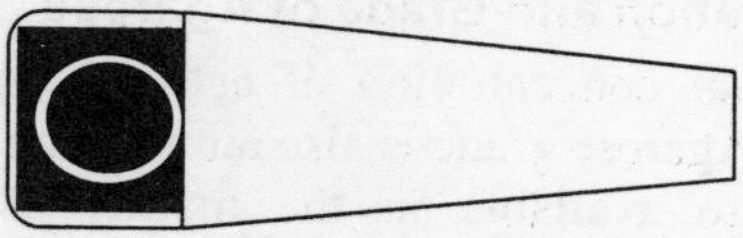

Fig. 2.5. Single sample applicator

Gel Scrapper

Made of Perspex is used for leveling the gel surface after pouring.

Leveling Table/ Gel Slicer

Fitted with four adjustable feet and circular spirit level. It is fitted with a fine slicing wire tensioned across the table between two pillars, which are adjustable in height and allow gel cakes to be sliced to the required thickness.

Cooled Platen

It is used when higher voltages are being employed in the interest of rapid results or when the nature of the sample demands protection against excessive heat.

PROTOCOL 2.1

AGAROSE GEL ELECTROPHORESIS FOR DNA SEPARATION

Buffers for Electrophoresis

Two buffers are commonly used for DNA electrophoresis; they are Tris-acetate with EDTA and Tris-borate with EDTA. The pH of these buffers is basic, therefore the DNA, because of negatively charged phosphate backbone migrates towards anode. For smaller DNA fragments (less than 12 to 15 Kb) either the 1X TAE or TBE (1X or 0.5X) is suitable for use. For larger DNA fragments the best buffer to be used is TBE with combination to low field strength (1-2 V/cm). The depth of buffer over the gel in a horizontal electrophoretic system should be 3-5 mm. Less buffer may cause dry out during electrophoresis whereas excess buffer depth may cause decreased DNA mobility and eventually distortion of bands.

Buffer depletion is also an important parameter for selection of the buffer system. Depletion rate is influenced by the type and buffering capacity of buffer used. A 0.5X TBE buffer has greater buffering capacity than a 1X TAE buffer and the pH used because the pKa of borate is closer to the initial buffer pH than that of acetate. Standard sized electrophoresis chambers (15 x 30 cm) with a 1.5 to 2 litre capacity will tolerate 40 to 50 watt-hours before buffer depletion, however buffer depletion does not occur in mini-electrophoresis chambers for 10 to 13 watt-hours. Buffer depletion is checked by gel melting, smearing of DNA and or overheating of chamber. In such instances buffer is recirculated intermittently. Tris-phosphate buffer is also used for DNA electrophoresis. Like TBE buffer, TPE buffer has a high buffering capacity but DNA recovery is difficult. This buffer is suitable when recovered DNA is used in a phosphate sensitive reaction (Table 2.1).

Concentration and Grade of Agarose

The optimal concentration of agarose depends on the size of the DNA fragments to be resolved. Agarose grade is also an important parameter in such separation. Different grades of agarose are available in the market like NuSieve® Agarose, NuSieve GTG Agarose, MetaPhor® Agarose, SeaPlaque® and SeaPlaque GTG Agarose, SeaKem® GTG and SeaKem

LE Agarose. Table 2.2 enlists some of the grade of agarose and their concentration in respect of the size of DNA to be resolved.

Table 2.1. Composition of buffers for electrophoresis

Buffer	Working solution	Concentrated stock solution (per litre)
Tris-acetate (TAE)	1X : 0.04 M Tris-acetate 0.001M EDTA	50X: 2.42 g Tris base 57.1 ml glacial acetic acid 100 ml 0.5 M EDTA (pH 8.0)
Tris-phosphate (TPE)	1X : 0.09 M Tris-phosphate 0.002 M EDTA	10X: 108 g Tris base 15.5 ml 85% w/v phosphoric acid) 40 ml 0.5 M EDTA (pH 8.0)
Tris-borate (TBE)	0.5X : 0.045 M Tris-borate 0.001 M EDTA	5X: 54 g Tris base 27.5 g boric acid 20 ml 0.5 M EDTA (pH 8.0)
Alkaline	1X : 50 mN NaOH 1 mM EDTA	1X: 5 ml 10 N NaOH 2 ml 0.5 M EDTA (pH 8.0)

Optimal Voltage and Electrophoretic Times

The distance between the electrodes is used for the determination of voltage gradient, not the length of the gel. If the voltage is too high, band streaking may result whereas too low voltage may result in broadening of the bands due to dispersion and diffusion.

Optimum voltage is required to achieve sharp bands. The gel should be run until the band of interest migrates 40-60% down the length of the gel. For various agarose gel systems the optimal voltage to run DNA is recommended in Table 2.3.

Gel Loading Buffers

Gel loading buffers serve three purposes in DNA electrophoresis

- Increase the density of the sample and ensure even application of DNA into every well.
- Add colour to the sample and thereby simplifies loading
- Add mobility dyes, which enable one to monitor the rate of electrophoresis process.

Loading buffers are prepared in 6 to 10 fold concentrated solutions (Table 2.4). For performing alkaline gel electrophoresis alkaline phosphate buffer is used. To increase the sharpness of bands of ficoll polymer is used as a sinking agent instead of glycerol.

Agarose Preparation for Electrophoresis

Agarose undergoes a series of steps when it is dissolved; dispersion, hydration and melting/dissolution. Dispersion simply refers to the separation of the particles by the buffer without clumping. Clumping occurs when the agarose starts to dissolve before it is completely dispersed, coating itself with a gelatinous layer which inhibits the penetration of water and keeps the powder inside from dispersing. Dissolution then becomes a long process. Hydration is the surrounding of agarose particles by a solution (e.g. water or running buffer). Problems are sometimes encountered with hydration when using a microwave oven to dissolve agarose. In part, this occurs because hydration is time dependent and microwave ovens bring the temperature up rapidly.

Table 2.2. Concentration and grade of agarose

Agarose grade	Size of DNA (base pairs)	Final agarose concentration % (W/V)	
		1X TAE buffer	1X TBE buffer
NuSieve® 3:1 Agarose	500-1000	3.0	2.0
	100-500	4.0	3.0
	10-100	6.0	5.0
NuSieve® GTG Agarose	500-1000	2.5	2.0
	150-700	3.0	2.5
	100-450	3.5	3.0
	70-300	4.0	3.5
	10-100	4.5	4.0
	8-50	5.0	4.5
MetaPhor® Agarose	150-800	2.0	1.8
	100-600	3.0	2.0
	50-250	4.0	3.0
	20-130	5.0	4.0
	<80	—	5.0
SeaPlaque® and SeaPlaque GTG Agarose	500-25000	0.75	0.70
	300-20,000	1.0	0.85
	200-12000	1.25	1.0
	150-6000	1.5	1.25
	100-3000	1.75	1.5
	50-2000	2.0	1.75
SeaKem® GTG and SeaKem LE Agarose	1000-23000	0.60	0.50
	80-10,000	0.80	0.70
	400-8000	1.0	0.85
	300-7000	1.2	1.0
	200-4000	1.5	1.25
	100-3000	2.0	1.75

Table 2.3. Optimal voltage for agarose gel systems

Size	Voltage	Recovery	Buffer analytical
< or = 1kb	5 Vcm^{-1}	TAE	TBE
1 to 2kb	4-10 Vcm^{-1}	TAE	TAE, TBE
> 12kb	1-2 Vcm^{-1}	TAE	TAE

The problem is exacerbated by the fact that the agarose is not being agitated to help dilute the highly concentrated solution around each particle and dissolution is slowed. The final stage in dissolving the agarose is the melting and dissolution of a high concentration gel. Melting can be done in either a microwave oven or on a hot plate. As the particles hydrate, they become small, highly concentrated gels. Since the melting temperature of a standard agarose gel is about 93°C, merely heating a mixture to 90°C will not completely dissolve agarose. Even low-melting-temperature agarose should be boiled when preparing gels to ensure that the solution is degassed and all agarose is fully dissolved.

Table 2.4. Composition and storage temperature of loading buffers

Loading buffer	6 X Solution (w/w)	Storage temperature
Sucrose based	40% Sucrose	4°C
	0.25% Bromophenol Blue	
	0.25% Xylene Cyanol FF	
Glycerol based	30% Glycerol in distilled water	4°C
	0.25% Bromophenol Blue	
	0.25% Xylene Cyanol FF	
Ficoll® based	15% Ficoll (type 400) polymer in distilled water	Room temperature
	0.25% Bromophenol Blue	
	0.25% Xylene Cyanol FF	
Alkaline	300 mM NaOH	4°C
	6 mM EDTA	
	0.15% Bromophenol Green	
	0.25% Xylene Cyanol FF	

Materials

Microwave oven or hotplate, Beaker that is 2-4 times the volume of the solution, Teflon® coated magnetic stir bar, Plastic wrap

Reagents

1X TAE, 1X TBE or 0.5X TBE electrophoresis buffer

Agarose powder

Agarose preparation in microwave (gel concentration < 2% w/v)

- Choose a beaker that is 2-4 times the volume of the solution.
- Add room-temperature 1X or 0.5X buffer and a stir bar to the beaker.
- Sprinkle in the premeasured agarose powder while the solution is rapidly stirred.
- Remove the stir bar if not Teflon coated.
- Weigh the beaker and solution before heating.
- Cover the beaker with plastic wrap.
- Pierce a small hole in the plastic wrap for ventilation.
- Heat the beaker in the microwave oven on high power until bubbles appear.
  Note: Any microwaved solution may become superheated and foam over when agitated.
- Remove the beaker from the microwave oven
- Gently swirl the beaker to resuspend any settled powder and gel pieces.
- Reheat the beaker on high power until the solution comes to a boil.
- Hold at boiling point for 1 minute or until all of the particles are dissolved.
- Remove the beaker from the microwave oven.

- Gently swirls the beaker to thoroughly mix the agarose solution.
- After dissolution, add sufficient hot distilled water to obtain the initial weight.
- Mix thoroughly.
- Cool the solution to 50-60°C prior to casting.

Agarose preparation in microwave (gel concentrations of > 2% w/v)

- Choose a beaker that is 2-4 times the volume of the solution.
- Add room temperature or chilled buffer (MetaPhor® and NuSieve® GTG® agaroses) and a stir bar to the beaker.
- Sprinkle in the premeasured agarose powder while the solution is rapidly stirred to prevent the formation of clumps.
- Remove the stir bar if not Teflon coated.
- Soak the agarose in the buffer for 15 minutes before heating. This reduces the tendency of the agarose solution to foam during heating.
- Weigh the beaker and solution before heating.
- Cover the beaker with plastic wrap.
- Pierce a small hole in the plastic wrap for ventilation.

  For agarose concentrations > 4%, the following additional steps will further help prevent the agarose solution from foaming during melting/dissolution:
- Heat the beaker in the microwave oven on medium power for 1 minute.
- Remove the solution from the microwave.
- Allow the solution to sit on the bench for 15 minutes.
- Heat the beaker in the microwave oven on medium power for 2 minutes.

  Note: Any microwaved solution may become superheated and foam over when agitated.
- Remove the beaker from the microwave oven.
- Swirl gently to resuspend any settled powder and gel pieces.
- Reheat the beaker on high power for 1-2 minutes or until the solution comes to a boil.
- Hold at the boiling point for 1 minute or until all of the particles are dissolved.
- Remove the beaker from the microwave oven.
- Swirl gently to mix the agarose solution thoroughly.
- After dissolution, add sufficient hot distilled water to obtain the initial weight.
- Mix thoroughly.
- Cool the solution to 50-60°C prior to gel casting.

Preparation of agarose on hot plate

- Choose a beaker that is 2-4 times the volume of the solution.
- Add chilled buffer (MetaPhor® or NuSieve® GTG® agarose) and a stir bar to the beaker.
- Sprinkle in the premeasured agarose powder while the solution is rapidly stirred to prevent the formation of clumps.
- Weigh the beaker and solution before heating. Cover the beaker with plastic wrap.
- Pierce a small hole in the plastic wrap for ventilation.
- Bring the solution to a boil while stirring.

- Maintain gentle boiling until the agarose is dissolved (approximately 5 minutes).
- Add sufficient hot distilled water to obtain the initial weight.
- Mix thoroughly.
- Cool the solution to 50-60°C prior to casting.

Casting Agarose Gels

Horizontal gel of 3-4 mm thick usually gives optimal resolution. The volume of gel solution needed can be estimated by measuring the surface area of the casting chamber, then multiplying by the gel thickness. For casting thinner gels a GelBond® film can be used.

Horizontal gel casting

- Allow the agarose solution to cool to 50-60°C. While the agarose solution is cooling, assemble the gel casting tray.
- Level the casting tray prior to pouring the agarose solution.
- Check the comb(s) teeth for residual dried agarose.
- Dried agarose can be removed by scrubbing the comb teeth with a lint-free tissue soaked in hot distilled water.
- Allow a small space (approximately 0.5-1 mm) between the bottom of the comb teeth and the casting tray.
- Pour the agarose solution into the gel tray. Replace the comb(s).
- Allow the agarose to gel at room temperature for 30 minutes.
- Low-melting-temperature agarose and MetaPhor® agarose require an additional 30 minutes of gelling at 4°C to obtain the best gel handling. The additional cooling step is essential for obtaining fine resolution in MetaPhor® agarose.
- Once the gel is set, flood with running buffer.
- Slowly remove the comb and place the gel casting tray into the electrophoresis chamber.
- Fill the chamber with running buffer until the buffer reaches 3-5 mm over the surface of the gel.
- Gently flush the wells out with electrophoresis buffer using a Pasteur pipette to remove loose gel fragments prior to loading the samples.
- Load DNA and electrophorese.

Notes

The thickness of the comb in the direction of the electric field can affect the resolution. A thin comb (< 1 mm) will result in sharper DNA bands. With a thicker comb, more volume can be added to the well but the separated DNA bands may be broader.

Vertical gel casting

This procedure is divided into the following segments: cassette assembly, cassette sealing, gel casting and preparation for electrophoresis.

Materials

Vertical electrophoresis apparatus, Combs and side spacers, Whatman 3 mm chromatography paper, Clamps, Silicone tubing or electrical tape, Two 60 ml syringes with 16-gauge needles, Heat gun or 55°C oven, Scalpel or razor blade

Cassette assembly

- Use clean glass plates. Clean with soap and water, rinse with distilled water and dry.
- Wipe the plates with ethanol and a lint-free tissue.
- Unlike polyacrylamide gels, agarose gels do not adhere to glass plates and may slide out during electrophoresis. To prevent this from happening, frosted glass plates can be used or the steps as given below may be followed.
- Place two side spacers on the back plate.
- For 1 mm thick which is considered standard-size gels, cut a strip of Whatman 3 mm chromatography paper (1 mm thick and 5-10 mm wide) long enough to fit between the two spacers.
- Wet with running buffer. Place at the bottom of the back plate in contact with the spacers on each side.
- Put on the front plate. Clamp the glass plates together.
- Seal the cassette against leaks with silicone tubing or tape.

Note

Alternatively, use Gel Bond film as a support for the gel, which obviates the need for the use of Whatman 3 mm chromatography paper to hold the gel in the cassette during electrophoresis. Gel Bond film is put into the casting cassette and the gel attaches to the film during the gelling process. After electrophoresis, the gel may be dried down on the Gel Bond film and kept as a permanent record. However, Gel Bond film blocks UV light below 300 nm and exhibits background fluorescence. To overcome these problems, gels cast on Gel Bond film may be photographed inverted (gel side down) on the UV light box. Background fluorescence can be screened using red, orange UV filters.

Cassette sealing

Follow one of the methods below to seal the cassette prior to casting the gel.

Silicone tubing Method

- Use silicone tubing, which should be of the same diameter as the spacer thickness.
- Cut a piece long enough to extend along the bottom and up both sides of the cassette.
- Place the tubing across the bottom of the back plate below the blotting paper strip.
- Place the top plate over the bottom plate and clamp the glass plates together at the bottom.
- Run the tubing up either side of the plates and finish clamping the plates together.

Tape method

- Place the top plate over the bottom plate.
- Tape the sides of the cassette with separate pieces of tape.
- Tape the bottom of the cassette with a separate piece of tape. This way the tape on the bottom can be removed for electrophoresis without disturbing the tape at the sides of the gel. Clamp the plates together.

Casting a vertical agarose gel

- Prepare agarose solution.
- Pre-warm the assembled cassette and a 60 ml syringe for 15 minutes by placing in a 55°C oven or by using a heat gun.

- Cool the dissolved agarose to 60°C. Pour into a pre-warmed 60 ml syringe fitted with a 16-gauge needle.
- Wedge the needle tip between the plates in the upper corner of the cassette with the needle opening directed towards the back plate.
- Inject the agarose solution at a moderate, steady rate. Keep a constant flow to prevent air bubble formation.
- Angle the cassette while pouring so the agarose solution flows down one side spacer, across the bottom and up the other side. Fill until the agarose solution goes just above the glass plates.
- Insert one end of the comb, then slowly insert the rest of the comb until the teeth are at an even depth. Insert the comb into the agarose to the minimal depth necessary to accommodate samples.
- Place extra clamps on the side of the glass plates to hold the comb in place. Cool the gel at room temperature for 15 minutes.
- Place the gel at 4°C for 20 minutes. Remove the clamps at the top of the gel.
- Remove any excess agarose with a scalpel or razor blade.
- Squirt running buffer in the spaces between the comb and the gel. Slowly and gently lift the comb straight up.
- Allow air or buffer to enter the well area to release the vacuum, which forms between the agarose and the comb. The wells can be further cleaned by flushing with running buffer.
- The gel can be stored overnight in a humidity chamber or in a sealed bag with a buffer-dampened paper towel.

Preparation for electrophoresis

- Remove the silicone tubing or tape at the bottom of the cassette and place the cassette into the chamber at an angle to minimize the number of bubbles, which can collect in the well area.
- Since agarose does not adhere well to glass, leave as many clips in place as possible.
- For some electrophoresis chambers, it is helpful to seal the spacers at the top of the gel with molten agarose

Vacuum Drying Agarose Gels

For drying the agarose gel, sandwich the gel between two sheets of porous cellophane or between Whatman 3 mm electrophoresis paper and plastic wrap. Place several sheets of Whatman 3 mm paper on the vacuum dryer, followed by the gel and plastic wrap. If the gel is cast on gel bond film, set up the sandwich so the film is not between the vacuum source and the gel. Turn on vacuum dryer. A rheostat may be used to control the temperature of gel dryer. If heat is to be applied, do not exceed 55°C as the gel may melt. Drying times depend upon the thickness of the gel. Times listed in Table 2.5 are approximate when drying at 55°C.

Table 2.5. Drying time for agarose gel

Gel thickness (mm)	Drying time (hours)
1mm	1-1.5
3-4mm	4

Sample Application

- After maturation of gel, remove the plastic sheet from the gel surface and measure length from cathode end and cut with the help of sharp wide razor blade. Then apply the sample to the solution and seal slit with soft paraffin wax or thin strip of glass. Carefully place the gel plate to the electrophoresis tank either in the horizontal or vertical position.
- Place the double layer of buffer soaked double layer of Whatman filter paper No. 3 between the gel and buffer compartments. Cover the gel with PVC sheet previously coated with liquid paraffin to reduce the evaporation during the run.
- In vertical gel electrophoresis prepare slot by removing slot former carefully and then apply sample in casted slots.
- Application of sample should be dome with utmost care using Pasteur pipettes so that sample does not leak in other slots.
- Seal the sample with molten/ soft vaseline or agar. After the slots get set place the gel on the vertical stand and connect to electrode bridge buffer with filter paper.
- Run the gel. After completion of run, remove the gel and place on glass plate.
- Slice the gel : for separation purpose
- Stain the gel : for identification purpose

Gel Staining

SYBR® Green I, Ethidium Bromide, Silver and acridine orange and methylene blue are commonly used stains for DNA. Detection limit and applications are summarized in table 2.6.

Table 2.6. Commonly used stains for DNA with their detection limit and applications

Stain	Limits of detection		Application
	dsDNA	ssDNA	
SYBR® Green I	60 pg	1 ng	For high detection sensitivity
SYBR Green II	5 ng	1 ng	High detection sensitivity for ssDNA and for RNA
Ethidium bromide	1-5 ng	5 ng	Carcinogenic
Silver stain for agarose	1 ng	5 ng	Better sensitivity for polyacrylamide gels
Methylene blue	40-200 ng	N/A	Non-toxic For staining large amounts of DNA
Acridine orange	50 ng	100 ng	To distinguish ssDNA from dsDNA

DNA staining with SYBR Green I or II

Materials

Clear polypropylene container, SYBR Green photographic filter or an equivalent, Microcentrifuge, UV transilluminator

Reagents

Buffer between pH 7.5-8.5 (TAE, TBE or TE)

SYBR Green I stain stock solution

Procedure

For optimal resolution, sharpest bands and lowest background, stain the gel with SYBR Green I stain following electrophoresis. Alternatively, SYBR Green I stain can be included in the agarose gel. When the dye is incorporated into the agarose, the gel is more sensitive to DNA overloading, and the electrophoretic separation of DNA may not be identical to that achieved with ethidium bromide.

Gel staining with SYBR Green I following electrophoresis

- Remove the concentrated stock solution of SYBR Green I stain from the freezer.
- Allow the solution to thaw at room temperature.
- Spin the solution in a microcentrifuge to collect the dye at the bottom of the tube.
- Dilute the 10,000X concentrate to a 1X working solution, in a pH 7.0-8.5 buffer, in a clear plastic polypropylene container.
- Prepare enough staining solution to just cover the top of the gel.
- Remove the gel from the electrophoresis chamber.
- Place the gel in staining solution.
- Gently agitate the gel at room temperature.
- Stain the gel for 15-30 minutes.
- The optimal staining time depends on the thickness of the gel, concentration of the agarose, and the fragment size to be detected. Longer staining times are required as gel thickness and agarose concentration increase.
- Remove the gel from the staining solution and view with a 300 nm UV transilluminator or 254 nm epi-illuminator.

Gel staining when included agarose gel

- Remove the concentrated stock solution of SYBR Green I stain from the freezer and allow the solution to thaw.
- Spin the solution in a microcentrifuge tube.
- Prepare the agarose solution.
- Once the agarose solution has cooled to 70°C, add SYBR Green I stain by diluting the stock 1:10,000 into the gel solution prior to pouring the gel.
- Slowly swirl the solution. Pour the gel into the casting tray. Load DNA onto the gel and run the gel.
- Remove the gel from the electrophoresis chamber. View with a 300 nm UV trans-illuminator or 254 nm epi-illuminator.

Staining Vertical Gels with SYBR Green I stain

SYBR Green I stain is not incorporated into the gel or prestaining the DNA in a vertical format. The dye apparently binds to glass or plastic plates and DNA may show little to no signal. Gels should be post-stained as already described.

Notes

New clear polypropylene containers should be obtained for use with SYBR Green I stain. When stored in the dark in polypropylene containers, the diluted stain can be used for up to 24 hours and will stain 2 to 3 gels with little decrease in sensitivity. The containers should be rinsed with distilled water (do not use detergents) after each use and dedicated to SYBR

Green I stain use only. SYBR Green I stain binds to glass and some non-polypropylene (polystyrene) plastics resulting in reduced or no signal from the nucleic acid.

A 1X working solution of SYBR Green I stain should be prepared from the 10,000X stock solution by diluting in a pH 7.0 to 8.5 buffer (e.g., TAE, TBE or TE).

Agarose gels should be cast no thicker than 4 mm. As gel thickness increases, diffusion of the stain into the gel is decreased, lowering the efficiency of DNA detection.

Optimal sensitivity of SYBR Green I stain-bound DNA is achieved with the SYBR Green Photographic Filter. This filter is of deep yellow colour and is 3 x 3 inches (75 x 75 mm). For photographing gels use a filter that will allow a 525 nm transmission.

SYBR Green I stained gels do not require destaining. The dye's fluorescence yield is much greater when bound to DNA than in solution form.

When the dye is incorporated into the agarose, the gel is more sensitive to DNA overloading. It is recommend that no more than 1 to 5 ng of DNA per band or making serial dilutions of a DNA marker to determine the optimal DNA loading level. Electrophoretic separation of DNA in the presence of SYBR Green I stain may not be identical to that achieved with ethidium bromide. The effect of SYBR Green I stain on DNA mobility is dependent on the DNA band's size and quantity, resulting in variable mobility shifts.

SYBR Green I stain is removed from double-stranded DNA by using ethanol precipitation of nucleic acids.

Gels previously stained with ethidium bromide can subsequently be stained with SYBR Green I stain post-staining. There will be some decrease in sensitivity when compared to a gel stained with only SYBR Green I stain.

The inclusion of SYBR Green I stain in cesium chloride density gradient plasmid preparations is not recommended as effect of the dye on the buoyant density of DNA is unknown. Addition of 0.1 to 0.3% SDS in the prehybridization and hybridization solutions is recommended when performing Southern blots on gels stained with SYBR Green I stain.

Double-stranded DNA-bound SYBR Green I stain fluoresces green under UV trans-illumination. Gels that contain DNA with single-stranded regions may fluoresce orange rather than green.

For Decontamination of staining solutions, pass them through activated charcoal followed by incineration of the charcoal. SYBR Green nucleic acid gel stains should be handled with care and disposed of properly. Gloves should be worn when handling solutions of this dye and stained gels. Avoid skin and eye exposure to UV light.

Photography of stained gel

Gels stained with SYBR Green I stain exhibit negligible background fluorescence, allowing long film exposures when detecting small amounts of DNA. When used with 300 nm transillumination and Polaroid® type 57 film, a 0.5-1 second exposure at f-4.5 is adequate. In the photographs, the DNA appears as bright bands against a gray gel. For Polaroid type 55 film, a 15-45 second exposure at f-4.5 is adequate. When used with 254 nm epi-illumination (especially with a handheld UV lamp), exposures of the order of 1-1.5 minutes may be required for maximal sensitivity. With 254 nm epi-illumination, the DNA appears as bright bands against a black background. SYBR Green I stain is also compatible with CCD imaging systems.

DNA detection using ethidium bromide

Materials

Staining vessel larger than gel, UV transilluminator, Magnetic stir plate, Magnetic stir bar

Reagents

Ethidium bromide stock solutions (10 mg/ml)

1g Ethidium bromide
100 ml Distilled water
Stir on magnetic stirrer for several hours
Transfer the solution to a dark bottle
Store at room temperature
Electrophoresis buffer or distilled water

Procedure

For optimal resolution, sharpest bands and lowest background, stain the gel with ethidium bromide following electrophoresis. Ethidium bromide can also be included in the gel and electrophoresis buffer (0.5 μg/ml) with only a minor loss of resolution. The electrophoretic mobility of DNA gets reduced by approximately 15%.

Procedure to stain DNA after electrophoresis

- Prepare enough working solution of ethidium bromide (0.5-1 μg/ml of ethidium bromide in distilled water or gel buffer) to cover the surface of the agarose gel.
- Remove the gel from the electrophoresis chamber.
- Submerge it for 20 minutes in the ethidium bromide solution then remove the gel from the solution.
- Submerge the gel for 20 minutes in a new container filled with distilled water. Repeat in fresh distilled water.
- Gels can be viewed with the help of a hand-held or tabletop UV light.

Notes

For gel concentrations of 4% or greater, destaining time may need to be doubled. If after destaining the background is still too high, continue to destain.

Procedure for including ethidium bromide in the agarose gel

- Prepare agarose solution. While the agarose solution is cooling, add ethidium bromide to a final concentration of 0.1 to 0.5 μg/ml to the solution. Slowly swirl the solution.
- Pour the gel into the casting tray. Add ethidium bromide to the running buffer to a final concentration of 0.5 μg/ml.
- Load and run the gel. Destain the gel by submerging the gel in distilled water for 20 minutes. Repeat in fresh distilled water.
- Gels can be viewed with a hand-held or tabletop UV light during or after electrophoresis.

DNA detection using silver stain

Materials

Gel Bond® film, Forced hot air oven, Staining vessels larger than the gel, Clean glass plate larger than the gel, Blotting paper, Rubber roller or tissue, Magnetic stir plate, Magnetic stir bar, Clamps or Clips

Reagents

Distilled water

Fixative Solution (Silver Stain)

500 ml Methanol
120 ml Glacial acetic acid
50 g Glycerol
Bring volume to 1 litre with distilled water
Prepare fresh

Solution A

50 g Sodium carbonate
Bring volume to 1 litre with distilled water
Stable for 2 to 3 weeks at room temperature

Solution B

2.0 g Ammonium nitrate
2.0 g Silver nitrate
10 g Tungstosilic acid
8.0 ml 37% Formaldehyde
Bring volume to 1 litre with distilled water
Stable for 1 week when stored in the dark at room temperature.

Stop Solution

1% Glacial acetic acid in distilled water
Prepare fresh

Procedure for silver staining

- Fix the dried gels for 30 minutes in the Fixative solution. Wash it three times in distilled water for 20 minutes.
- Vigorously stir solution A on a magnetic stir plate. To prepare the staining solution, add an equal volume of solution B to solution A.
- Place the staining solution in a staining vessel.
- Place the gel into the staining solution.
- Allow it to stay in the stain until the bands appear.
- Place the gel in the stop solution for 5 minutes and rinse the gel in distilled water.
- Allow the gel to air dry.

DNA detection using methylene blue

Materials

Staining vessel larger than the gel, Distilled water

Reagents

Methylene blue stain solution

0.02% Methylene blue in distilled water

Procedure

- Remove gel from electrophoresis chamber.
- Stain gel for 15 minutes in staining solution.
- Destain gel for 15 minutes in distilled water.

DNA detection using acridine orange

Materials

Enamel staining container larger than the gel, UV transilluminator

Reagents

Acridine orange

10 mM Sodium phosphate buffer or distilled water

95% Ethanol

Acridine orange stock staining solution

10 mg/ml acridine orange in distilled water

Store protected from light at 4°C

Procedure

- Dilute the acridine orange stock solution to 30μg/ml in 10 mM sodium phosphate buffer or distilled water. Remove the gel from the electrophoresis chamber.
- Stain the gel in the dark for 30 minutes in the diluted staining solution.
- Destain the gel in the dark for 30 minutes in distilled water or 10 mM sodium phosphate buffer.
- Removal of high background fluorescence can be achieved by destaining overnight at 4°C in the dark.
- View under 300 nm UV light.
- Clean the enamel staining container by washing with 95% ethanol.

Notes

If destaining is incomplete, the background will appear dark green, and the red bands will appear dull, or even black. Faint bands may not be visible at this stage. Photography of gels stained with acridine orange is best carried out with a red photographic filter. The red filter enhances the ability to discriminate the red bands against a green background

PROTOCOL 2.2

ONE DIMENSIONAL AGAROSE GEL ELECROPHORESIS

Materials

Agarose solution in TBE or TAE (generally 0.7-1%), 1X TBE or TAE, Gel loading dye 10 mg/ml ethidium bromide

Procedure

- To prepare 100 ml of a 0.7% agarose solution measure 0.7 g agarose into a glass beaker or flask and add 100 ml 1X TBE or TAE.
- Microwave or stir on a hot plate until agarose is dissolved and solution is clear.
- Allow solution to cool to about 55°C before pouring. (Ethidium bromide can be added at this point to a concentration of 0.5 μg/ml).

- Prepare gel tray by sealing ends with tape or other custom-made dam. Place comb in gel tray about 1 inch from one end of the tray and position the comb vertically such that the teeth are about 1-2 mm above the surface of the tray. Pour 50°C gel solution into tray to a depth of about 5 mm. Allow gel to solidify. It takes about 20 minutes at room temperature.
- To run, gently remove the comb, place tray in electrophoresis chamber, and cover (just until wells are submerged) with electrophoresis buffer (the same buffer used to prepare the agarose).
- To prepare samples for electrophoresis, add 1 µl of 6X gel loading dye for every 5 µl of DNA solution. Mix well. Load 5-12 µl of DNA per well (for mini gel).
- Electrophorese at 50-150 volts until dye markers have migrated an appropriate distance, depending on the size of DNA to be visualized.

Notes

If the gel was not stained with ethidium bromide during the run, stain the gel in 0.5 µg/ml ethidium bromide until the DNA has taken up the dye and becomes visible under short wave UV light, if the DNA is not to be used further, or with a hand-held long-wave light if the DNA is to be cloned.

Compositions of Various Reagents

50X TAE
- 242 g Tris base
- 57.1 g Glacial acetic acid
- 100 ml 0.5 M EDTA

10X TBE
- 108 g Tris base
- 55 g Boric acid
- 40 ml 0.5 M EDTA, pH 8.0
- Distilled water to 1 litre

6X Gel loading buffer
- 0.25% Bromophenol blue
- 0.25%Xylene cyanol FF
- 15% Ficoll Type 4000
- 120 mM EDTA

PROTOCOL 2.3

TWO DIMENSIONAL (2-D) AGAROSE GEL ELECTROPHORESIS OF DNA REPLICATION INTERMEDIATES

In the 2-D gel electrophoresis polypeptides are separated on different conditions on each direction. The first dimension gel is run at low voltage in low percentage agarose to separate DNA molecules in proportion to their mass. The second dimension is run at high voltage in a gel of higher agarose concentration in the presence of ethidium bromide so that its shape drastically influences the mobility of a non-linear molecule (Fig. 2.6). In comparison to SDS-PAGE, 2 D-gel electrophoresis gives better resolution to complex protein samples.

First Dimension

Materials

1X TBE

0.089M Tris-borate, 0.089 M boric acid 0.002 M EDTA

Electrophoresis buffer

0.4% Agarose in 1X TBE

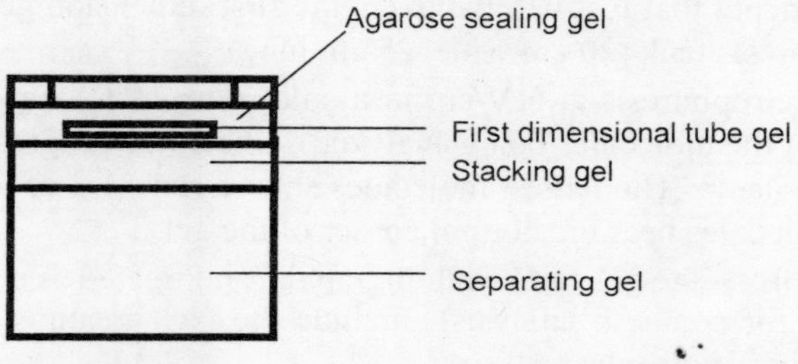

Fig. 2.6. Positioning of tube gel on top of slab gel for second dimensional run

Procedure

- Pour agarose in horizontal slab gel apparatus with a comb ~1.5 mm from the bottom support plate. The dimensions of the slab are somewhat arbitrary; convenient dimensions are 13 cm wide, 20 cm long, and ~0.6 cm thick..
- Use a comb with narrow, thin teeth (for example, 4 mm wide and 1.2 mm thick) to produce a narrow first dimension gel lane with tight, sharp bands. Load alternate lanes of the gel. The empty lanes prevent accidental cross-contamination when the lanes are excised for the second dimension.
- Carry out the electrophoresis, with the gel submerged by a few mm, at 0.7 to 1 V/cm for 15 to 30 hours. (If a voltmeter is not available, estimate the voltage required by measuring the distance between the electrodes of the gel box and set the voltage accordingly). Stain the first dimension slab gel in 1X TBE with 0.3 μg/ml ethidium bromide for ~20 minutes. Examine the gel on long wave UV light box and mark lanes to be run in the second dimension.

Notes

Do not expose the gel to excessive doses of UV light as the DNA will become nicked and replicating structures can be lost. Excise the lanes of interest with a clean razor blade, making at least one edge very straight, vertical, and close to the lane of interest. It is through this cut edge that the DNA will run in the second dimension. The lane can be trimmed which contains the size range of interest. When possible, include the entire lane from the well to at least 1cm beyond the band of interest.

Second Dimension

Materials

1.0-1.2% Agarose gel in 1X TBE

0.3 μg/ml Ethidium bromide

Electrophoresis buffer: 1X TBE with 0.3 μg/ml ethidium bromide (2-3 litre total) circulated from anode to cathode at 50 to 100 ml/minute.

Procedure

- Place the lane on a clean gel support at 90°C to the direction of electrophoresis. Convenient dimensions for the second gel are 10 cm wide (or the length of the first dimension gel lane) by 13 cm long.
- Permit the agarose to cool to ~55°C and then pour the agarose around the first dimension lane, to a final depth that just barely covers the first dimension gel lane. Submerge the gel in an electrophoresis tank (20 cm wide, 25 cm long).
- Perform the electrophoresis at 5 V/cm in a cold room (4°C) for 4-8 hours (depending on the size range of the molecules being analyzed). Check the progress of electrophoresis with a hand-held UV lamp. The largest molecules should run ~1/3 of the length of the gel with the smallest molecules near the bottom corner of the gel.
- After electrophoresis the gel can be photographed and treated as a gel for Southern analysis (see procedure for southern analysis). Include the HCl treatment to facilitate transfer of large and branched molecules.

Notes

Some restriction enzymes have non-specific single-stranded nucleases as contaminants. These will destroy branched molecules. Check with manufacturer, or incubate the enzymes with single-stranded circles of M13 or PhiX174 DNA and assay on gels for breakage or degradation. Avoid using Spermidine in restriction enzyme digestions. Spermidine remains associated with the DNA during electrophoresis and reduces the charge on the DNA. The result is that the proportion of the fragments trail during the first dimension electrophoresis. In the second dimension the retarded DNA produces horizontal streaks across the gel. Manipulating the 0.4% agarose gel slab can be tricky since it has so little gel strength and also slippery. Handle it with plastic support sheets.

PROTOCOL 2.4

ELECTROPHORETIC SEPARATION OF PLASMA PROTEINS

In this experiment, proteins obtained from human plasma by salt precipitation are separated by electrophoresis.

Materials

1% Alcoholic solution of bromophenol blue

Sodium nitrite solution 12%

Normal saline solution (0.9% NaCl)

Barbitone buffer 0.07 M, pH 6.8

Acetic acid solution 0.5%

Procedure

Fractionation of human plasma

- Mix 9.5 ml sodium nitrite solution in 0.5 ml collected human plasma.
- Allow to stand at room temperature for 10-15 minutes.
- Collect the precipitate by centrifugation at 3000g for 10 minutes and store. At this concentration of salt, fibrinogen is precipitated.
- Decant the supernatant, measure the volume and add to it, sufficient amount of sodium nitrite so that the final concentration is 15%. At this stage the α-globulins precipitate out.
- Collect the precipitate by centrifugation as before and store.
- The γ-globulins in the supernatant, are precipitated out by raising the salt concentration upto 20% and the precipitate is collected. Save the supernatant also.
- Dissolve the precipitates in 0.5 ml saline (0.9% NaCl).

Electrophoresis of samples

- Fill the tanks with barbitone buffer (0.07 M, pH 6.8) to equal level.
- Moisten a filter paper strip (Whatman 1 mm; 9 cm x 3 cm) with the buffer, drain off the excess fluid by slightly folding in between blotting papers, and lay it on a solid support (a glass plate) between the two tanks. The two ends should dip in the buffer solution.
- Alternately, paper wicks can be used to bring about contact between the buffer and the paper.
- Now carefully streak 10 μl of unfractionated plasma across the breadth, midway between the tanks.
- Cover the set-up. Switch on the power supply and adjust the voltage to 36 V (4V/cm).
- Leave the set-up undisturbed for about 6 hours and at the end of the period turn off the power supply.
- Remove the strip and dry by placing in an oven for a few minutes.
- Repeat for various fractions obtained from plasma.
- In some instruments it is not possible to use 3 or 4 strips at the same time, in that case the voltage has to be increased correspondingly.

Detection of protein bands

- The dry strips are soaked in a 1% alcoholic solution of bromophenol blue, when the protein gets stained.
- After soaking for 15 minutes, the strips are removed and soaked in another tray containing 0.5% acetic acid solution. The acid treatment removes the excess dye, which remains unabsorbed to the protein.
- The acid washing is carried out till a clear background is obtained with the blue bands of proteins.
- Give a quick wash with water to remove acid and dry the strips in air.
- Compare the bands obtained with the whole plasma and those from the fractionated samples and comment on the results.

PROTOCOL 2.5

SDS-POLYACRYLAMIDE GEL ELECTROPHORESIS

SDS gel electrophoresis is widely used for the analysis and characterization of protein samples. It is useful in molecular weight determination, relative estimation of purity and amino acid sequencing of proteins.

Stock Solution

Monomer solution

Acrylamide	97.5 g
Bis	2.5 g
Distilled water	q.s. to 200 ml. Store at 4°C in the dark.

Running gel buffer

Tris	36.3 g
Distilled water	q.s. to 200 ml. Adjust to pH 8.8 with HCl.

Stacking gel buffer

Tris	6.0 g
Distilled water	q.s. to 50 ml. Adjust to pH 6.8 with HCl

10% SDS

SDS	50 g
Distilled water	q.s. to 500 ml

Initiator

Ammonium persulphate	0.75 g
Distilled water	q.s. to 50 ml

Running gel overlay

Tris	25 ml solution
SDS	1.0 ml solution
Distilled water	q.s. to 100ml

2X Treatment buffer

Tris	2.5 ml solution
SDS solution	4.0 ml
Glycerol	2.0 ml
2-Mercaptoethanol	1.0 ml
Distilled water	10 ml

Tank buffer

Tris	12 g
Glycine	57.6 g
SDS	40 ml solution
Distilled water	q.s. to 4.0 litre

Stain stock

Coomassie blue	2.0 g
Distilled water	q.s. to 200 ml

Stir and filter

Preparation of the Separating Gel (Table 2.7)

- In a sidearm vacuum flask mix 40 ml of separating gel solution with the help of magnetic stirrer.
- Apply a vacuum to the flask for several minutes.
- Add the TEMED and ammonium per sulphate.
- Swirl the flask to mix.
- Pipette the solution into the sandwich to a level about 4.0 cm from the top.
- With the help of smooth running syringe layer the slab with water.
- Formation of a very sharp water gel interface will indicate the completeness of gelling.
- Remove the water layer by tilting casting stand.
- Rinse the surface of the gels once with distilled water.
- Add about 1.0 ml of running gel overlay solution.
- Allow the gel to set for several hours.
- Leave out the ammonium persulphate and the TEMED.
- Stir by using small magnetic stirrer.

Preparation of the Stacking Gel (Table 2.8)

- Pour the liquid to the surface of the gels
- Degas the stacking gel solution as described before.
- Add the ammonium persulphate and TEMED.
- Gently swirl the flask to mix.
- Add 1-2 ml of stacking gel solution to each sandwich to rinse the surface of the gel.
- Rock the casting stand and pour off the liquid.
- Fill each sandwich with stacking solution.
- Insert a comb into each sandwich. Take care not to trap any bubbles below the teeth of the combs.
- Allow the gel to set for at least half an hour.
- Combine equal parts of protein sample and treatment buffer in a test tube.
- Put the tube in a boiling water bath for 90 seconds.
- Remove the sample and put it on ice until ready to use.
- This treated sample can be put in the freezer for future runs.

Loading and Running the Gels

- Slowly remove the combs from the gels. Be careful to pull the comb straight up, to avoid disturbing the well dividers.
- Rinse each well with distilled water. Carefully invert the casting stand to drain the wells.
- Fill each well with tank buffer.
- Using a Hamilton syringe under layer the sample in each well.
- Add a spinner to the lower buffer chamber.
- Place the chamber on a magnetic stirrer.
- When the lower bubble is circulated, the temperature of the buffer remains uniform. This is important, because uneven heating distorts the banding pattern of the gel.

- Put a drop of 0.1% phenol red (tracking dye) in the upper buffer chamber.
- Set the power supply to constant voltage.
- Turn the power supply on and adjust the voltage so that proteins stack better.
- Run the separating gel at 100-150 Volts.
- When the dye reaches the bottom, turn the power supply off and disconnect the power cables.

Table 2.7. Composition of SDS polyacrylamide separating gels

Acrylamide stock (%)	4.0	6.0	8.0	10.0	12.0
Running gel buffer	15.0	15.0	15.0	15.0	15.0
Water	19.7	17.7	15.7	13.7	11.7
10% SDS	0.4	0.4	0.4	0.4	0.4
1.5% Ammonium persulphate	0.9	0.9	0.9	0.9	0.9
TEMED	0.02	0.02	0.02	0.02	0.02

Table 2.8. Composition of staking gel

Final acrylamide concentration (%)	3.0	6.0
Acrylamide stock	0.6	1.0
Stacking gel buffer	1.25	1.25
Water	7.55	7.15
10% SDS	0.1	0.1
1.5% Ammonium persulphate	0.5	0.5
TEMED	0.005	0.005

Staining and Destaining the Gels

Composition of staining solution

Coomassie blue	62.5 ml stain stock
Methanol	250 ml
Acetic acid	50 ml

Composition of destaining solution

Acetic acid	700 ml
Methanol	500 ml
Water	10 litres

Procedure

- Disassemble the sandwiches.
- Put the gel into stain.
- Gently shake the gels for 4-8 hours
- Remove the gels and put them in destaining solution.
- Shake for one hour.
- Use destaining solution for further destaining.

PROTOCOL 2.6

SOUTHERN ANALYSIS

In order to determine the sequences of DNA restriction fragments, which are transcribed in RNA or able to map hybridization to restriction fragments, the technique named as southern blot is used. In this method DNA restriction fragments on an agarose gel are denatured into single stranded form by alkali treatment and the gel is then laid on the top of the buffer saturated filter paper. The top of the surface of the gel is covered with a nitrocellulose membrane and this membrane is itself overlaid with many layers of dry filter paper. Due to capillary action the buffer passes though the gel accompanying the progressive wetting of the dry filter and in so doing elutes out the denatured DNA from the gel, after blotting a special pattern of bands on the surface of membrane is achieved.

Stock Solution

Southern transfer depurination solution

0.3 M HCl

Procedure

- Prepare the gel and pour in suitable container. Trim away unused portion. Submerge the gel in excess volume of 0.3 M HCl for 30 minutes.
- At room temperature submerge the gel in several volumes of 0.4 M NaOH for 30 minutes under constant agitation.
- Saturate the Whatman No. 3 paper with 0.4M NaOH.
- Invert the gel carefully so that its original underside makes the uppermost layer and then place on previously saturated Whatman No. 3. Place thicker plastic wrap around the gel to prevent short circuit.
- Squeeze out any bubbles between the gel and filter paper wick.
- Carefully align one side of the nitrocellulose membrane keeping marked side down. Remove the bubbles in between gel and nitrocellulose membrane.
- Wet two pieces of Whatman No. 3 filter paper in double distilled water and align wetted filters on top of the nitrocellulose membrane.
- Align the dry pieces of Whatman No. 3 filter paper on top of wet filter. Remove air bubbles carefully.
- Immediately align the stack of paper towels on top of filter paper and on top, place glass plate and keep an evenly distributed weight of 500 g on top of the paper towels.
- Allow the transfer to proceed for 6-8 hours at room temperature and carefully remove the cellulose membrane from the transfer apparatus.
- Submerge the membrane in 0.5 M Tris HCl-1.5 M NaCl (pH 8.0) for 5 minutes. Transfer the membrane to a dish containing 2 X SSC and submerge for 2 minutes.
- Dry the membrane in an vacuum oven at 80°C for 1 hour (keep the membrane in between two sheets of Whatman No. 3 filter paper prior to drying).
- Store the membrane overnight by covering with a Whatman No. 3 filter paper at dry place at room temperature.

PROTOCOL 2.7

IMMUNOBLOT (WESTERN BLOTTING)

Western blotting is most commonly used for identifying specific proteins recognized by antibodies. The blotting membrane is the solid phase of immunoblotting and it serves as an immobilized matrix capable of adsorbing and retaining the transferred molecules in the original separation pattern during the subsequent detection steps. Nitrocellulose is commonly used for immobilization of transferred proteins as it is easy to handle and has a high binding capacity. For the detection of the specific proteins, blocking is essential by using either proteins or detergents. The proteins for blocking include bovine serum albumin, fetal calf serum, casein and animal serum. Commonly used detergents are polyoxyethylene alcohols or polyoxyethylene sorbitan alcohol (Tween 20).

Stock solution

Transfer buffer

Tris	12 g
Glycine	57.6 g
Methanol	800 ml
Water	q.s. to 4 litre

Procedure

- After completion of SDS run, remove the gel from the glass plate sandwich. Place the gel in a tray containing 200 to 300 ml of transfer buffer and incubate the gel for 10 minutes.
- Pour about 1 inch of transfer buffer in a second tray. Fill the transfer tank with 4 litres of transfer buffer.
- Place the gel on the cassette with foam and a blotter paper between the gel and the cassette. Place the nitrocellulose on top of the gel so as not to trap any air bubbles between the gel and the membrane. Now place two sheets of blotter paper over the gel. It is important to use two sheets of paper at this step in order to position the gel near the center of the cassettes where the electrical field is most uniform. Place the second half of the cassette on the top and hook it together.
- Quickly lift the cassette out of the tray of buffer and transfer it to one of the center slots in the buffer chamber. Be certain that the cassette is oriented with the nitrocellulose membrane on the fast side, or anode side of the gel. Tap the cassette to dislodge any bubbles that may be trapped by the cassette grid.
- Place the power lid on the unit. Turn on the power supply to 50 Volts. Run the unit for 4-5 minutes or as required.

Proteins detection by the use of antibodies

- Incubate the blot in 2% Bovine Serum Albumin (BSA) and 0.05% Tween 20 in PBS (PBT) for 30 minutes.
- Following blocking, the blot should be washed two times in PBT. First antibody incubation should be carried out either for 2 hours at room temperature or overnight at 4°C.
- Following first antibody incubation, wash the blot extensively with PBT.

- Second antibody could either be directly conjugated to peroxidase or it could be biotinylated by application of avidin conjugation to peroxidase
- For colour development 33 mg of 4 chloronaphthol is dissolved in 10 ml of methanol and the volume made up to 50 ml with PBS is used. 10 µl of H_2O_2 is added to the blots, which are incubated in this solution and develop colour. Colour could be intensified by addition of a pinch of imidazole. Blots can be dried and stored between two sheets of paper.

PROTOCOL 2.8

ANTI-PHOSPHOTYROSINE WESTERN BLOTTING

Materials

5% Milk
20 mM Tris pH 7.4
150 mM NaCl
1 mM Vanadate
0.1% Tween
Antiphosphotyrosine antibody
Anti-mouse-HRP conjugated secondary antibody

Procedure

- After SDS-PAGE, set up transfer as usual.
- Block for 1 hour at room temperature before probing (Table 2.9).

Table 2.9. Blocking solution

Material	Quantity
20 mM Tris pH 7.4	2 ml 1 M Tris pH 7.4
150 mM NaCl	3 ml 5 M NaCl
10% Milk	10 g Skim milk powder
1% BSA	1 g BSA
0.1% Tween 20	100 µl Tween-20
1 mM Vanadate	1 ml 100 mM Vanadate
Double distilled water	to 100 ml

- The remaining steps are performed at room temperature in 5% milk, 20 mM Tris pH 7.4, 150 mM NaCl, 1 mM Vanadate, 0.1% Tween (no BSA). Composition are given in Table 2.10.
- Add antiphosphotyrosine antibody at 1/5000 (2 µl/10ml) for 2 hours. Wash 6 times for 15 minutes.
- Incubate with anti-mouse-HRP conjugated secondary antibody for 1 hour. Wash 5 times for 10 minutes with 20 mM Tris pH 7.4, 150 mM NaCl and 0.1% Tween with no milk).

Table 2.10. Composition of stock solution

Stock solution	For 500 ml	For 1 litre
1M Tris pH 7.4	10 ml	20 ml
5M NaCl	15 ml	30 ml
Skim milk powder	25 g	50 g
Tween 20	0.5 ml	1 ml
Sodium orthovanadate	0.09 g	0.18 g
Double distilled water to	500 ml	1 litre

- Blot membrane on 3 mm paper.
- Place membrane in ECL mix for 1 minute Blot dry on 3 mm paper.
- Expose to film for 5 minutes and develop. Re-expose for various times as necessary.

SUGGESTED READINGS

Carmichael, G.G. and McMaster, G.K., Methods in Enzymology, Academic Press, Inc. 1980.

Flores, N., *BioTechniques*, 13(2), 203-225, 1992.

FMC BioProducts, Resolutions, Vol. 11(2), 1995.

Heidcamp, W. H., Cell Biology Laboratory Manual, 1996.

Jayaraman, J., Laboratory Manual in Biochemistry, New Age International Publication, New Delhi, India, 1999.

McMaster G.K. and Carmichael, G.G., *Proc. Natl. Acad. Sci.* 74: 4835-4848, 1977.

Peats, S., *Anal. Biochem.*, 140, 178-182, 1984.

Sadasivam, S. and Manickem, A., Biochemical Methods, 2nd Edition, New Age International Publishers, New Delhi, India, 1997.

Sambrook, J., Fritsch E. F. and Maniatis, T., Molecular Cloning: A Laboratory Manual, 2nd Edition, Cold Spring Harbor Press, NewYork, USA, 1989.

Talwar, G. P. and Gupta, S. K., A Handbook of Practical and Clinical Immunology, 2nd Edition, CBS Publishers and Distributors, New Delhi, 1992.

Vyas, S. P. and Dixit, V. K, Pharmaceutical Biotechnology, CBS Publishers, New Delhi, India, 1998.

CHAPTER 3

Conjugation Techniques

- Introduction
- Glutaraldehyde based hapten-carrier conjugation
- Conjugation of proteins to liposomes
- Carbodiimide based conjugation to phosphatidylethanolamine lipid derivatives
- Glutaraldehyde based conjugation to phosphatidylethanolamine lipid derivatives
- Avidin-biotin system
- Preparation of avidin-HRP or streptavidin-HRP conjugates
- Preparation of colloidal gold-labeled proteins
- Radiolabeled antibodies
- Cascade blue conjugation of antibodies
- Preparation of antibody- toxin conjugates
- PE conjugation of antibodies

INTRODUCTION

The technology of bioconjugation has affected nearly every discipline in the life sciences. It includes the linking of two or more molecules to form a novel complex having the combined properties of its individual components. Natural or synthetic compounds with their individual activities can be chemically combined to create unique substances possessing carefully engineered characteristics. The application of the available cross-linking reactions and reagent systems for creating novel conjugates with peculiar activities has made possible the assay of minute quantities of substances, the *in vivo* targeting of molecules, and the modulation of specific biological processes. Modified or conjugated molecules have been used for purification, for detection or localization of specific cellular components, and in the treatment of diseases.

Cross-linking and modifying agents produced with the help of conjugation techniques can be applied to alter the native state and function of peptides and proteins, sugars and polysaccharides, nucleic acids and oligonucleotides, lipids and almost any other imaginable molecule that can be chemically derivatized. The structure and function of natural and synthetic molecules can be investigated and receptor-ligand interactions can be revealed with the help of modification or conjugation strategies.

Bioconjugate Chemistry

Modification and conjugation techniques are based on two interrelated chemical reactions: the reactive functional groups present on the various cross linking or derivatizing reagents and functional groups present on the target macromolecules to be modified. Without both types of functional groups being available and chemically compatible, the process of derivatization would be impossible. Reactive functional groups on cross-linking reagents, tags and probes provide the means to label specifically certain target groups on ligands, peptides, proteins, carbohydrates, lipids, synthetic polymers, nucleic acids, and oligonucleotides. Knowledge of the basic mechanisms by which the reactive groups couple to target functional groups provide the means to design intelligently a modification or conjugation strategy. Choosing the correct reagent systems that can react with the chemical groups available on target molecules, forms the basis for successful chemical modification.

Bioconjugate Reagents

The principal reactive functional groups commonly encountered on bioconjugate reagents are now commercially available. These reagents are used to solve almost any conceivable modification or conjugation problem.

Zero-length cross-linkers are smallest available reagent systems for bioconjugation. These compounds mediate the conjugation of two molecules by forming a bond containing no additional atoms. Thus, one atom of a molecule is covalently attached to an atom of a second molecule with no intervening linker or spacer. In many conjugation schemes, the final complex is bound together by virtue of chemical components that add foreign structures to the substances being cross-linked, i.e., EDC [1-Ethyl-3-(3-dimethylaminopropyl)carbodiimide hydrochloride], EDC plus N-Hydroxysulphosuccinimide, CMC [1-Cyclohexyl-3-(2-morpholinoethyl) carobodiimide], N,N' -Carbonyldiimidazole.

Homobifunctional cross-linkers are used for modification and conjugation of macromolecules consisted of bioreactive compounds containing the same functional group at both ends. Most of these homobifunctional reagents are symmetrical in design with a carbon chain spacer connecting the two identical reactive ends, i.e., formaldehyde, glutaraldehyde, carbohydrazide, DST (disuccinimidyl tartarate) etc.

Heterobifunctional cross-linkers contain two different reactive groups that can couple to two different functional targets on macromolecules, the result is the ability to direct the cross-linking reaction to selected parts of target molecules, thus garnering better control over the conjugation process. i.e., SPDP [(N-Succinimidyl 3 - (2-pyridyldithio)propionate], ABH [p-Azidobenzoyl hydrazide], APG [p-Azidophenyl glyoxal] etc.

Trifunctional cross-linkers are relatively new form of conjugation reagents, possessing three different reactive or complexing groups per molecule. i.e., 4-Azido-2-nitrophenyl-biocytin-4-nitrophenyl ester.

Tags and probes are relatively small modifying agents and are used to label proteins, nucleic acids, and other molecules. These compounds often contain groups that provide sensitive detectability by virtue of some intrinsic chemical or atomic property such as fluorescence, visible chromogenic character, radioactivity, or bioaffinity towards another protein. Most probes can be designed to contain a reactive portion capable of coupling to the functional groups of biomolecules. After modification of a protein via this reactive part, the probe becomes permanently attached, thus permanently tagging it with a unique detectable property. Subsequent interactions that the protein is allowed to undergo can be followed through tag's visibility, i.e., fluorescent labels such as fluorescein derivatives, rhodamin derivatives; biotinylation reagents such as D-biotin, biotin-hydrazide, photobiotin; iodination reagents such as chloramine-T, Iodo-beads, Iodo-Gen.

Bioconjugate Applications

Bioconjugation techniques are used in the preparation of unique conjugates and labeled molecules for use in particular application areas. These include hapten-carrier immunogen conjugates and antibody-enzyme conjugates.

Hapten-carrier immunogen conjugates i.e., carbodiimides mediated hapten carrier conjugates and glutaraldehyde-mediated hapten carrier conjugates, are used in antibody production, in immune response research and in the creation of vaccines.

Antibody-enzyme conjugates i.e., NHS ester-maleimide-mediated conjugates, glutaraldehyde mediated conjugates are used in immunoassays, targeting and detection techniques. since the development of enzyme-linked immunosorbent assay (ELISA) systems and the ability to make conjugates of specific antibodies with enzymes has provided the means to quantify or detect hundreds of important analytes. The use of enzymes as labels in immunoassay procedures surpassed radioactive tags as the means of detection, primarily due to the long-term stability potential of an enzyme system and the hazards and waste problems associated with radioisotopes.

In addition to labeling immunoglobulins with enzymes to provide detectability through their catalytic action on a substrate, antibody molecules also can be labeled or tagged with small compounds that can provide indigenous traceable properties. Labeled antibodies i.e., fluorescently labeled antibodies, radiolabeled antibodies and biotinylated antibodies are also having immense uses in immunoassays, targeting and detection techniques. Antibody-liposomes conjugates may possess encapsulated components that can be used for detection of therapy. Liposomes possessing antibodies directed against tumour cell antigens can deliver encapsulated toxins or drugs to the associated cancer cells, affecting toxicity and cell death (Fig. 3.1). Biotin, avidin and proteins can also be appended on to the surface of liposomes with the help of various conjugation techniques for different types of therapeutic applications.

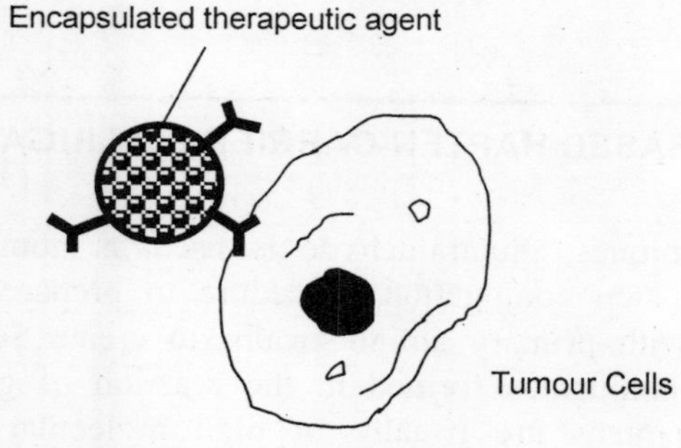

Fig. 3.1. Antibody-liposomes immunotherapeutic system

Avidin or streptavidin conjugates are used in immunoassays. The specificity of antibody molecules provides the targeting capability to recognize and bind particular antigen molecules. If there are biotin labels on the antibody molecule, it creates multiple sites for binding of avidin and streptavidin. If avidin or streptavidin in turn labeled with an enzyme, fluorophore, etc., then a very sensitive antigen-detection system is created. The potential for more than one labeled avidin to become attached to each antibody through its multiple biotinylation sites is the key to dramatic increase in assay sensitivity over that obtained through the use of antibodies directly labeled with a detectable tag (Fig. 3.2).

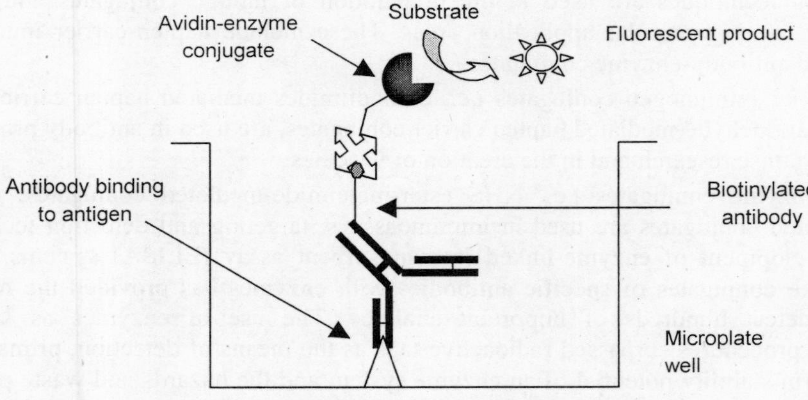

Fig. 3.2. The basic design of the labeled avidin-biotin (LAB) assay system

Enzymatic labeling of DNA and chemical modification of nucleic acids and oligonucleotides can be done effectively with the help of bioconjugation techniques. To modify the unique chemical groups on nucleic acids, novel methods have been developed that allow derivatization through discrete sites on the available bases, sugars, or phosphate groups. These conjugation methods can be used to add a functional group or a label to an individual nucleotide or to one or more sites in oligonucleotide probes or full-sized DNA or RNA polymers.

PROTOCOL 3.1

GLUTARALDEHYDE BASED HAPTEN-CARRIER CONJUGATION

In bioconjugation techniques, glutaraldehyde is used as homobifunctional cross-linking reagent in one or two step conjugation procedure to prepare hapten-carrier conjugates. Glutaraldehyde reacts with primary amino groups to create Schiff bases or double-bond addition product. The conjugates formed in the reaction of glutaraldehyde with protein carriers and peptide haptens are usually of high molecular weight and may cause precipitation products. Various types of procedures are discussed in the literature to form glutaraldehyde conjugates. In some methods neutral pH environment in phosphate buffer (pH 6.8-7.5) is used while in others alkaline conditions in carbonate buffer (pH 8-9) are used. In general, the higher pH conditions will be more effective to form Schiff base intermediates and result in greater conjugation yields with higher molecular weight conjugates. One step glutaraldehyde method is utilized in the following procedure in which by varying the pH and the amount of glutaraldehyde added to the reaction, the yield and molecular weight of the conjugate formed can be controlled.

Materials, Chemicals and Buffers

Materials

For column separations, following pre-poured column can be used:

For 1.25 ml to 2.5 ml sample volumes: Sephadex G-50.

Chemicals

Glutaraldehyde
Sodium borohydride
Sodium bicarbonate
Sodium carbonate
Sodium chloride

Buffers

Phosphate buffer saline (PBS pH 7.4)

Disodium hydrogen phosphate	2.80 g
Potassium dihydrogen phosphate	0.19 g
Sodium chloride	8.0 g
Distilled water	to 1000 ml

Procedure

- Carrier protein (or another carrier that contains amino groups) is dissolved in 0.1 M sodium carbonate, 0.15 M NaCl, pH 8.5, at a concentration of 2 mg/ml. Peptide hapten is added to the carrier solution to obtain a concentration of about 2 mg/ml. Alternatively, the molar ratio of peptide to carrier is determined. 20:1 to 40:1 (peptide: carrier) ratio result in good immunogens.
- Fresh glutaraldehyde is added and thoroughly mixed with the peptide/carrier solution to obtain a 1% final concentration. It is allowed to react for 2-4 hours at 4°C. Solution is mixed periodically on a rotary flask shaker. (Caution: Use of fume hood is recommended when working with glutaraldehyde. Avoid contact with skin and clothing.)
- The conjugation may be stabilized by the addition of a reductant e.g., sodium borohydride or sodium cynoborohydride which is usually recommended for specific reduction of Schiff bases, but since the conjugate has already been formed at this point, sodium borohydride reduces the Schiff bases and eliminates any remaining aldehyde group as well. Sodium borohydride is added to the final concentration of 10 mg/ml and allowed to react for 1 hour at 4°C.
- Finally, conjugate is purified by gel electrophoresis using Sephadex G-25 or dialysis to remove excess reagent. Some precipitation may occur in the final product due to the presence of high molecular weight conjugates. If turbidity is evident, dialyze against PBS at pH 7.4 instead of gel filtering.

CONJUGATION OF PROTEINS TO LIPOSOMES

Conjugation of liposomes with proteins may be done through reactive functional groups on the head groups of phospholipids with homobifunctional or heterobifunctional cross-linking reagents, with carbodiimides, by reductive amination, by NHS ester activation of carboxylates, or through the noncovalent use of avidin-biotin interaction. The resultant protein-liposomes composition is highly dependent on the size of each liposome, the amount of protein charged to the reaction, and the molar quantity of reactive lipid present in the bilayer construction. Liposome protein coupling occasionally induces vesicle aggregation due to unique properties or concentration of the protein used, or it may be a result of liposome to liposome cross-linking during the conjugation process hence amount of protein charged to the reaction has to be adjusted to solve an aggregation problem.

PROTOCOL 3.2

CARBODIIMIDE BASED CONJUGATION TO PHOSPHATIDYLETHANOLAMINE LIPID DERIVATIVES

Liposomal membrane is composed of underivatized PE that contains an amino group that participates in the carbodiimide reaction with carboxylate groups of proteins. Carboxylate groups are activated by water-soluble carbodiimide EDC to form active ester intermediate that can react with PE to form an amide linkage (Fig. 3.3). Unfortunately, since abundance of both amide and carboxylates present on proteins, EDC coupling of proteins to the surface of liposomes often results in considerable protein to protein cross-linking. Sometimes vesicle aggregation also occurs due to protein coupling to more than one liposomes. This polymerization problem can be avoided by first blocking the amino groups of the protein with citraconic acid, which has been used successfully with antibodies.

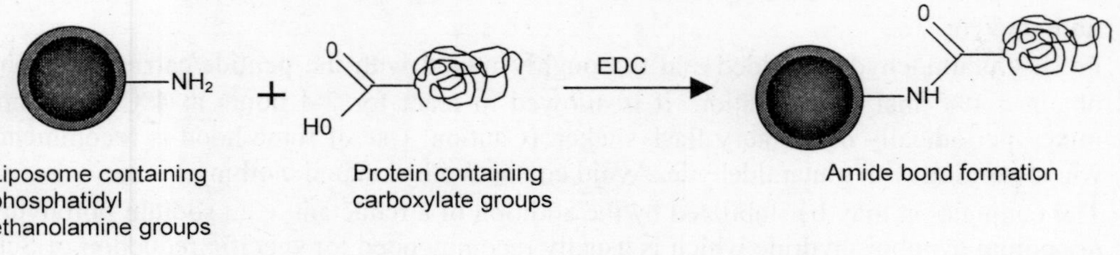

Fig. 3.3. Reaction showing the conjugation of protein with a liposome containing PE groups using a carbodiimide reaction with EDC

Materials, Chemicals and Buffers

Materials

For column separations, following pre-poured column can be used:
For 1.25 ml to 2.5 ml sample volumes: Sephadex G-75.

Chemicals

Phosphatidylcholine (PC)
Phosphatidylethanolamine (PE)
Phosphatidylglycerol (PG)
Cholesterol
1-Ethyl-3-(3-dimethylaminopropyl)carbodiimide hydrochloride (EDC)
Sodium phosphate
Sodium chloride

Buffers

Phosphate buffer saline (PBS pH 7.2)

Disodium hydrogen phosphate	2.38 g
Potassium dihydrogen phosphate	0.19 g
Sodium chloride	8.0 g
Distilled water	to 1000 ml

Procedure

- Liposomal suspension containing PE are prepared by mixing PC:cholesterol:PG:PE in a molar ratio of 8:10:1:1 by any suitable method. Concentration is adjusted to about 5 mg lipid/ml buffer. The final liposomal suspension should be in 10 mM sodium phosphate, 0.15 M NaCl, pH 7.2.
- Protein is dissolved in PBS, pH 7.2, and an aliquot is added to the liposomal suspension. The amount of protein to be added can vary considerably, depending on the abundance of protein and the desired final density required. From 1mg protein/ml to 20 mg protein/ml liposome suspension can be reacted.
- 10 mg EDC/ml of lipid/protein mixture is added and solubilized using a vortex mixer. It is allowed to react for 2 hours at room temperature. Scale back the amount of EDC added to the reaction if liposomes aggregation or protein precipitation occurs during the cross-linking process. Conjugate is purified by gel filtration using a column of Sephadex G-75.

PROTOCOL 3.3

GLUTARALDEHYDE BASED CONJUGATION TO PHOSPHATIDYLETHANOLAMINE LIPID DERIVATIVES

Glutaraldehyde, a homobifunctional cross-linker reacts with PE residues present on the liposome surface to form an activated surface reactive aldehyde group. A two-step conjugation reaction via glutaraldehyde is a suitable method when working with liposomes, since precipitated protein would be difficult to remove from vesicle suspension (Fig. 3.4).

Materials, Chemicals and Buffers

Materials

For column separations, following column can be used:
For 1.25 ml to 2.5 ml sample volumes: PD-10 (Sephadex G-50).

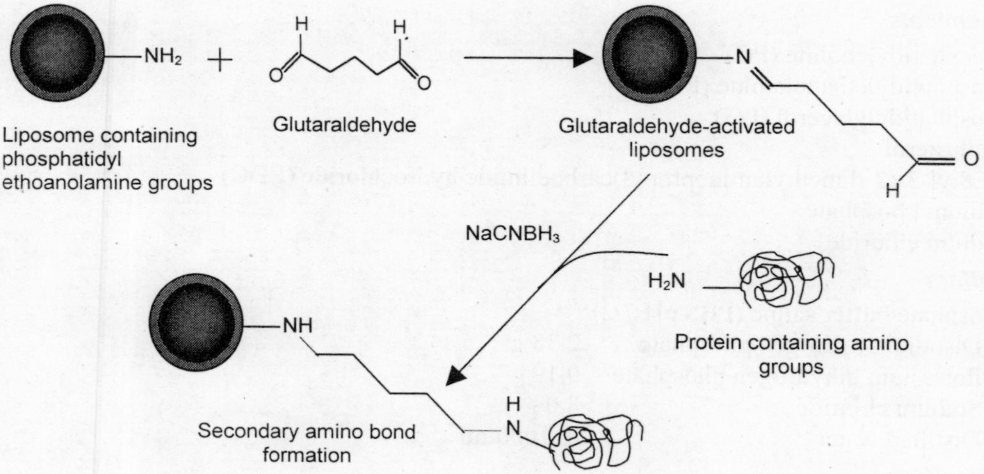

Fig. 3.4. Reaction showing glutaraldehyde activation of PE-containing liposomes used to couple protein molecules

Chemicals

Phosphatidylcholine
Phosphatidylethanolamine
Phosphatidylglycerol
Cholesterol
Glutaraldehyde
Sodium borohydride
Sodium bicarbonate
Sodium carbonate
Sodium chloride

Buffer

Phosphate buffer saline (PBS pH 6.8)

Disodium hydrogen phosphate	2.80 g
Potassium dihydrogen phosphate	0.19 g
Sodium chloride	8.0 g
Distilled water	to 1000 ml

Procedure

- Liposomal suspension containing PE are prepared by mixing PC:cholesterol:PG:PE in a molar ratio of 8:10:1:1 by any suitable method. Concentration is adjusted to about 5 mg lipid/ml buffer. The final liposomal suspension should be in 10 mM sodium phosphate, 0.15 M NaCl, pH 7.2.
- Glutaraldehyde is added to the liposomal suspension to obtain final concentration of 1.25% v/v and allowed to react overnight at room temperature under a nitrogen blanket. Activated liposomes are purified to remove excess glutaraldehyde by gel filtration (using Sephadex G-50) or by dialysis against PBS, pH 6.8.

- Protein or peptide solution is prepared in 0.5 M sodium carbonate, pH 9.5 at a concentration of 10 mg/ml.
- This protein or peptide solution is mixed with activated liposomal suspension for conjugation reaction to be accomplished. Usually 4 mg of protein per milligram of total lipid is required for acceptable conjugation.
- It is allowed to react overnight at 4°C under an atmosphere of nitrogen. Sodium borohydride is added to the final concentration of 10 mg/ml for reduction of resultant Schiff bases and any excess of aldehyde.

AVIDIN-BIOTIN SYSTEM

Avidin-biotin system is one of the most popular conjugation techniques of noncovalent conjugation, which is used, in specific targeting applications and assay designs. Avidin is a glycoprotein that contains four identical subunits and each subunit contains one binding site for biotin and one for oligosaccharide modification. This interaction may be used to enhance the signal strength of immunoassay systems. The only disadvantage is the tendency of avidin molecule to bind non-specifically to components other than biotin due to its high pI (isoelectric point) and carbohydrate content. Streptavidin is another biotin binding protein isolated from *Streptomyces avidinii* having less nonspecificities of avidin. Streptavidin, similar to avidin, contains four subunits, each with a single biotin binding site. Avidin and streptavidin are used in bioconjugation techniques to conjugate other proteins or label with various detection reagents without loss of biotin binding activity.

There are various basic immunoassays based on avidin-biotin interaction. Biotinylated antibody creates multiple sites for the binding of avidin or streptavidin. If avidin or streptavidin is labeled with enzyme or fluorophore etc. then a very sensitive antigen detection system can be created. Some of the assay systems are, labeled avidin-biotin (LAB) assay system, bridged avidin-biotin system (BRAB), and avidin-biotin complex (ABC) system. Similar techniques are used to develop avidin-biotin system for detection of nucleic acid hybridization in which avidin labeled complexes are used to detect DNA probes labeled with biotin after binding with their complementary DNA target. Avidin-biotin system can also be used in the nonenzyme assay systems in which labeled avidin molecules can be utilized for detection of biotinylated molecule after it has bound to its target. Similarly, in radioimmunoassay designs, radiolabeled avidin can be employed as a universal detection reagent. In the tumour imaging techniques, avidin labeled ^{125}I can be used to localize biotinylated monoclonal antibodies directed against tumour cells *in vivo*.

PROTOCOL 3.4

PREPARATION OF AVIDIN-HRP OR STREPTAVIDIN-HRP CONJUGATES

Horseradish peroxidase can be conjugated with avidin or streptavidin by periodate oxidation and reductive amination. Periodate oxidation of polysaccharide components of the glycoprotein molecule (HRP and avidin) produces reactive aldehyde groups. Another protein (biotin) can be conjugated with these reactive aldehyde groups by reacting the aldehyde with amines to form Schiff bases with subsequent reduction using sodium cynoborohydride to create stable secondary amino bonds (Fig. 3.5).

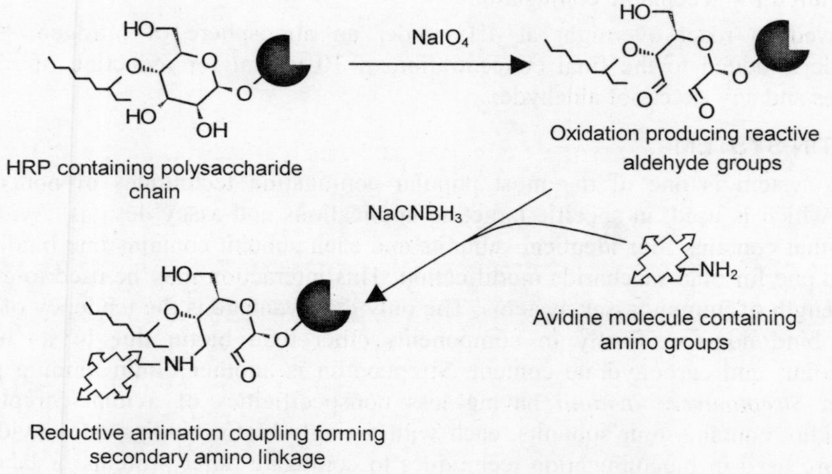

Fig. 3.5. Schematic diagram showing the conjugation of HRP with avidine by the process of reductive amination and periodate oxidation.

Materials and chemicals

Materials

For column separations, following pre-poured column can be used:

For 1.25 ml to 2.5 ml sample volumes: Sephadex G-25.

Chemicals

Horseradish peroxidase (HRP)
Sodium periodate
Ethanolamine
Sodium cynoborohydride
Sodium bicarbonate
Sodium phosphate
Sodium carbonate
Sodium chloride

Procedure

- HRP is dissolved in water or 0.01 M NaCl, pH 7.2, at a concentration of 10-20 mg/ml. Sodium periodate solution is prepared in water at a concentration of 0.088 M. It must be protected from light.
- Immediately, 100 µl of sodium periodate solution is added and mixed to each ml of the HRP solution.
- It is allowed to react in the dark for 20 minutes at room temperature. As the reaction proceeds, the colour changes will be apparent from brownish/gold to green.

- Oxidized enzyme must be purified immediately by gel filtration using column of Sephadex G-25. Fractions (0.5 ml) are collected and monitored for protein at 280 nm. HRP may also be detected at 403 nm.
- Fractions are pooled and enzyme concentration is adjusted to 10mg/ml for the conjugation step. HRP is stored freeze-dried for a long period without loss of activity. It should not be stored at room temperature due to the risk of polymerization.
- Avidin or streptavidin is dissolved in 0.2 M sodium bicarbonate at a concentration of 10 mg/ml, pH 9.6 at room temperature. The high pH buffer results in high molecular weight conjugates. Lower molecular weight conjugates can also be prepared by using lower pH value e.g., protein can be dissolved at a concentration of 10 mg/ml in 0.1 M sodium phosphate, 0.15 M NaCl, pH 7.2.
- The periodate activated HRP is finally purified with 0.01 M sodium phosphate, 0.15 M NaCl, pH 7.2. HRP can be used directly at 10 mg/ml for the conjugation using lower pH environment. For conjugation using higher pH environment, HRP should be dialyzed against 0.2 M sodium carbonate, pH 9.6 for 2 hours at room temperature prior to use.
- Avidin or streptavidin solution is mixed with enzyme solution at a ratio of 1:6 (v/v). This ratio of volumes will result in molar ratio of HRP: avidin equal to 4:1. Amount of enzyme solution can be increased for the preparation of greater enzyme: avidin ratio. It is allowed to react for 2 hours at room temperature to form initial Schiff bases.
- In the fume hood, 10 µl of 5 M sodium cyanoborohydride is added per millilitre of reaction solution. Caution: Cyanoborohydride is extremely toxic. All operations should be done in fume hood. It is allowed to react for 30 minutes at room temperature (in a fume hood).
- Unreacted aldehyde sites are blocked by the addition of 50 µl of 1 M ethanolamine, pH 9.6, per millilitre of conjugation solution. It is allowed to react for 30 minutes at room temperature. Conjugate is then purified from excess reactants by gel filtration using Sephadex G-25.

PROTOCOL 3.5

PREPARATION OF COLLOIDAL GOLD-LABELED PROTEINS

The labeling of targeting molecules, especially proteins, with gold nanopoarticles have been used in the visualization of cellular or tissue components by electron microscopy. Gold labeling of immunoglobulin binding proteins are used as a universal probe for detection and visualization of any antibody-antigen interaction in tissue sections, cells and blots (Fig. 3.6).

The labeling of macromolecules with gold particles depends on the several interactions such as the electrostatic attraction between the positively charged gold particles and negatively charged sites on the protein molecule, adsorption phenomenon and the potential for covalent binding of gold to free sulphydryl groups (dative binding). Mono-dispersed colloidal gold suspensions are used for protein labeling which can be produced by a variety of chemical methods in which reductive processes on chlorouric acid ($HauCl_4$) are used to create the spheroidal gold particles.

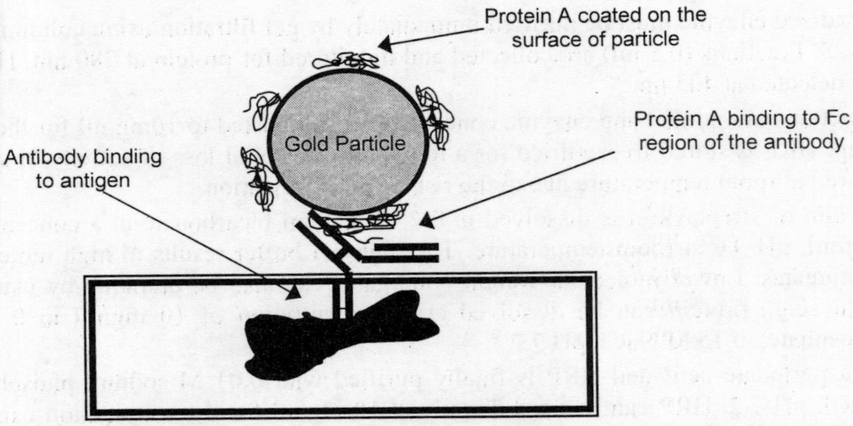

Fig. 3.6. Schematic diagram showing protein A-gold complex for Visualization of tissue components in electron microscopy

Materials and chemicals

Chlorouric acid
Polyethylene glycol
Potassium carbonate
Sodium borohydride
Sodium bicarbonate
Sodium phosphate

Procedure

Preparation of gold particle sol

- 1 ml of 4% $HauCl_4$ solution is prepared in deionized water. 375 µl of chlorouric acid solution and 500 µl of 0.2 M K_2CO_3 is added to 100 ml deionized water, cooled on ice to 4°C and mixed well. Sodium borohydride ($NaBH_4$) is dissolved in 5 ml of water at a concentration of 0.5 mg/ml. It should be freshly prepared.
- Five 1ml aliquot of the sodium borohydride solution is added to the chlorouric acid/carbonate suspension with rapid stirring. As the reaction completes, the reddish-orange colour becomes visible. After the completion of sodium borohydride addition, suspension is stirred for 5 minutes.

Preparation of complex

- The minimum amount of protein A required to stabilize the colloidal gold sol being used is determined. The suspension should be adjusted, if needed, with 0.1 M K_2CO_3, to pH 6-7.
- Stabilizing amount of protein A and an additional 10% is mixed with the appropriate volume of colloidal gold. After 1 minute, 250 µl of 1% PEG (MW 20,000) per 10 ml of gold sol is added.
- Suspension is stirred for an additional 5 minutes. Centrifuge the preparation at a minimum of 50,000g for 30 minutes to several hours (4°C) to remove excess protein A. Supernatant is discarded and protein A-gold pellet is resuspended in 0.01M sodium phosphate, pH 7.4, containing 1% PEG.

RADIOLABELED ANTIBODIES

Radioactive labels can be attached onto an antibody molecule, which is a powerful means of detection in immunoassay procedures, tracking of analytes, for *in vivo* diagnostic procedures, and for detection or therapy of numerous types of malignancies. Radioactive iodine can be labeled to an antibody using number of techniques. ^{125}I supplied as sodium salt, is used in most of the procedures by virtue of its comparably 60 days long half life, easy availability and relatively low-energy photon emission. It must be oxidized to electrophilic species capable of modifying molecules. Chloramine-T, Iodo-beads and Iodo-gen are commonly used oxidizing agents causing an iodination reaction to occur at available tyrosine residues within the polypeptide chain. Some other cross-linking or modification reagents containing an activated aromatic ring may also be iodinated to label at other conjugation site within protein molecule, if tyrosine can not be labeled. For example, Bolton-Hunter reagent may be used to add radioactive iodine to antibody molecule by modifying the primary amines within the antibody. It can also be used in the absence of tyrosine residue on the molecule (Fig. 3.7).

PROTOCOL 3.6

CASCADE BLUE CONJUGATION OF ANTIBODIES

Cascade Blue, a UV-excitable dye, can be used for immunofluorescence labeling. When used with the 351/361 nm excitation lines of an Argon laser, it is not very bright; usually only extremely high density antigens can be well-resolved by Cascade Blue. However, when used with the 405 nm excitation line of a Krypton laser, it becomes a useful dye with a brightness approaching that of fluorescein. Emission is collected at 440 nm (see the flourescence spectra).

Conjugation Method

The conjugation can be performed in two steps:

- Covalent conjugation
- Preparation of antibody

The antibody at a concentration of at least 2 mg/ml is also needed in addition to the materials given below. The extent of the dye conjugation to the antibody may depend on the concentration of antibody in solution. Therefore a consistent concentration of antibody should be used for consistent conjugation. One should know how to use a desalting column and how to take absorbance spectra.

The reactive Cascade Blue molecule is unstable. Solution of the Cascade Blue is solubilized, it should be used almost immediately. When first conjugating an antibody, a range of Cascade Blue to antibody concentrations should be compared. The protocol suggests 150 μg per mg of antibody; for a first-time titration of Cascade Blue, try a range of 40 to 600 μg Cascade Blue per mg of antibody. Compare each conjugate by staining (a titration of antibody on cells for each reagent to determine the optimal staining concentration should be performed). Then the conjugate with the brightest "positive" cells should be chosen.

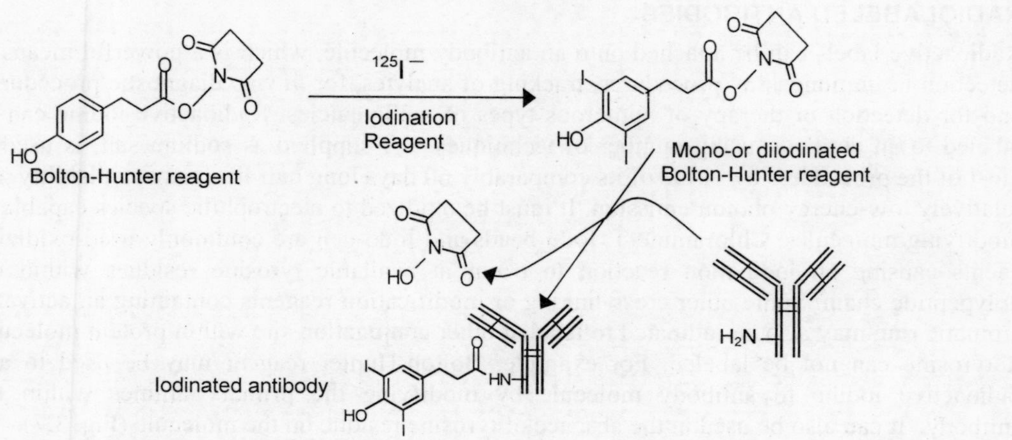

Fig. 3.7. Radioactive iodine labels added to antibody molecule using Bolton-Hunter reagent by modification of amines

Materials, Chemicals and Buffers

Materials

For column separations, one of the two types of pre-poured columns can be used:
For 1.25 ml to 2.5 ml sample volumes: PD-10 (Sephadex G-25M).
For 0.5 to 1.5 ml sample volumes: KwikSep dextran desalting columns.

Chemicals

Cascade Blue acetyl azide trisodium salt
pHix - 5 mg/ml Pentachlorophenol in 95% ethanol (use as 10,000X, or 3-4 drops per litre)
DMSO - Anyhydrous dimethyl sulphoxide
Note: Keep the DMSO absolutely dry at all times and the bottle in a dessicator. Pour out an amount of DMSO sufficient for the need and then pipette that; don't pipette directly into the bottle.
Sodium bicarbonate
Sodium chloride
TRIZMA 8.0 - Combination of Tris base and Tris HCl

Buffers

Two buffers are used:
B Reaction Buffer

$NaHCO_3$	84 g

Make the volume to 1 litre with distilled water and maintain pH to 8.4.

Storage-Buffer

TRIZMA 8.0	1.42 g
NaCl	8.77 g
pHix	3-4 drops

Make the volume up to 1 litre and maintain pH to 8.2

Procedure

- Cascade Blue is covalently coupled to primary amines (lysines) of the immunoglobulin. Dissolve Cascade Blue (5 mg) in anhydrous dimethyl sulphoxide (500 µl) immediately before use. Add Cascade Blue to give a ratio of 150 µg per mg of antibody; mix immediately.
- Wrap the tube in foil, incubate and rotate at room temperature for 4 hours. Remove the unreacted Cascade Blue and exchange the antibody into "Storage Buffer" by gel filtration or dialysis.
- The unreacted dye will have the apparent colour on the column; usually, the antibody conjugate will be in too low concentration to be coloured: do not make the mistake of collecting the antibody by colour visualization. (a hand-held UV lamp in a darkened room should be used to visualize the conjugate, which will appear faintly blue in comparison to the buffer).

Preparation of antibody

- Dialyze or exchange antibody over a column in the "B Reaction Buffer". Measure the antibody concentration after buffer equilibration. (1 mg/ml IgG has absorbance 1.4 at 280 nm).
- If the antibody concentration is less than 1 mg/ml, the conjugation will probably be sub-optimal. If necessary, dilute the antibody to a concentration of 4 mg/ml.

Note

It is critical that sodium azide be completely removed from any antibody.

PROTOCOL 3.7

PREPARATION OF ANTIBODY- TOXIN CONJUGATES

Purification of Toxins

Ricin

This galactose-binding toxic lectin may be readily purified by a two-stage chromatographic process based on the method of Nicolson and Blaustein. Galactose-binding proteins are first isolated on an agarose matrix and then subjected to a gel filtration step.

- Untoasted castor bean cake (pomace) may be obtained from castor bean processors. It should be further defatted by extraction three times with 5 volumes (v/w) 40-60°C petroleum ether. The air-dried material (500 g) is then extracted overnight by stirring it in 4 litres PBS (pH 7.4).
- The supernatant is partially clarified by filtration through nylon gauze followed by centrifugation at 1500 g for 1 hour. The supernatant is subjected to ammonium sulphate precipitation at 4°C, the fraction precipitating between 40 and 60% saturation being collected by centrifugation (1500 g, 1 hour), redissolved in about 500 ml PBS and dialyzed against three changes of 6 litres PBS.

- This solution, clarified by centrifugation if necessary, is then applied to a column (bed volume~800 ml) of Sepharose 4B running in PBS. The gel should be pretreated with 2 M propionic acid at room temperature for at least 2- 3 weeks to enhance its binding capacity to lectins. The column should be jacketed and run at a temperature of <10°C to optimize lectin binding. After application of the sample, the column is washed with at least 4 bed volumes of PBS. Some sources of castor beans, especially those of Chinese origin, contain two species of toxins differing in isoelectric point. The prolonged elution of the column ensures that the species with higher pH (~8.2), which binds only feebly to Sepharose, is washed through together with all nonbinding proteins. When the UV absorbance (280 nm) of the elute has reached a stable, low value, the strongly binding lectins are displaced from the column with 100 mM galactose in PBS. The toxin and lectin elute together as a single sharp peak.
- This mixture is resolved by gel filtration on Sephacryl S-200, also running in PBS. The sample size should be restricted to 3-4% of the bed volume of the column, under these conditions the lectin of molecular weight 120,000 and the toxin of molecular weight 60,000 are fully resolved. The material recovered from the affinity column (second step) must be concentrated by ultrafiltration to ~20 mg/ml before applying to the gel filtration medium. Some sources of beans contain quantities of a material, which has a molecular weight about 90,000 and is both toxic and a haemagglutinin. Toxin fractions should be selected so as to avoid contamination with this material. Five hundred grams of defatted pomace should yield about 1250 mg toxin,
- $E^{1\%}_{1cm}$ = 11.8, at 280 nm. Sterile solutions of holotoxin may be stored at 4°C for at least 12 months without any detectable loss of activity or deep frozen (–30°C) for several years.

Abrin

- Abrin may be purified from seeds of *Abrus precatorius* by essentially similar methodology.
- The seeds (500 g), which should be bright scarlet, are grounded and extracted overnight with 4 litres of PBS at 4°C. The yield may be increased by reextracting the pellet of softened stroma from the first centrifugation with a further quantity (2 litres) of PBS for 4-6 hours at room temperature after homogenization.
- The combined extracts are then subjected to ammonium sulphate precipitation, and the material precipitated between 40 and 70% saturation is collected.

Other procedures are identical to those for ricin, but it may be noted that material of intermediate molecular weight (i.e., 90,000) is not seen in the galactose-binding proteins of Abrus extracts. 500 g of ground beans will yield about 800 mg of toxin, $E^{1\%}_{1cm}$ 15.9 at 280 nm.

Diphtheria Toxin

Partially purified diphtheria toxin may be purified by the method given by Collier and Kandel.

- A dialyzed solution of 500 mg crude diphtheria toxin in 0.01 M sodium phosphate buffer, pH 7.0, is applied to a column (2.6 x 34 cm) of DADE-cellulose equilibrated in the same buffer. The column is washed at 100 ml per hour with a sequence of sodium phosphate buffer (pH 7.0) of increasing molarity (300 ml of 0.01 M buffer, 300 ml of 0.05 M buffer, 700 ml of 0.1 M buffer and 300 ml of 0.25 M buffer respectively).

- The toxin elutes as a major peak with a trailing shoulder during the 0.1 M buffer step. The toxin may be identified by means of its precipitation reaction with horse antitoxin in Ouchterlony immunodiffusion assays.
- The toxin solution is concentrated by ultrafiltration to 25 ml and applied to a column (5 x 76cm) of Sephadex G-100 (super fine grade) equilibrated in 0.05 M sodium borate buffer, pH 8.5. Elution with the same buffer removes the toxin as a component (~90%) of approximate molecular weight 65,000. A minor component (~20%) of approximate molecular weight 130,000, probably dimeric toxin, may also be seen. The toxin should be concentrated to 20 mg/ml ($E^{1\%}_{1cm}$, 12.3 at 280 nm) and stored in aliquots at 30°C.

Isolation of Toxin A Chains

Abrin and ricin

The A chains may be conveniently prepared by cleaving the disulphide bond while the toxins are immobilized on an agarose matrix via the binding site of the B chain.

Procedure

- Apply Toxin (100-150 mg) to a column of acid treated Sepharose 4B, bed volume 24 ml. This represents about half to maximal loading of the gel. Equilibrate sample and column with 0.1M phosphate buffer, pH 8.0, containing 0.1 mM EDTA.
- Immediately, after the sample has been run onto the column, allow it to run 15 ml buffer containing 5% 2-mercaptoethanol and allow the column to stand for 2 minutes at room temperature.
- Liberated A chain with the phosphate buffer, B chain and residual holotoxin being retained on the column. Dialyze the eluted peak against three changes of 0.1 M phosphate buffer, pH 8.0, containing 0.1 mM each of EDTA and dithiothreitol to prevent oxidation of the sulphydryl group.
- Remove the traces of B chain or holotoxin by absorption twice with asialofetuin immobilized on Sepharose: approximately 2 mg asialofetuin per millilitre of gel, 1 ml of settled gel per 20 ml of A chain solution. Yield of recovered A chain should be between 75 and 95% of theoretical yield.
- Free A chains should not be frozen (freezing tends to cause loss of enzymatic function) but rather stored at 4°C. They are particularly prone to surface denaturation and manipulations such as concentration by ultrafiltration should be avoided where possible.
- The addition of 20% glycerol is recommended to stabilize sample before transport. In general, it is desirable to prepare A chains as and when required.

Diphtheria toxin

- To 1 ml of a 25 mg/ml solution of purified diphtheria toxin in 0.05 M borate buffer, pH 8.6, add 1 ml of a 2 μg/ml solution of trypsin in the same buffer containing 2 mM EDTA.
- Incubate the mixture for 2 hours at 25°C to cleave any single chain toxin proteolytic to its nicked (i.e., A and B chain) form; 500 μl of a 10 μg/ml solution of soyabean trypsin inhibitor is added to terminate the reaction.
- Reduce the nicked diphtheria toxin by addition of 500 μl of 0.6 M dithiothreitol and incubate for 90 minutes at 37°C. Liberated B chain sediments as a dense, elute the precipitate.

- Centrifuge and apply the clear supernatant to a column (2.6 x 50cm) of Sephadex-G-100 (Superfine grade) equilibrated with 0.05 M borate buffer, pH 8.5, containing 1 mM EDTA and 0.1M 20 ml mercaptoethanol. Eluting with the same buffer solution removes the A chain as the major peak (MW~22,000).
- Concentrate the A chain to 5 ml by ultrafiltration and further purify by gel filtration on a column (2.6x 80 cm) of Sephadex G-75 equilibrated with the same buffer.
- Heat the A chain to 80°C for 10 minutes to destroy any residual traces of toxin or B chain.

Coupling of Antibodies and Intact Toxins

Heterobifunctional agents have two reactive groups that are different and which react with amino acids in proteins under different conditions. These reagents permit for greater control over the coupling reaction and reduce the risk of forming intra- and intermolecular cross-links. Coupling reaction protocols for three such heterobifunctional reagents are as follows;

N-hydroxysuccinimidyl ester of chlorambucil

- To 30 mg immunoglobulin at a concentration of 10mg/ml in borate saline buffer (0.05 M borate, 0.3 M NaCl, 0.5% n-butanol, pH 9.0) is added 1 mg of the N- hydroxysuccinimidyl ester of chlorambucil dissolved in 0.5 ml dry dimethyl sulphoxide.
- After stirring on ice for 1 hour, the solution is applied to a jacketed column (1.6 x 36 cm) of Sephadex G-25 equilibrated with borate saline buffer and maintained at 4°C.
- The column is washed with borate saline buffer and the derivatized globulin, which elutes first, is added immediately to an ice cold solution of 50 mg toxin in 5 ml of the same buffer.
- This solution (~20 ml) is concentrated to 5.0 ml in a cooled Amicon ultrafiltration cell using a PM10 membrane. The concentrated solution is then warmed to room temperature and left for 48 hours to react before its resolution by gel filtration.

N-succinimidyl-3-(2-pyridyldithio)propionate

- To 10 mg of toxin in 1.0 ml borate saline buffer is added 150 µg SPDP in 25 µl dry dimethylformamide.
- After stirring for 30 minutes at room temperature, the solution is applied to a column (1.6x 22 cm) of Sephadex G-25F equilibrated with phosphate saline buffer (0.1 M phosphate, 0.1 M NaCl, 1 mM EDTA, 0.02% NaN_3, pH 7.5). The derivatized toxin is collected in a volume of 10 to 12 ml.
- To a solution of 25 mg of immunoglobulin in 2.5 ml borate saline buffer is added 185 µl dry dimethylformamide. After stirring at room temperature for 30 minutes, the solution is applied to a column (1.6x36 cm) of G-25 Sephadex equilibrated with NaN_3, pH 4.5.
- The derivatized antibody is collected in a volume of 10-12 ml. 10 ml of this solution is concentrated to 2.5 ml by ultrafiltration and 22 mg dithiothreitol in 500 µl acetate buffer is added.
- After stirring for 30 minutes at room temperature, the solution is applied to a column (1.6 x 36 cm) of Sephadex G-25 equilibrated in nitrogen flushed phosphate saline buffer. The emergent protein peak is immediately added to 10 ml of the derivatized toxin.
- The reaction mixture is then concentrated to 5 ml by ultrafiltration and left at room temperature for 18 hours before resolution by gel filtration.

N-hydroxysuccinimidyl ester of iodoacetic acid

- To a solution of 20 mg ricin in 1.5 ml borate saline buffer is added 300 µg of the N-hydroxysuccinimidyl ester of iodoacetic acid in 200 µl of dry dimethylformamide.
- After stirring for 30 minutes at room temperature, the solution is applied to a column (1.6 x 22 cm) of Sephadex G-25 equilibrated with phosphate saline buffer and the derivatized ricin is collected in a volume of 10-12 ml.
- Immunoglobulin (45 mg) is derivatized with SPDP and then concentrated to 3.0 ml. This intermediate is reduced by the addition of 22 mg of dithiothreitol in 500 µl acetate buffer.
- After stirring for 30 minutes at room temperature, the solution is applied to a column (1.6 x 20 cm) of Sephadex G-25 equilibrated with nitrogen flushed phosphate saline buffer.
- The protein that elutes at the void volume is added immediately to 11 ml of the derivatized ricin solution.
- The reaction mixture is then concentrated to 5.0 ml by ultrafiltration and left at room temperature for 18 hours.
- N-ethylmaleimide (1 mg) dissolved in dimethylformamide is added to inactivate any remaining free sulphydryl groups and the reaction mixture stirred gently for an hour before resolution by gel filtration.

Coupling of Antibodies and Toxin A Chains

- To 26 mg antibody at a concentration of 10 mg/ml in phosphate saline buffer is added 220 µg SPDP in 100 µl dry dimethylformamide.
- Stir for 30 minutes at room temperature and apply to a column (1.6 x 30 cm) of Sephadex G-25 equilibrated in the same buffer; the derivatized antibody elutes in the void volume in about 10-12 ml.
- Concentrate the product to about 3.5 ml by ultrafiltration. To it add 15 mg of toxin A chain in 7 ml of nitrogen flushed phosphate saline buffer and mix the solution for 10 minutes and then leave at room temperature for 18 hours before resolution by gel filtration.

Note: An antibody (i.e. immunoglobulin or Ig) is a protein molecule with two identical heavy (H) chains and two identical light (L) chains. Both the H and L chains consist of a variable (V) region that constitutes the antigen combining site and a constant (C) region that determined the isotype F(e.g., IgG, IgM, IgA, IgD and IgE for H chains; κ, λ for H L chains) of an antibody. T cell receptors (TcR) have a heterodimeric protein structure which exists either as a α/β or a γ/δ form, each (TcR) polypeptide subunit (ie, α, β, γ, δ) also carries an antigen recognizing V region and a C region of unknown function.

PROTOCOL 3.8

PE CONJUGATION OF ANTIBODIES

Phycoerythrin (PE) is one of the most commonly-used fluorescent dyes for FACS analysis. PE is a large protein (approximate molecular weight 240 KD) containing 25 fluors. Typically, only one PE molecule is conjugated to an antibody. Nonetheless, by virtue of its huge absorption coefficient and almost perfect quantum efficiency it is one of the brightest dyes used today. It emits at about 570 nm, and can be excited by common Argon laser lines. Direct PE conjugates are relatively easy to make. Phycoerythrin can be purchased from several vendors, or isolated from the algae directly. There is a conjugation kit available from Prozyme Inc., which uses essentially this protocol. The entire procedure takes about 2 hours to complete (the kit eliminates steps I and II in the conjugation protocol given below).

Materials

For column separations, use one of two types of pre-poured columns:
For 1.25 - 2.5 ml sample volumes: PD-10 (Sephadex G-25).
For 0.5 - 1.5 ml sample volume: KwikSep dextran desalting columns.

Chemicals

Sodium chloride
5 mg/ml pentachlorophenol in 95% ethanol (pHix), (3-4 drops per litre)
Succinimidyl 4-(N-maleimidomethyl) cyclohexane-1-carboxylate (SMCC)
Anyhydrous dimethyl sulphoxide (DMSO)
Dithiothreitol (DTT)
Ethylenediaminetetraacetic acid (EDTA), (Disodium salt: dihydrate)
[2-(N-morpholino)ethanesulphonic acid] (MES)
TRIZMA 8.0 - Combination of Tris base and Tris HCl

Buffers

Dialysis Buffer (50 mM Sodium phosphate, 1 mM EDTA, pH 7.0)

Sodium phosphate dibasic ($7H_2O$)	13.41 g
EDTA	0.37 g

Make the volume up to 1 litre with distilled water.

Exchange Buffer (50 mM MES, 2 mM EDTA, pH. 6.0)

MES	10.90 g
EDTA	0.74 g

Make the volume up to 1 litre with distilled water and adjust the pH to 6.0

Storage Buffer (10 mM Tris, 150 mM NaCl, pHix, pH 8.2)

TRIZMA 8.0	1.42 g
NaCl	8.77 g
pHix	3-4 drops

Make the volume up to 1 litre with distilled water and adjust the pH to 8.2

Conjugation Methods

- Preparation of PE
- Derivatization of PE
- Reduction of IgG
- Covalent conjugation

Procedure

The entire conjugation can be performed in a single day. However, dialysis of stored PE prior to conjugation can take 24-48 hours. In addition, a solution of antibody at a concentration of at least 2 mg/ml is also required for conjugation.

Preparation of PE

- Dialyze or exchange the PE into "Dialysis Buffer". PE concentration before derivatization is typically 5-10 mg/ml. Note: PE is most stable as a SAS (sodium ammonium sulphate) precipitate prior to coupling. If the PE is stored as a SAS precipitate, it must be extensively dialyzed prior to use.
- Dialyze against 2 changes of 1 litre per ml PE of PBS before dialyzing against 1 litre per ml of "Dialysis Buffer".
- Use 3.5 mg of R-PE per mg of IgG to be modified; this includes an extra 10% for loss during buffer exchanges.
- To check the PE purity and concentration, measure the absorbance at 280, 565 and 620 nm. (1 mg/ml of PE has an optical density at 565 nm of 8.2). A 565/620 ratio > 50 indicates adequate removal of contaminating phycocyanin; a 565/280 ratio > 5 indicates adequate removal of all other proteins.

Derivatization of PE

The amino groups on the phycoerythrin (PE) react with the succinamide to yield a maleimide-labeled PE.

- Prepare a 10 mg/ml stock solution of SMCC in dry DMSO immediately prior to use.
- Add 11 μl of SMCC per mg of PE while vortexing.
- Wrap the reaction tube in aluminum foil and rotate at room temperature for 60 minutes.
- Pass the derivatized PE over a gel filtration column pre-equilibrated with "Exchange Buffer".
- The SMCC-derivative is stable and may be stored at 4°C for several weeks; a high concentration of PE (> 4 mg/ml) is desirable for such longer-term storage.

Note: for conjugations, which fail or are poor, it may help to increase or decrease the amount of SMCC with respect to PÈ, or to use an alternative heterobifunctional crosslinking reagent.

Reduction of IgG

The hinge disulphide bonds are reduced to yield free sulphydryls.

- Prepare a fresh solution of 1 M DTT (15.4 mg/100 μl) in distilled water. IgG solutions should be at 4 mg/ml or higher for best results. The reduction can be carried out in almost any buffer; MES, phosphate, and TRIS buffers (pH range 6 to 8) have been used successfully. The antibody should be concentrated if the concentration is less than 2 mg/ml. Include an extra 10% for losses on the buffer exchange column.
- Make each IgG solution 20 mM in DTT by adding 20 μl of DTT stock per ml of IgG solution while mixing.
- Allow it to stand at room temperature for 30 minutes without additional mixing (to minimize reoxidation of cysteines to cystines).
- Pass the reduced IgG over a filtration column pre-equilibrated with "Exchange Buffer". Collect 0.25 ml fractions off the column; determine the protein concentrations and pool the fractions with the majority of the IgG. This can be done either spectrophotometrically or colorimetrically.
- Carry out the conjugation as soon as possible after this step.

Note: for conjugations, which are poor or fail, it may help to reduce the DTT concentration.

Covalent conjugation

The PE is covalently coupled to the IgG through reaction of the maleimide groups with the free sulphydryl on the IgG. Do not delay this step since the IgG sulphydryls will reoxidize.

- Add 3.2 mg of SMCC-PE per mg of IgG. Wrap the reaction tube in aluminum foil and rotate for 60 minutes at room temp. Note: These molar ratios (~2 PE per IgG) have worked very well. For conjugations, which fail or are poor, different other molar ratios may help.
- After 60 minutes, unreacted free sulphydryls on the IgG must be blocked.
- Prepare a fresh solution of 10 mg NEM in 1.0 ml dry DMSO.
- Add 34 µg (3.4 µl) per mg of IgG. Wrap and rotate for 20 minutes at room temperature.
- The product can be either dialyzed or exchanged over a column into an appropriate buffer (e.g. storage buffer). It is best to keep the product at high concentration (> 1 mg/ml) for optimal stability. Never freeze the conjugates. It may be useful to spin PE conjugates prior to use in staining, especially if background seems to be a problem (e.g., at 10,000g in a microcentrifuge, at 4°C).

SUGGESTED READINGS

Hardy, R.R., Handbook of Experimental Immunology, 4th Edition,. Blackwell Scientific Publications, Boston, 1986.

Hermanson, G.T., Bioconjugate Techniques, Academic Press, Inc., San Diago, California, 1995.

Talwar, G. P. and Gupta, S. K., A Handbook of Practical and Clinical Immunology, 2nd Edition, CBS Publishers and Distributors, New Delhi, 1992.

CHAPTER 4

Fermentation

- Introduction
- Yogurt fermentation with lactobacillus cultures
- Cheese production from milk
- Batch submerged fermentation of baker's yeast
- Wine production by yeast
- Study of variables in wine fermentation
- Fermentation products

INTRODUCTION

Fermentation may be defined as the process of growing a culture of microorganisms in a nutrient media and thereby converting feed into desired end product. Fermentation is an anaerobic reaction which occurs in some of the less complex organisms such as bacteria and yeasts. Anaerobic reactions involve cellular food products and/or glucose sugar as their reactants and without oxygen they can produce combinations of ethyl alcohol, carbon dioxide and lactic acid as their products.

Yeasts are used as tiny "fermentation units" for the production of carbon dioxide and alcohol. Certain bacteria and moulds ferment milk, producing carbon dioxide and lactic acid. It is well realized that the fermentation is the result of growth of bacteria, yeasts, moulds, or combinations of these. Stated more precisely, the changes that occur are caused by the enzymes liberated by these microorganisms. Some foods usually said to be fermented, are actually cured by the enzymes naturally present in the foods. Throughout the centuries fermentation has been one of the most important methods for preserving food and it still remains one of the most important methods. Relatively few people, however, are aware that many food products consumed regularly are prepared and/or preserved by fermentation processes. It is essential to understand that the lactic acid bacteria produce acid that in effect inhibits the growth of many other organisms. Most species convert sugars to acids, alcohol, and carbon dioxide. The fermentative yeasts produce ethyl alcohol and carbon dioxide from sugars. They require oxygen for growth but not for fermentation. The changes that occur during fermentation of foods are the result of the activity of enzymes. The enzymes arise from three sources viz., from the microorganisms that are involved in the fermentation, from the food, and from the microbial flora present upon the unfermented food. A good use of fermentation is in those processes, where the enzymes produced by the fermentative microorganisms play the primary role.

There are relatively few pure culture fermentations. An organism that initiates fermentation will develop until its byproducts inhibit further growth and fermentation. During this initial growth period other organisms grow simultaneously. They in turn are followed by other more tolerant species. This succession of growth of different species may be referred to as a natural sequence of growth. In general, growth is initiated by bacteria, followed by yeasts and then moulds, if conditions are suitable for growth of these microorganisms. Bacteria, yeasts, and moulds have been used for centuries to produce a host of fermented foods including buttermilk, yogurt, sour cream, butter, cheese (over 700 kinds), pickles, sauerkraut, sausages, breads, crackers, pretzels, doughnuts, grape nuts, wines, beer, spirits, coffee, cacao, vanilla, tea, citron, ginger, and more.

The new technologies have allowed researchers to target the genetics of plants, animals, and microorganisms and to manipulate them to our food production advantage. The predicted improved products may include

- Environmentally hardy food-producing plants that are naturally resistant to pests and diseases and capable of growing under extreme conditions of temperature, moisture, and salinity.
- An array of fresh fruits and vegetables, with excellent flavour, appealing texture, and optimum nutritional content, that stay fresh for several weeks.
- Custom designed plants with defined structural and functional properties for specific food-processing applications.
- Cultures of microorganisms that are programmed to express or shut off certain genes at specific times during fermentation in response to environmental triggers.
- Strains engineered to serve as delivery systems for digestive enzymes for individuals with reduced digestive capacity.
- Cultures capable of implanting and surviving in the human gastrointestinal tract for delivery of antigens to stimulate the immune response or protect the gut from invasion by pathogenic organisms.
- Microbially derived, high-value, natural food ingredients with unique functional properties.
- Microsensors that accurately measure the physiological state of plants; temperature-abuse indicators for refrigerated foods; and shelf-life monitors built into food packages.
- On-line sensors that monitor fermentation processes or determine the concentration of nutrients throughout processing.
- Biotechnologically designed foods to supply nutritional need; meat with reduced saturated fat and milk with improved calcium bioavailability.

Microbes are now designed to produce various bioactive proteins such as human type insulin, enzymes, vitamins and specific antibiotics on a large industrial scale (Table 4.1).

Table 4.1. Various fermentation products

S. No.	Fermentation Product	S. No.	Fermentation Product
1	Foods and beverages	7	Alcohol
2	Antibiotics	8	Carbohydrates
3	Vitamins	9	Enzymes
4	Amino acids	10	Single cell protein
5	Organic acids	11	Biological pesticides
6	Solvents	12	Miscellaneous products

The Fermentation Process and Optimization

Process of fermentation is based upon utilization of metabolic and enzymatic activities of various microorganisms so as to transform organic compounds to desired end product. Therefore, proper understanding of the kinetics of microbial, animal or plant cell growth kinetic is imperative for the design of maximal capacity fermenter. Cell production kinetics revolves around the cell-growth rate and it is affected by various physicochemical conditions. Cell kinetics is the consequential interaction of numerous complicated biochemical reactions and transport phenomenon, involving multiple stages of multicomponent systems. The complete mathematical modeling of growth kinetics is not possible as a heterogeneous mixture of young and old cells continuously transforms and adapts to a changing environment during growth phase. Hence, in order to derive simpler models of fermentation operation and performance that can accommodate mathematical modeling, assumptions must be made regarding the involvement of various cellular components and population dynamics. Table 4.2 shows various fermentation models.

Table 4.2. Various fermentation models

Population	Cell component unstructured	Cell component structured
Distributed	Cell represented by single component, which is uniformly distributed throughout the culture	Multiple cell components uniformly distributed throughout the culture, interact with each other
Segregated	Cell represented by single component, but form a heterogeneous mixture	Cells composed of multiple component and form a heterogeneous mixture

Among the models suggested, the simplest model is unstructured distributed model (Table 4.2), which is based upon two basic assumptions.

- All the cells can be represented by single component such as cell mass, cell number etc.
- Cellular mass is distributed throughout the culture.

In addition to the cells, the medium should be formulated such that 'one component may limit the reaction rate'. All components should be present at sufficiently high concentrations so that the minor changes do not affect the growth significantly. Growth rates based on the cell weight and on the number of cells are not necessarily the same, as the average cell size may vary considerably from one stage to another. For example, when the mass of an individual cell increases without division, the growth rate based on cell weight increases while growth rate based upon number of cells remains constant. However, during exponential growth phase, cell number based growth rate and growth rate based on cell weight is proportional. Sometimes growth rate is confused with division rate.

A vessel in which all the cells at time t = 0 ($Cn = Cn_0$) have divided once after a certain period of time, the cell population will have increased to $Cn_0 \times 2$. All the cells are divided X times after time t, the total number of cells will be:

$$Cn = Cn_0 \times 2M \quad \text{------------------------------------} [1.1]$$

Cn versus t curve represents a relationship between growth and time where the growth rate is expressed as the slope of the curve (Fig. 4.1). If the sterile medium is inoculated and the cell density is measured deriving subsequent growth as against time, the result could be distinguished as six stages in batch growth cycle.

- Latent period: The phase in which the cell number does not vary.
- Accelerated growth: The cell number starts increasing and cell division rate accelerates.
- Exponential growth: It is the phase of exponential increase in cell number.
- Decelerated growth: The phase where growth rate is maximum and during this period growth and division rates starts decreasing.
- Static period: Any further proliferation of cells is stopped and cell number reaches to a maxima point.
- Death period: The period where limiting growth substances have depleted and cells begin to die.

The major applications of kinetic growth data and models are to predict the length of fermentation stage in order to estimate the necessary fermenter size before considering other more complex factors. Furthermore, the same models could be utilized in designing batch fermentation processes as well as to predict the fermentation size necessary for continuous culture fermentation.

The foremost objective of the fermentation is to support the growth of specific culture and to promote high end point yield. In certain conditions excess of essential nutrients concentration could extensively inhibit growth, hence essential nutrients should not always be supplied in excess. It is precisely to correlate that the nutrient concentration in the broth should appropriately be optimized with respect to the requirement of the micro-organisms involved in the fermentation process.

The prediction of kinetics for single cell growth is quite simple

$$\mu = \frac{dX}{d\theta} \quad \text{------------------------------------} [1.2]$$

Where θ is time factor

μ is specific growth rate and

X is the concentration of cells

For complex cell growth a Monod equation is utilized. It projects an empirical and simplified model for complex cell-growth.

$$\mu = \mu_m \frac{[C_1]}{[C_1 + K_1]} \frac{[C_2]}{[C_2 + K_2]} \qquad \text{--[1.3]}$$

The two limiting component C_1 and C_2 are the concentration.

$$\mu = \mu_m \frac{[C_i]}{[C_i + K_i]} \frac{[C_p]}{[C_p + K_p]} \qquad \text{--[1.4]}$$

Where K_p is the saturation constant for the products K_i and C_p is the product concentration. For an optimum fermentation design it is the foremost requirement that the latent state as has been pointed earlier should be shortened. Hence, following three points are to be considered:

- Inoculum should be as active as possible.
- Inoculum medium should correspond as closely as possible to the fermenter.
- Reasonably large volume of inoculum should be used to minimize the loss of key metabolic intermediates by diffusion.

A proper consideration of all kinetics related factors and appropriate modeling of the fermentation unit should be considered for development and design of a fermenter.

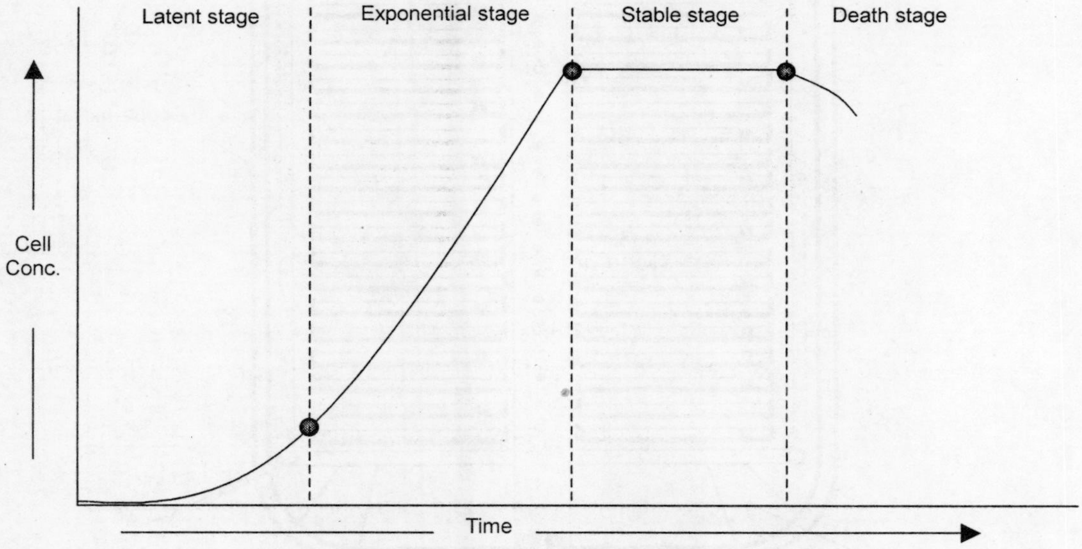

Fig. 4.1. Batch fermentation stages

The heart of fermentation process is the fermenter, which is a container in which a favourable environment is maintained for the operation of desired biological process. Fermentation is typically either batch operated or continuous mode. Broadly, the fermenters could be grouped under two classes.

Submerged fermenters (suspended-growth systems)

In submerged fermenters, the organisms are immersed in and dispersed throughout there nutrient medium and their movement follows that of nutrient liquid. These types of fermenter tenks are being successfully utilized in brewing industry. Some of the examples represent this class are mechanically stirred fermenters and forced convection fermenters and fermenter with pneumatic operations.

Surface fermenters (supported-growth systems)

In the case of supported growth systems, the organisms grow as a layer or a film on a surface in contact with a nutrient medium. Tray reactors (Fig. 4.2) and film reactors represent this class.

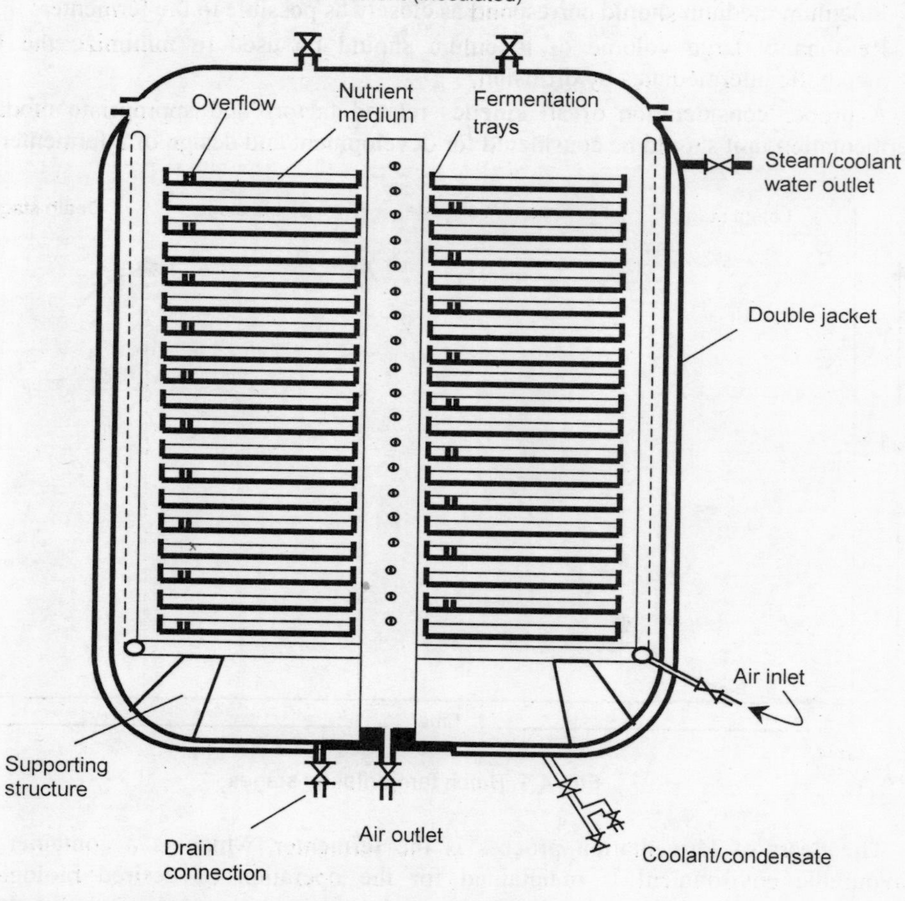

Fig. 4.2. Schematic diagram showing tray fermenter as a continuous process

PROTOCOL 4.1

YOGURT FERMENTATION WITH LACTOBACILLUS CULTURES

Principle

The mushy substance formed during the prolonged procuring process in cheese manufacturing in which the natural action of lactose fermenting culture originally resident in butter milk was utilized to acidify milk. This custard-textured substance was called as yogurt.

Other than cheese, buttermilk and yogurt, lactic starter cultures are also useful in manufacturing of a wide variety of food products such as sour dough bread, pickles, and sausages. As the name implies, they belong to a category of microorganisms that can digest the milk sugar lactose and convert it into lactic acid. For the cells to utilize lactose, deriving carbon and energy from it, they must also possess the enzymes needed to break lactose into two component sugars: glucose and galactose. Some representative strains are *Streptococcus lactis, S. cremoris, thermophilus, Lactobacillus bulgaricus, L. acidophilus,* and *L. plantarum.* The tablets containing micro-organisms are prescribed to be taken orally during the intake of dairy products by those people who have digestive tract disorder and cannot tolerate lactose. The major steps involved in a large-scale production of lactic starter cultures are the following: media preparation (constitution, mixing, straining, sterilization), inoculum preparation, fermentation, cell concentration by centrifugation, liquid nitrogen freezing, and packaging.

In summary, commercial yogurt production is composed of the following steps: pretreatment of milk (standardization, fortification, lactose hydrolysis), homogenization, heat treatment, cooling to incubation temperature, inoculation with starter, fermentation, cooling, post-fermentation treatment (flavouring, fruit addition, pasteurization), refrigeration/freezing, and packaging. For set yogurt, the packaging into individual containers is carried out before fermentation.

Equipment

Beakers, Heat source, Incubator, Thermometer, Reagent, Milk, Starter culture or plain yogurt from local stores.

Procedure

- Heat 1 litre of milk in a beaker slowly to 85ºC and maintain at that temperature for 2 minutes. This step kills undesirable contaminant microorganisms. It also denatures inhibitory enzymes that retard the subsequent yogurt fermentation.
- Cool milk in a cold water bath to 42-44ºC. The cooling process should take about 15 minutes.
- Add 5 g of starter culture to the cooled milk and mix with a glass rod.
- Cover the container to minimize the possibility of contamination.
- Incubate at 42ºC for 3 to 6 hours undisturbed until the desired custard consistency is reached. Yogurt is set when the mixture stops flowing as the container is tipped slowly. Fluid yogurt results if the mixture is stirred as the coagulum is being formed.
- The freshly made yogurt is ready for consumption when it is set.

- For the use of *Lactobacillus acidophilus,* grind 4 yogurt tablets (about 1 g) into fine powder and repeat previous steps.

Notes

The yogurt in the local market usually contains an active culture. Thus, if a starter culture is not readily available, it can be easily derived from plain store-bought yogurt. In this case, a few teaspoonfuls of the store-bought yogurt will adequately act as the starter culture. The culture in fresh yogurt is healthier and more active than that in an outdated one.

A stale one is also more likely to be contaminated with undesirable microorganisms. If possible, choose the "All-Natural" variety, because stabilizers and additives, included to suppress microbial activities, are generally harmful to the culture.

A household electric or gas oven is an ideal substitute for the incubator. The middle shelf, slightly away from the direct heat, usually gives the most even temperature. The temperature can be controlled better if a pan of warm water is placed on the bottom rack.

Favorite fruits, fruit preserves, puree, jam, or sweeteners can be added to enhance the taste. Many types of yogurt differ mainly in the post-incubation processing. For example, the yogurt may be frozen, spray-dried or freeze-dried, carbonated, or concentrated.

The window of proper fermentation is quite small, i.e. from 42°C to 44°C. In general, as the temperature is raised up to 44°C, the rate of culture metabolism is higher, and the yogurt is sweeter. Faster growth also prompts the yogurt to set faster. When the desired acidity is reached, yogurt is quickly cooled to halt further fermentation and metabolic activity. This cooling step is quite critical in industrial yogurt production and must be done quickly to control the acidity of the yogurt, which has a profound effect on the taste.

PROTOCOL 4.2

CHEESE PRODUCTION FROM MILK

Principle

Cow's milk is rich in a wide range of chemical compounds that can be processed into various dairy products such as cheese, butter, and yogurt. Specifically the milk component involved in cheese production is a soluble protein called casein. The enzyme rennet can be used to catalyze the conversion of casein in milk to para-casein by removing a glycopeptide from the soluble casein. Para-casein further clots, i.e. coagulates, in the presence of calcium ions to form white, creamy lumps called the *curd*, leaving behind the supernatant called the *whey*.

$$\text{Casein} \xrightarrow{\text{Rennet}} \text{Para-casein (aq.)} \xrightarrow{Ca^{++}} \text{Para-casein (ppt)}$$

The precipitate is soft at this point and can be separated from the whey by the use of cheesecloth. Filtration does not work very well as filter paper clogging is a recurrent problem.

There is no standard method of cheese making as limitless variations exist for all stages of the process e.g. pre-ripening, curdling, addition of artificial ingredients and salt for flavour, and aging. This variation in processing accounts for the wide range of cheeses commercially available, differing in texture and flavour. The curd can also be processed with other techniques to make a variety of products. However, all processes have one thing in common: the separation of the curd from the whey.

Procedure

- To prepare milk for curdling three different ways are being introduced for this experiment. Industrially, adding a starter culture of *Streptococci* or *Lactobacilli* to the milk and fermenting at 32°C for 10 to 75 minutes increases the lactic acid level in the milk. In addition to biologically converting the lactose present in the milk to lactic acid, these strains of microorganisms also greatly affect the flavour of the final product. Thus, the selection of a suitable strain, the amount of starter culture, and the length of pre-ripening, is of the utmost importance in creating the subtle differences in the final color and aroma that distinguishes an expensive cheese from a cheap one.
- In second approach the existing *Lactobacillus* culture in buttermilk is used as the starting culture. 1 ml of buttermilk is added per 100 ml of milk and the mixture is then fermented at room temperature for 4-12 hours. At the end of fermentation, the temperature of the mixture is raised to 32°C, and artificial coloring is added to the mixture prior to curdling.
- The third way to prepare the milk in a short time frame is to add acid (HCl) and to heat to 32°C. After rennet is added to the pre-cured milk, the coagulation process is started. In cheese making, as coagulation comes to completion, the temperature is gradually raised to about 38°C. This slightly elevated temperature facilitates the separation of the curd from the whey. A higher temperature also hardens the curd. The curd may be hardened further by cooking it for a longer period of time, either with or without the whey.
- After the curd is separated from the whey, salt, seasoning, and other curing and flavouring ingredients are added. The curd is wrapped in cheesecloth and pressed for 12 to 18 hours to remove the additional whey soaked in the curd. The curd hardens and forms a cheese block in the shape of the press as the whey is squeezed out. Finally, the cheese block is dried for 6 hours.
- It is now ready for consumption, or it may be left to age in a controlled cool environment (2-13°C). Although a higher temperature promotes faster curing, there is also a higher chance of spoilage due to undesirable microbial activities at elevated temperatures. Prior to aging, the cheese block is usually wrapped tightly to exclude air and microbial contaminants from entering and spoiling the cheese.
- One way to accomplish this is to dip the cheese block in a pot of melted wax. During the aging process, many complicated microbial and chemical actions continue to take place in the cheese block.
- Thousands of techniques exist to develop various distinctive flavours. These reactions are not well characterized; thus, cheese making is still an art rather than a science. Depending on the technique employed, this final aging process takes anywhere from 2 weeks to 6 months (Fig. 4.3).

Procuring at a warm temperature (acidify the milk)

⇩

Colouring

⇩

Coagulation by rennet

⇩

Separation of the whey

⇩

Flavour addition

⇩

Compression of the curd

⇩

Aging

⇩

Finished cheese

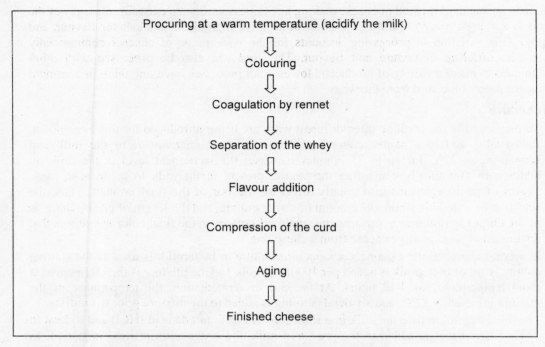

Fig. 4.3. Steps involved in cheese making

PROTOCOL 4.3

BATCH SUBMERGED FERMENTATION OF BAKER'S YEAST

Principle

The proper procedure for batch fermentation is first to inoculate a small flask of nutrient broth with a pure culture from a Petridish, a culture tube (containing liquid nutrient), or a slant tube (containing solid gel). The inoculated flask is constantly agitated in a temperature controlled flask shaker. A small amount of the culture in the original flask is pipetted out during the *exponential growth phase*, or *log phase*, and is used to inoculate the next flask. This process is repeated a few times to ensure that the culture is acclimated before it is employed to study the fermentation kinetics.

A similar process of repeated inoculation is carried out in the fermentation industry to build up enough inoculum needed to seed a larger fermenter. To reduce the shock resulting from a drastic change in the growth environment, the composition of the media used in preparing the inoculum should optimally be identical as that used in the main process. When working with a pure culture, one must operate under the assumption that contaminating microorganisms are present everywhere in the open environment. It is important to know intuitively when sterile tools or glassware must be used and when sterilization is not necessary. This requires the ability to distinguish clearly the sterile side from the nonsterile side.

In this experiment, the interior of the shaker flask is the sterile portion of the system. Anything that is that part of the system and anything that ever comes in direct contact with that part of the system must be sterile. Thus, the nutrient in the shaker flask before inoculation must be sterile, which in turn requires that the reservoir storing the filtered nutrient is sterile and that the entire process of dispensing the nutrient from the medium jar to the shaker flask is carried out aseptically. In addition, items that enter the shaker flask such as the cotton plug, inoculation loop, sampling pipettes, and even air must all be sterile.

Most practical industrial fermentation processes are based on complex media because of the cost and the choice of the nutrients and the ease of nutrient preparation. For example, complex media for yeast fermentation can be easily prepared in a lab by following the same recipe as that used in the YPG agar, minus the agar: 0.5% yeast extract, 1.0% peptone, and 0.5% glucose. However, the use of complex media is discouraged in the fundamental studies of fermentation kinetics because of the possibility of variations in the nutrient composition from run to run. For example, the exact content of a yeast extract preparation is not known, and its nutritional quality may vary from batch to batch. On the other hand, a defined medium can be reproduced time after time to ensure the reproducibility of biochemical experiments.

The disadvantage of a defined medium is that there is always the possibility of missing some important growth factors. The formulation of a defined medium is often a tedious process of trial and error. However, a defined medium can support the healthy growth and maintenance of cells as effectively as, or sometimes superior to, a complex one. A defined medium will be used in this experiment.

Equipments

Erlenmeyer flasks with cotton plugs, Graduated cylinders, Nutrient jar with rubber stoppers, In-line filters (0.2 μm, for nutrient and vent), Temperature controlled flask shaker, Thermometer, Bunsen burner, Inoculation loop, Autoclave, Balance, Magnetic stirrer, Sterile Pipettes (1ml and 10ml), Sampling vials (8 ml), Centrifuge or filtration setup for dry cell mass measurement, In-line filter holder (25 mm, 0.45μm) for sample clarification. Syringe

Materials

Baker's yeast, Nutrients, Sucrose, Glucose, Ethanol, 100%

Procedure

Nutrient preparation (defined medium)

- The overall nutrient composition is shown in Table 4.3.
- To facilitate nutrient preparation and to minimize the chance of making the fatal mistake of omitting one or two trace components, two concentrated (100 fold) stock solutions can be made according to the formula given in Table 4.4 to 4.6.
- Mix the concentrated mineral stock solution.
- Adjust the quantity according to the need.
- Bottled solutions can be stored on a shelf for more than six months.

- A yellowish colour may develop upon prolonged storage; however, yellowing of the solution seems to impart no harmful effect.
- Mix the concentrated vitamin stock solution.
- Keep the stock solution in the dark at 4°C.
- Discard the solution if mould growth can be visually detected. The storage life of the stock solution is approximately 2-3 months.
- To obtain a working nutrient solution, add to 750 ml of stirred deionized water the components of Table 4 in the order listed.
- Precipitate may form if the order is not strictly followed. KOH pellets are used to neutralize the phosphoric acid and bring the pH close to the desired value.
- Add water to 1 litre. Finally, adjust the pH to the desired value by dropwise adding 1N KOH solution. (pH 5 will be used in this experiment.)

Table 4.3. Composition of defined medium for baker's yeast

Compound	Concentration
$MgCl_2.6H_2O$	0.52 g/l
$(NH_4)_2SO_4$	12 g/l
H_3PO_4 (85%)	1.6 ml/l
KCl	0.12 g/l
$CaCl_2.2H_2O$	0.2 g/l
NaCl	0.06 g/l
$MnSO_4.H_2O$	0.024 g/l
$CaSO_4.5H_2O$	0.0005 g/l
H_3BO_3	0.0005 g/l
$Na_2MoO_4.2H_2O$	0.002 g/l
NiCl	0.0025 mg/l
$ZnSO_4.7H_2O$	0.012 g/l
$CoSO_4.7H_2O$	0.0023 mg/l
KI	0.0001 g/l
$FeSO_4(NH_4)_2SO_4.6H_2O$	0.035 g/l
Myo-Inositol	0.125 g/l
Pyridoxine-HCl (Vitamin B_6)	0.00625 g/l
Ca-n-Pantothenate	0.00625 g/l
Thiamine-HCl (Vitamin B_1)	0.005 g/l
Nicotinic Acid	0.005 g/l
D-Biotin (Vitamin H)	0.000125 g/l
Carbon source (e.g. Glucose)	0.5 g/l
EDTA	0.1 g/l

Nutrient sterilization

The prepared nutrient is sterilized by autoclaving. However, autoclaving is not a suitable sterilization method for this formulation because of two reasons. First, the heat of autoclaving will caramel the sugar and darken the nutrient to a brown color. Secondly, the heat will destroy vitamins. Furthermore, the loss of liquid due to boiling during the autoclaving process will change the concentration of various nutrient components, including the rate limiting carbon source. Evaporation loss is especially severe when ethanol is the designated carbon source. Instead, membrane filtration will be used to sterilize the nutrient in this experiment. This can be accomplished by drawing the nutrient from a mixing jar and forcing it through an in-line filter (0.2 μm pore size) either by gravity or with a peristaltic pump. The sterilized medium is fed into an autoclaved nutrient jar with a rubber stopper fitted with a filtered vent and a hooded sampling port. Care must be taken in filling the nutrient jar as overfilling will forced out of the nutrient from venting filter and wet it.

A wet venting filter must be aseptically replaced with another dry sterile one. Otherwise, the wet filter will support the unwarranted proliferation of a wide range of microorganisms, which will soon destroy the filter membrane and enter into the nutrient jar and contaminate the broth. For the same reason, soon after the filling process is completed, disconnect the in-line nutrient filtration unit, and wash the residual nutrient. If the nutrient filter is to be reused, wash and autoclave it before it is destroyed by the microbial growth either due to clogging or breaking of the membrane.

Table 4.4. Mineral stock solution (100X)

Compound	Weight-volume
H_3PO_4 (85%)	160 ml
KCl	12 g
$CaCl_2.2H_2O$	20 g
NaCl	6 g
$MnSO_4.H_2O$	2.4 g
$CaSO_4.5H_2O$	0.05 g
H_3BO_3	0.05 g
$Na_2MoO_4.2H_2O$	0.2 g
NiCl	0.25 mg
$ZnSO_4.7H_2O$	1.2 g
$CoSO_4.7H_2O$	0.23 mg
KI	0.01 g
Add water to	1 litre

Table 4.5. Vitamin stock solution (100X)

Compound	Weight-volume
Myo-Inositol	12.5 g
Pyridoxine-HCl	0.625 g
Ca-n-Pantothenate	0.625 g
Thiamine-HCl	0.5 g
Nicotinic Acid	0.5 g
D-Biotin	0.0125 g
Add water to	1 litre

DELAWARE VALLEY COLLEGE LIBRARY

Table 4.6. Normal strength working nutrient solution

Compound	Weight-volume
Phthalic acid, monopotassium salt	0.2 g
$MgCl_2.6H_2O$	0.52 g
EDTA	0.1 g
$(NH_4)_2SO_4$	12 g
Mineral Stock Solution	10 ml
$FeSO_4(NH_4)_2SO_4.6H_2O$	0.035 g
Vitamin stock soution	10 ml
Carbon Source (e.g. Glucose)	0.5 g
KOH (for pH 5)	1.62 g
Add water to	1 litre
Adjust pH to 5 with 1N KOH and 1N HCl	

The hooded sampling port consists of a tubing reaching into the bottom of the nutrient jar and a rubber bulb on the side. Normally, a sampling bottle is attached to the sampling port to keep its tip airtight and sterile. When the rubber bulb is squeezed, the air in the sampling bottle is forced into the nutrient jar. When the bulb is released, nutrient equal to the volume of the displaced air is sucked up the sampling tube and is collected in the sampling bottle. A sterile medium bottle with the same cap size may be attached to the sampling port in place of a sampling bottle if fermentation is to be conducted directly in the medium bottle or if it is more convenient to store the media in smaller bottles, each holding enough for one or two shaker flasks. The content from the media bottles may later be poured into shaker flasks as needed. Alternatively, a sterilized flask may be placed under the exposed sampling tube. Applying pressure to the vent will force liquid out from the jar into the flask. Flame both the sampling port and the mouth of the sterile sampling bottle before screwing on the sampling bottle. Although the turbidity in the nutrient jar may be due to the precipitation of some of the nutrient components, it is almost always due to the presence of contaminants. At the first sign of contamination, either totally kill the contaminants by autoclaving or reduce the viability by adding bleach solution. Discard the contents only after sanitization.

Shaker flask preparation

- Make cotton-gauze plugs to fit the mouth of 250 ml shaker flasks. Plug the flask and cover the plug with a piece of aluminum foil before autoclaving. The aluminum foil will prevent dust from directly settling on the cotton plug while standing on the shelf waiting to be used. This is generally the case where many flasks are simultaneously autoclaved for later use.
- After autoclaving the flasks, cool them to room temperature. Pour sterile nutrient into the flasks aseptically.

Inoculum preparation

- Find a single isolated colony of yeast on the petridish from which the culture is to be transferred. Following the aseptic plate streaking techniques introduced in the previous weeks, lift a small loopful of the creamy culture off the agar plate. Dip the loop into a 250 ml flask containing 100 ml of 0.5% glucose. Swirl the loop in the nutrient solution to dislodge the selected culture from the loop.

- Flame the neck of the flask and the cotton plug before inserting the plug back on the flask. Also, flame the loop to kill the residual microorganisms.
- Place the flask in a temperature controlled shaker at 37°C. The exponential growth phase will last from 2 to 24 hours after inoculation. The exact time and duration depend on the physiological conditions of the inoculum. An exponentially growing culture should be provided.

Shaker flask inoculation

- Follow the same procedure described previously to prepare nutrient solutions with the following carbon sources (Table 4.7):
- Sterilize the nutrient through filtration as described above. Autoclave 1000 ml flasks and transfer 500 ml of the nutrient into each of them. Inoculate the flask with 10 ml of suspended actively growing yeast culture obtained at the end of Step* (refer previous page) with a sterile 10 ml pipette.

Table 4.7. Carbon sources for fermentation

Run	Carbon source	Weight g/l
A	Ethanol	5
B	Glucose	5
C	Sucrose	5
D	Glucose	2.5
E	Sucrose	2 5

Batch fermentation monitoring

- Remove the flask from the shaker and draw a sample at 90-120 minutes intervals. The fermentation should last for approximately 24-36 hours before the culture enters the stationary phase (*See Notes*).
- Although a 10 ml sample is more than adequate to analyze for optical density, glucose/sucrose concentration, and ethanol concentration, an extra 10 ml will ensure the availability of a sufficient quantity of sample broth, if the quantitative analysis fails.
- Immediately after taking a 20 ml aliquot with a sterile pipette, flame the neck of the flask and place the plug back in the mouth.
- Record the pH of the sample just taken.
- Save a drop of the sample on a slide for microscopic examination later.
- Initially, when the cell density is still low, the optical density of the sample can be measured without dilution with water. Perform this step quickly with a spectrophotometer at 550 nm.
- Filter out the cells from the sample. After the optical density is over 0.5, save 1 ml of the sample by pipetting it into a test tube for optical density measurement. Force the remaining sample through a filter.

- The clear filtrate is collected in a tightly capped sampling vial for later analysis. Freezing the filtrate will better preserve the existing condition.
- If a 1 ml sample is saved for the optical density measurement, dilute the sample with 5 ml of water.
- Record the optical density.
- Clean the filter unit, test tubes, and pipette.
- Return the flask back to the shaker and get ready for the next sampling.

Dry cell weight measurement

- Terminate the experiment when the stationary phase is reached. Obtain a calibration curve for the cell concentration in g/l as a function of the optical density.
- Measure the volume of the remaining culture. Weight an empty aluminum weighing pan or a sheet of dried filter paper stored in a desiccator.
- Separate the cells from the broth either by centrifugation or by filtration.
- After drying the cell paste in an oven set at 100°C for 24 hours. Measure the weight of the weighing pan or the filter paper.

Quantitative analysis

After the experiment is concluded for each sample, measure the glucose concentration with the DNS reagent, the sucrose concentration and ethanol concentration according to official procedure given in I.P, 1966.

Notes

The shaking action should be stopped prior to door is opened. Pump the syringe twice to let the dead volume in the sampling tube recirculate back into the flask, because it is the residual broth from the previous sampling and is not representative of the prevailing condition in the shaker flask.

Withdraw approximately 7 ml of sample in the syringe, and disconnect the syringe from the rubber stopper by twisting it counterclockwise, not by pulling it. Do not contaminate the syringe tip by touching it. Inject the sample into a small beaker. Twist the syringe back onto the rubber stopper and collect another 7 ml of sample. At the end of sampling, twist the syringe back onto the rubber stopper.

Close the shaker door. A total of 15-20 ml should be enough to carry out all the required analysis. Save a drop of the sample on a slide glass. Visually inspect for the presence/absence of contaminants under a microscope at the end of the procedure. Measure and record the pH.

Measure the optical density at 550 nm. Dilute just enough sample with water as needed (probably 1 ml of sample with 5 ml of water) to keep the reading below 0.5; keep the remainder undiluted, because doing so will make the subsequent glucose/ethanol analysis very difficult. Report the OD. Example: if an absorbance of 0.123 after diluting 1 ml of sample with 5 ml of water and if the absorbance of the supernatant from the next step, i.e., the background, was 0.214 then:

$$OD = 0.123 \text{ X } 6 - 0.214 = 0.524$$

Centrifuge the undiluted sample at 10,000 rpm for 5 minutes to collect the supernatant. Avoid resuspending cells back into the supernatant. Measure the absorbance of the clear supernatant, and use it in calculation of the cell optical density above. Supernatant should be colorless; however, this is not always true if other media, e.g., YPG formulation used to prepare plates last week, are used.

Save the supernatant in a clean properly labeled sampling bottle and store it in the freezer. This frozen cell-free sample will be thawed. Analyze the sample quantitatively for glucose and ethanol. Repeat the procedure for other flasks.

PROTOCOL 4.4

WINE PRODUCTION BY YEAST

Principle

Wine making is still very much an art rather than science. The procedures of making grape wine at home are quite straightforward. Grape juice is simply inoculated with a package of commercially available yeast starter culture. Primary fermentation lasts for approximately one week; during that time most of the sugar originally present in the juice is converted to ethanol and yeast cells, with the evolution of carbon dioxide. The excess yeast cells are then removed from the juice along with other sediment, and a slower secondary fermentation is allowed to proceed to develop the final flavour. Sugar may be added to the original to achieve the desired alcohol content or to modify the flavour. The type of wine can be classified according to the colour of the wine. Another classification is based on the starting sugar content, as listed in Table 4.8.

Table 4.8. Classification of wines according to the sugar content.

Type	Specific gravity	Sugar content (wt. %)
Dry wine	1.085-1.100	21 - 25
Medium sweet wine	1.120 - 1.140	29 - 33
Sweet wine	1.140 - 1.160	33 - 37

Wine on large scale is produced by fermentation of the juices of grapes and other fruits such as peaches, pears, and plums. This biochemical conversion of the juice to wine is carried out by the action of yeast cells which degrades the fruit sugars, fructose and glucose by enzymatic action. The commercial production of wine is a long and exacting process. First, the grapes are crushed or pressed to express the juice, which is called, must. Potassium metabisulphite is added to the must to retard the growth of acetic acid bacteria, moulds and wild yeast that are endogenous to grapes in the vineyard. A wine-producing strain of yeast, *Saccharomyces cerevisae* var. ellopsoideus is used to inoculate the must which is then incubated for 3 to 5 days under aerobic conditions at 21°C to 32°C. this is followed by an anaerobic incubation period. The wine is then aged for a period of 1 to 5 years in aging tanks or wooden barrels. During this time, the wine is clarified of any turbidity, thereby producing volatile esters that are responsible for characteristic flavours. The clarified product is then filtered, pasteurized at 60°C for 30 minutes and bottled.

Materials

Culture

50 ml of grape juice broth culture of *Saccharomyces cerevisiae* var. ellipsoideus incubated for 48 hours at 25°C.

Media

500 ml of pasteurized grape juice.

Equipment

1 litre Erlenmeyer flask, one holed rubber stopper containing a 2 inch glass tube plugged with cotton pan balance, spatula, glassine paper, 10 ml graduated cylinder, ebulliometer and burette or pipette for titration.

Procedure

- Pour 500 ml of the grape juice into the 1 litre Erlenmeyer flask. Add 20 gm of sucrose and 50 ml of *S. cerevisae* grape juice broth culture (10 % starter culture). Close the flask with the stopper containing cotton plugged air vent.
- After 2 to 4 days of incubation, add 20 g of sucrose to the fermenting wine.
- Incubate the fermenting wine for 21 days at 25°C.

PROTOCOL 4.5

STUDY OF VARIABLES IN WINE FERMENTATION

Materials

Graduated cylinder, Test tubes, Erlenmeyer flasks or bottles, Rubber stoppers, Tygon tubing, Hydrometer, Balance, Grape juice, Sucrose, Active dry wine yeast, Strains of *Saccharomyces ellipsoideus*

Procedure

Preparation of starter yeast culture

- Mix 1 g of dry wine yeast culture in 100 ml of grape juice.
- Grow the yeast in a loosely capped container at room temperature for 24 hours.

Primary fermentation

- Add enough sugar to grape juice to prepare the substrates A, B, C and D with concentration 0, 100, 200 and 300 respectively.
- Measure the specific gravity and PA value (potential alcohol value) for each of the starting substrates with a hydrometer. This is the initial PA value of alcohol.
- Inoculate each bottle with 20 ml of the starter yeast culture prepared in the previous step.
- Plug the juice bottle with a rubber stopper. A piece of Tygon tubing is extended from the stopper to provide a vent for the evolved carbon dioxide. The other end of the tubing is

dipped in water in a small test tube taped to the bottle. The water prevents the entry of oxygen, which alters the metabolism of the yeast and spoils the wine. At the same time, carbon dioxide can escape from the bottle.

- Ferment at room temperature for one week.

Secondary fermentation

- At the end of one week, decant the juice from the bottle to clean individual temporary containers.
- Measure the PA values for each of the substrate with a hydrometer.
- Estimate the alcohol content by subtracting the present PA value from the initial PA value.
- Discard the sediment and wash each bottle with water.
- Pour the juice back into the cleaned bottle.
- Put back the cleaned assembly of rubber stopper and Tygon tubing.
- Ferment slowly for another 4-6 weeks.
- Measure the PA values as before when it is ready for consumption.

Evaluation of Produced Wine

Measurement of density by hydrometer

A hydrometer is a floatation device used to measure the density of a liquid. Because the liquid exerts a buoyancy force equal to the weight of the volume displaced by the hydrometer, the meter will float higher in a denser fluid than in a lighter fluid. In general, a denser solution has more dissolved solids. A conventional hydrometer can easily measure the specific gravity of a liquid to an accuracy of 0.001. Many scales are available on a hydrometer. A typical one employed in the alcoholic beverage industry allows readings in the Balling/Brix scale and the Potential Alcohol (PA) scale, as well as the usual specific gravity scale.

The calibration of Balling or Brix, scale is based on the weight percent of sugar in solution. Whereas, the PA scale is an indication of the potential (volume) percent of alcohol that may be produced through fermentation based on the complete conversion of the sugar originally present in the solution. Of course, this represents the maximum value that is rarely reached. Usually, residual sugar is present and is sometimes desirable for taste. Note that for historical reasons, the alcohol content is commonly measured in units of volume percent or proof, while the sugar content is expressed in weight percent. Both units are widely used in wine industries.

The proper way of using a hydrometer is to spin it gently in the grape juice, must, or wine for which the specific gravity is to be measured. Twisting of the hydrometer removes most of the air bubbles from its surface, which can invalidate the measurement. The sugar content of the sample in weight percent is read from the meter, which in turn indicates the potentially achievable alcohol content in the final fermented product. Two readings are required to estimate the alcohol content in a fermented wine. The first reading is taken at the beginning of fermentation. The second reading will tell one the amount of the remaining sugar at the time of the reading. Thus, the current alcohol content is simply the present PA value minus the starting PA value. Because the density of a liquid is a function of the temperature, Table 4.9 gives the correction that one should add to the specific gravity readings to obtain the corresponding values at 60° F, the temperature at which the meter is calibrated.

Table 4.9. Temperature correction to the specific gravity reading.

Temperature(°F)	Correction (sp. g.)
50	0.000
70	+0.001
77	+0.002
84	+0.003
95	+0.005
105	+0.007

Notes

Fresh grapes may be crushed to obtain the juice. Most wineries add sulfur dioxide either as a gas or as a solid salt to prevent the growth of other yeast and bacteria, which cause spoilage. Sulfur dioxide is also produced by *Saccharomyces* during fermentation. Dry wine yeast may be directly added to grape juice from a package at the level of 1 g per 4 litre. For best results, first suspend 1 g of dry wine yeast in 10 ml of warm water at about 35ºC. Then add the suspended culture to grape juice.

FERMENTATION PRODUCTS

The list of very commonly in used food products with their material requirement and possible processing variable is given below.

Production of Sausages

Semi-dry fermented sausages

Summer sausages from *Pediococcus cerevesiae* and *Lactobacillus plantarum*

Dry fermented sausages

Sausages from *Pediococcus cerevesiae,Lactobacillus plantarum,Genoa salami, Micrococcus spp.* mixed with either *Pediococcus cerevesiae* or *Lactobacillus plantarum*

Processing variables

Lactic acid is produced, lowering the pH of the sausage to preserve and flavour.

Production of Some Enzymes

Chymosin

Replaces rennet in over 80% of the cheese produced. Rennet is extracted from the stomachs of milk-fed veal calves. The supply is linked to the veal market, causing wide shifts in availability of the rennet. An *E. coli* produces recombinant Chymosin. The gene for chymosin was transferred from a calf to *E. coli*.

Amylase

Amylase is the enzyme that will break starch into its separate glucose components. Amylase is used in the brewing industry for malting and used in baking.

Glucose isomerase

The enzyme glucose isomerase converts or isomerizes glucose (an aldehyde) to fructose (a ketone) which is a sweeter product.

Pectinase

Pectinase is the enzyme that breaks down pectin, a polysaccharide found in fruit. Pectinase is used to remove particulate matter, or clarify, fruit juices.

Glucose oxidase

Glucose oxidase is an enzyme used in the production of dried egg whites. When drying egg whites the glucose present in the white can react with amines in a reaction known as Maillard browning. This will cause the dried egg whites to turn brown. The addition of glucose oxidase will break down the glucose and prevent the glucose from reacting and causing the off color of the egg whites.

To produce these recombinant enzymes, the gene is first transferred into bacteria. The bacteria are then grown in fermenter. The enzyme is purified and sold.

Commercial Xanthan Gum

Xanthan gum is a polysaccharide produced by the bacterium *Xanthomonas campestris* on the cell wall. *Xanthomonas campestris* occurs naturally on the leaves of plants in the cabbage family. Commercial xanthan gum is produced by aerobic submerged fermentation. The bacteria are mixed with sugar, a nitrogen source, trace elements, and other growth factors in a large stainless steel tank. During fermentation aeration, agitation, pH and temperature are precisely controlled. After fermentation the solution is pasteurized to kill all bacteria. The gum is used in many products including cakes, muffins, ice cream, sherbet, sour cream, salad dressings, sauces, gravies, syrups, and toppings.

Materials

Bottles (washed and sterilized), Wine corks or caps and crowns, Stirring spoon, Large (20 litre), enamel kettle or pot (do not use aluminium vessels), Shillings root beer concentrate 59 ml, Sucrose, Chlorine-free water, Containers to measure out needed volumes of materials, Yeast

Possible variables

Flavorings other than shillings root beer Extract
Amount of sucrose
Amount of root beer extract
Quick rise in yeast versus normal
Amount of yeast
Different sources of sugar (i.e. dextrose)

Production of Kimchee

Materials

Chinese cabbage, Red hot chili pepper, Cloves garlic, non-iodized salt, soda bottle, Large plastic lid (Petri plate lid), pH indicator paper, Small plastic pipette

Processing Variables

Different cabbage types
Change seasonings or ingredients
Place bottles at various temperatures

Production of Sauerkraut

Materials

Cabbage sliced into thin strips, Non-iodized salt, Container (consider the fact that cabbage will require anaerobic conditions while fermenting in this container. Container should not be chipped or cracked. Food grade sturdy plastic pails are excellent containers. Do not use metal containers of any type.)

Processing variables

Different types of cabbage can be used

Cabbage can be cut into different sizes to see how size varies the resulting product

Spices or seasonings can be added for a variety of kraut flavours

Sauerkraut can be canned for long-term storage

Notes

Containers used in making kraut should be cleaned and rinsed well. Crocks should have shiny glaze to the surface, and not be cracked or chipped. Metal containers are definitely not to be used. If plastic is used, only use food- grade plastic.

Fermenting Power of Bread Yeast

Materials

50 or 100 ml graduated cylinder, 100 ml graduated cylinder, greased with vaseline, Flour, Two brands, A and B, of active dry yeast (either A or B should be a yeast cake), *Saccharomyces cerevesiae,* young streak culture (solid medium), Square sheets of brown wrapping paper, Buffered methylene blue stain :Mix 1 part of 1:5000 methylene blue and 1 part of a phosphate buffer solution (99.25 ml of 0.2 M KH_2PO_4 to 0.25 mL of 0.2 M Na_2HPO_4) to give pH 4.6, Microscope, Microscope slides and coverslips

Processing variables

Different brands of yeast

Different forms of yeast

Rapid rise versus normal

Different temperatures

SUGGESTED READINGS

Bailey, J. E. and Ollis, D. P., Biochemical Engineering Fundamentals, 2nd Edition, McGraw Hill, 1986.

Boyd, R. F., General Microbiology 2nd Edition, Times Mirror/Mosby College, 1988.

Cappuchino, J. G. and Sherman, N., Microbiology: A Laboratory Manual, 4th Edition, Addison-Wesley Longman, Inc. Harlow, England, 1993.

Driessen, F. M., Ubbels, J., and Stadhouders, J., *Biotech. Bioeng.,* 19, 821, 1977.

Frazier, W.C. and Westhoff, D.C., Food Microbiology, 3rd Edition. McGraw-Hill, Inc., New York, 1978.

Harley, J. and Prescott, L., Laboratory Exercise in Microbiology, William C. Brown Publishers, 1993.

Laboratory Experiments in Biotechnology and Related Areas, Vol. III, Department of Biological Sciences, Mankato State University, Mankato, MN, 1988.

Mennes, M., Food Science, Food Management Specialist, University of Wisconsin-Madison, UW-Extension.

Ough, C. S., Chemical Used in Making Wine, C and EN, 1987.

Oura, E., *Biotech. Bioeng.* 16, 1197, 1974.

Robinson, R. K., A Colour Guide to Cheese and Fermented Milks, Chapman and Hall, London.

Robinson, R. K., Dairy Microbiology, Vol. 2, Applied Science Publishers, New Jersey, 1981.

Rose, A. H., Fermented Foods, Academic Press, New York, 1982.

Tamime, A. Y. and Deeth, H. C., *J. Food Protection,* 43, 939, 1980.

The BioNet Booklet, Vol. 3, , Rod Johnson, Eau Claire North High School, Eau Claire, WI 54703, 1995.

Trehan, K., Biotechnology, Wiley Eastern Limited, New Delhi, India, 1991.

Vyas, S. P. and Dixit, V. K, Pharmaceutical Biotechnology, CBS Publishers, New Delhi, India, 1998.

Wagner, M., Bradley, R. and M. Mennes, *Agricultural Bulletin*, 53715, 608-262-3346.

CHAPTER 5

Biochemical Preparations

- Introduction
- Tyrosinase as a model enzyme
- Extraction of tyrosinase
- Preparation of standard curve of tyrosinase
- Assessment of optimum enzyme concentration for reaction kinetics
- Effect of pH on enzyme activity
- Effect of temperature on enzyme catalyzed reaction
- Kinetic analysis
- Determination of K_m and V_{max}
- Kinetic analysis for α- amylase activity
- Production of corn syrup using bacterial amylase
- Evaluation of Amino transferases activity
- Evaluation of phospholipases activity
- Determination of acetyl cholinesterase activity
- Cellulases ($c_x\beta_{(1-4)}$ gluconase) assay
- Evaluation of papain activity
- Evaluation of glucose oxidase activity
- Sucrose synthase
- Lipase enzyme activity determination
- Isolation of crystalline animal cytochrome c
- Digestion of protein into amino acid
- Amino acid assay by ninhydrin colorimetric method
- Determination of total carbohydrate by anthrone method
- Glucose assay by dinitrosalicylic acid colorimetric method
- Estimation of amylase in saliva
- Isolation of phospholipids from egg yolk
- Chromatography of phospholipids
- Estimation of serum cholesterol

INTRODUCTION

The enzymes are critical in the functioning of cells. Life is a dynamic process that involves constant changes in chemical composition. These changes are regulated by catalytic reactions, which are regulated by enzymes. At one time, the cell was actually conceived of as a sac of enzymes. It was believed that on the basis of the reactions and their rates of action, cell and indeed, life itself could be defined. Few biologists continue to think of this as a simple task, but we know that life could not exist without the function of enzymes. Ideally, enzymes could be examined within an intact cell, but this is difficult to control. Consequently, enzymes are studied *in vitro* after extraction from cells. In a simpler way enzymes can be defined as biocatalysts. Catalysts are the substances that accelerate the reaction but do not get itself modified in the process so that it can be used again and again. Enzymes are the largest and most specialized class of protein molecules. More than a thousand different enzymes have been identified, many of them have been obtained in pure and even in crystalline form.

An important feature of enzyme activity is its substrate specificity, i.e. a particular enzyme will act only on a certain specific substrate. Some enzymes have nearly absolute specificity for a given substrate and will not act on even very closely related molecules, as for example stereoisomers of the same molecule. Other enzymes have relative specificity, since they will act upon a variety of related compounds. Some enzymes require small non protein components called cofactors for their activity for example some enzymes are conjugated proteins having tightly bound prosthetic groups, as in case of cytochrome, which have an iron porphyrin complex. Other enzymes can not function without the addition of small molecules called coenzymes, which become bound during the reaction. When joined with a coenzyme, these inactive enzymes (also called apoenzymes) form active holozymes.

$$\text{Holozymes} \longrightarrow \text{Apoenzymes} + \text{Coenzymes}$$

Since all enzymes are proteins, and proteins are differentially soluble in salt solutions, enzyme extraction procedures often begin with salt (typically, ammonium sulphate) precipitation. On the simplest level, proteins can be divided into albumins and globulins on the basis of their solubility in dilute salt solutions. Albumins are considered to be soluble while globulins are insoluble. Solubility is relative, however, and as the salt concentration is increased, even proteins tend to precipitate.

Thus, if a tissue is homogenized in a solution that retains the enzyme in its soluble state, the enzyme can be subsequently separated from all insoluble proteins by centrifugation or filtration. The enzyme will be impure, since it will be in solution with many other proteins. If aliquots of a concentrated ammonium sulphate solution are then added serially, individual proteins will begin to precipitate according to their solubility. By careful manipulation of the salt concentrations, thus fractions, which contain purer solutions of enzymes, or at least are enriched for a given enzyme can be produced. In order to determine the effectiveness of the purification, each step in the extraction procedure must be monitored for enzyme activity. That monitoring can be accomplished in many ways, but usually involves a measurement of the decrease in substrate, or the increase in product specific to the enzyme.

It is important to remember that enzymes act as catalyst to a reaction and affect only the reaction rate. The general scheme for the action of an enzyme is given by the following equation:

$$E+S \underset{K_2}{\overset{K_1}{\rightleftharpoons}} ES \underset{K_4}{\overset{K_3}{\rightleftharpoons}} E+P \qquad \text{------------------------------------[5.1]}$$

Where

E = concentration of the enzyme

S and P = concentrations of substrate and product respectively
ES and EP = concentration of enzyme-substrate complex and enzyme-product complex
K_1 –K_4 = rate constants for each step.
From above equation 5.1, the rate (velocities) of each reaction can be given by:

$V_1 = K_1[E][S]$ Formation of enzyme-substrate complex
$V_2 = K_2[ES]$ Reformation of free enzyme and substrate
$V_3 = K_3[ES]$ Formation of product and free enzyme
$V_4 = K_4[E][P]$ Reformation of enzyme-product complex

At steady state, $(V_1–V_2) = (V_3–V_4)$ and, if all product is either removed or does not recombine with the enzyme, then $K_4 = 0$, then

$$K_1[E][S] - K_2[ES] = K_3[ES] \quad \text{--}[5.2]$$

This equation can then be rearranged to yield:

$$K_1[E][S] = (K_2+K_3)\ [ES] \quad \text{--}[5.3]$$

The left side of this equation can be given as a single constant, known as K, the rate constant, or the Michaelis constant. Note that the units for this constant will be that of concentration.

One of the important concepts of metabolism is that enzymes from differing sources may have the same function (i.e. the same substrate and product), but possess significantly different K values. Since biological function is as dependent on the rate of a reaction as it is on the direction of a reaction, it becomes necessary to measure the K value for any enzyme under study.

Enzymes act as catalysts because of their three dimensional protein structure. This structure is controlled by many factors, but is particularly sensitive to changes in pH, salts and temperature. Small changes in the temperature of a reaction can significantly alter the reaction rate, and extremely high temperatures can irreversibly alter both the three dimensional structure of the enzyme and its activity. It may even render the enzyme non-functional; that is, to denature the enzyme. Salts can also cause denaturation, but the effect of ammonium sulphate is usually reversible.

Active Sites

An enzyme works by binding to a substrate in a geometrical fashion so that the substrate is able to undergo the reaction (product formation) at a more rapid rate. This type of reaction is commonly referred to as the lock and key model for enzyme action. It implies that there is a particular part of the enzyme structure, the active site, which specifically binds sterically to a substrate. The enzyme does not actually react with the substrate but merely brings the substrate into the proper alignment or configuration for it to react spontaneously or in conjunction with another substance. Since a reaction proceeds normally by a random kinetic action of molecules colliding with each other. Any time molecules come in contact and react in a faster manner. Thus, for any given enzyme there will be a best-fit configuration to the protein in order to align the substrate and to facilitate the reaction. When the enzyme is in its ideal configuration, the reaction proceeds at its maximum rate, and the overall rate of action will depend on substrate concentration.

Maximum reaction rate assumes that an optimal pH, salt environment and temperature have been established. Maximum rate further assumes the presence of any co-enzymes and/or cofactors that the enzyme requires. Co-enzymes are organic molecules, which must bind to the protein portion of the enzyme in order to form the correct configuration for a reaction. Whereas cofactors are inorganic molecules which do the same.

To measure the concentration of an enzyme via its action rate (i.e. the velocity of the catalyzed reaction), the effect of temperature, pH, salt concentration, coenzymes, cofactors, and substrate concentration on reaction rate must be controlled. Each of these parameters affects the rate of an enzyme reaction. Thus, each must be carefully controlled if we attempt to study the effects of changes in the enzyme itself.

The relationship between substrate concentration and enzyme concentration was mathematically established by the work of two biochemists, L. Michaelis and M.L. Menten in 1913. In recognition of their work, the plots of enzyme activity vs. substrate concentration are known as Michaelis-Menten plots. These are relatively simple plots in which the substrate concentration is on the x-axis, and the velocity of reaction is on the y-axis. The plot demonstrates that as the substrate increases, the velocity increases hyperbolically, and approaches a maximum rate known as V_{max}. This is dependent upon saturation of the enzyme. At V_{max}, all enzyme molecules are complexed with substrate, and thus any additional substrate added to the reaction has no effect on the rate of reaction.

However, this situation becomes more complex on changing the enzyme concentration, V_{max} will also change. Thus, V_{max} is not a constant value, but is constant only for a given enzyme concentration. Consequently, the value of Vmax can not be used directly to infer enzyme concentration. It is dependent upon at least two variables, enzyme concentration and substrate concentration (assuming temperature, pH and cofactors have all been controlled). Michaelis and Menten gave a simple means of solving the equations for two variables. If multiple plots of enzyme activity vs. substrate concentration are made with increasing enzyme concentration, the value of V_{max} continues to increase, but the substrate concentration, which corresponds to $1/2V_{max}$, remains constant. This concentration is the Michaelis Constant for an enzyme. As mentioned, it is designated as K and is operationally the concentration of substrate, which will give exactly $1/2V_{max}$ when reacted with an enzyme with maximum pH, temperature and cofactors.

According to the Michaelis-Menten equation:

$$V = \frac{V_{max}\,[S]}{K_m + [S]} \qquad \text{------------}[5.4]$$

Above equation is derived from the formula for a hyperbola (c=xy)

Where $K_m = [S]\,(V_{max}/V-1)$

When $V = V_{max}/2$,

$K_m = [S][V_{max}/(V_{max}/2)-1] = [S]$, This confirms that the units of this constant is that of concentration.

A Michaelis-Menten plot thus provides an easy way to measure the rate constant for a given enzyme. An immediate difficulty is apparent, however, when Michaelis-Menten plots are used. V_{max} is an asymptote. Its value can only be certain if the reaction is run at an infinite concentration of substrate. In 1934, two individuals, Lineweaver and Burke made a simple mathematical alteration in the process by plotting a double inverse of substrate concentration and reaction rate (velocity).

The Lineweaver/Burke equation is:

$$\frac{1}{V} = \frac{K_m + [S]}{V_{max}\,[S]} \quad \text{------------------------------[5.5]}$$

On simplification

$$\frac{1}{V} = \frac{K_m}{V_{max}\,[S]} + \frac{1}{V_{max}} \quad \text{------------------------------[5.6]}$$

This equation fits the general form of a straight line, y=mx+b, where m is the slope of the line and b is the intercept. Thus, the Lineweaver/Burke plot for an enzyme is more useful than Michaelis-Menten, since as velocity reaches infinity, $1/V_{max}$ approaches 0. The slope of straight line is equal to K_m/V_{max}, the y intercept equals $1/V_{max}$ (1/[S]=0). Projection of the line back through the x-axis yields the value $-1/K_m$ (when 1/V=0). These values can easily be determined by using a linear regression plot and calculating the corresponding values for x=0 and y=0. The inverse of the intercept values will then yield V_{max} and K_m. The aim of all of these calculations is to determine the true activity and thus the concentration of the enzyme. If the reaction conditions are adjusted so that the substrate concentration is at K_m, then alterations in the rate of reaction are linear due to alterations in enzyme concentration. Kinetic analysis is the only means of accurately determining the concentration of active enzyme.

Specific Activity

Specific activity is defined in terms of enzyme units per mg enzyme protein. An enzyme unit is the amount of substrate converted to product per unit time under specific reaction conditions for pH and temperature. As generally accepted, an enzyme unit is defined as that which catalyzes the transformation of 1 μM of substrate per minute at 30°C with optimal chemical environment (pH and substrate concentration). Specific activity relates the enzyme units to the amount of protein in the sample. Though it is relatively easy to measure the protein content of a cell fraction, there may be a variable relationship between the protein content and a specific enzyme function. Remember that the initial extraction of an enzyme is accomplished by differential salt precipitation.

Many proteins may precipitate together due to their solubility, but have no other common characteristics. Determination of both protein content and enzyme activity requires two different procedures. One can measure the amount of protein, or one can kinetically measure the enzyme activity. Combining the two will give the specific activity.

TYROSINASE AS A MODEL ENZYME

Tyrosinase is the common name for an enzyme that is formally termed monophenol monooxygenase (Standard Enzyme Nomenclature 1.14.18.1). It is also known as phenolase, monophenol oxidase and as cresolase. Functionally it is an oxygen oxidoreductase enzyme. Enzyme tyrosinase was discovered in animal systems and named for its action on the amino acid tyrosine specifically for its ability to form dopaquinone (an intermediate metabolite) in the production of melanin. The same enzyme isolated from plant materials had been examined for its ability to oxidize phenolic residues, and thus the name phenolase, monophenol oxidase and cresolase were given. Since it has been extensively studied in melanin production and known commonly as tyrosinase. The enzyme tyrosinase is fairly ubiquitous and present in nearly all cells. It is isolated and purified from the fungi *N. crassa* by freezing fungal mycelia in liquid nitrogen, homogenizing the frozen tissue with a French Press, precipitating the proteins in ammonium sulphate, and purifying the enzyme chromatographically on Sephadex and Celite columns. Tyrosinase has also been extracted from hamster melanomas by modifying the technique and with the addition of acetone extractions as well as DEAE-cellulose (diethyl aminoethyl cellulose) chromatography and alumina treatments. Tyrosinase has also been separated from many plant tissues utilizing a far simpler technique based principally on ammonium sulphate precipitation of proteins.

The catalytic action of this enzyme is the conversion of tyrosine in presence of O_2 to yield dihydroxyphenylalanine (DOPA), which is then converted to dopaquinone and H_2O. Dopaquinone in turn can be readily converted to dopachrome, an orange to red pigment (found in human red hair), which can then be converted to the black/brown melanin pigments (found in virtually all human pigments).

$$\text{Tyrosine} + 1/2\ O_2 \longrightarrow \text{DOPA}$$

$$2\ \text{DOPA} + O_2 \longrightarrow 2\ \text{Dopaquinone} + 2\ H_2O$$

$$\text{Dopaquinone} \longrightarrow \text{Leukodopachrome}$$

$$\text{Leukodopachrome} + \text{Dopaquinone} \longrightarrow \text{Dopachrome} + \text{DOPA}$$

The enzyme takes part in catalysis of the first two of these reactions, which are the conversion of tyrosine and the conversion of DOPA. The formation of dopachrome from dopaquinone is spontaneous. Activity of the enzyme can be monitored by analyzing the disappearance of tyrosine and/or DOPA as substrates, the appearance of leukodopachrome or dopachrome as products, or by monitoring the use of oxygen. Natural pigment dopachorome could be measured at λ_{max} 475 nm. This absorbance allows us to use standard spectrophotometric analysis by analyzing the formation rate of dopachrome from the substrate DOPA. The summary reaction for tyrosinase activity, which makes the basis of its estimation in the reaction is

$$\text{DOPA} + 1/2\ O_2 \longrightarrow \text{Dopachrome}$$

To study the various parameters for the evaluation of an enzyme, tyrosinase is selected as model enzyme. This exercise involves the isolation (extraction) of the enzyme tyrosinase from potatoes and subsequent measurement of its activity.

PROTOCOL 5.1

EXTRACTION OF TYROSINASE

The enzyme tyrosinase is insoluble in 50% ammonium sulphate, but is soluble in the citrate buffer.

Equipment

Blender, Volumetric cylinders (50 ml, 100 ml, 250 ml) Cheesecloth, Beakers (100 ml, 250 ml), Chilled centrifuge tubes (30-50 ml), Refrigerated centrifuge, Glass stirring rod

Materials

Potatoes
0.1 M Sodium fluoride
0.1 M Citrate buffer (pH 4.8),
Saturated ammoniumsulphate (4.1 M at 25°C)

Procedure

- Peel a small potato and cut into pieces. Put 100 g of potato in a blender and add 100 ml of sodium fluoride (NaF). Homogenize for about one minute at high speed. Pour the homogenate (mixture) through several layers of cheesecloth.
- Measure the volume of the homogenate and add an equal volume of saturated ammonium sulphate and allow to stand till a flocculent white precipitate appears as many of the soluble potato proteins become insoluble. The enzyme tyrosinase is one of these proteins.
- Centrifuge at 1500g for 5 minutes at 4°C and collect the centrifuge tubes, and carefully discard the supernatant. Collect the pellets. Combine all of the pellets into a 100 ml beaker.
- Add 60 ml of citrate buffer (pH 4.8) to the beaker and break the pellet using glass rod. Again divide the solution into centrifuge tubes and recentrifuge at 300g for 5 minutes at 4°C. Collect the supernatant. Place it in an Erlenmeyer flask, label it as Enzyme Extract and keep it in an ice bucket in which tyrosinase is stable for about an hour. If enzyme is not to be used within this period then extract enzyme from fresh potatoes at the time of its use.

PROTOCOL 5.2

PREPARATION OF STANDARD CURVE OF TYROSINASE

Equipments

Test tubes, 5 ml Pipette, Spectrophotometer and cuvettes

Materials

8 mM DOPA
Enzyme extract
0.1 M Citrate buffer, pH 4.8

Procedure

- Prepare a standard solution of the orange colored dopachrome from L-DOPA. To 10 ml of 8 mM DOPA, add 0.5 ml of enzyme extract and keep the solution to stand for 15 minutes at room temperature. During this period, all of the DOPA gets converted to dopachrome, and solution contains 8 mM dopachrome. Dopachrome is somewhat unstable in the presence of light and should be stored in an amber bottle in a dark place.
- Prepare dilutions of the 8 mM dopachrome to yield the concentrations 8.0, 4.0, 2.0, 1.0, 0.5, 0.25, 0.125 mM of dopachrome. One tube containing no dopachrome is used as blank.
- Take 3.0 ml of each indicated concentratrion in tubes. As the units of concentration are millimolar (mM). A 1.0 mM solution contains 0.001 moles per litre or 0.000001 moles per ml. Thus, with a volume of 3.0 ml, there are 0.000003 moles of dopachrome, or 3 μM. Correspondingly, tubes 2 to 8 contain 1 to 24 μM of dopachrome.
- Measure the absorbance of each solution at 475 nm using content of the tube 1 as blank. Average the values of obtained absorbance that is the average extinction coefficient and can be used in subsequent determinations of dopachrome concentrations according to the Beer-Lambert law.
- One more accurately determine the extinction coefficient is by performing a linear regression analysis of the data, and computing the slope and Y-intercept. The slope of the linear regression will represent the extinction coefficient for a sample. Plot a scattergram of the absorbance value against the concentration of dopachrome. The known concentration of dopachrome is taken on the x-axis, while absorbance on the y-axis. Plot the computed slope and intercept of the linear regression as a straight line overlaying the scattergram. The equation for a straight line is $y = mx + b$, where m is the slope and b the intercept.

Note

Since tyrosinase catalyzes the conversion of L-DOPA to dopachrome, this exercise measures the conversion of colorless DOPA to the dark orange dopachrome. Substrate and product are in a 1:1 ratio for this reaction, thus the amount of product formed equals the amount of substrate used. The optical density of dopachrome at 475 nm is directly proportional to the intensity of orange colour formation in solution (Beer-Lambert Law).

PROTOCOL 5.3

ASSESSMENT OF OPTIMUM ENZYME CONCENTRATION FOR REACTION KINETICS

Equipments

10 ml Pipette, Ice bath, Spectrophotometer and cuvettes

Materials

Enzyme extract

0.1 M Citrate buffer, pH 4.8

8 mM DOPA

Procedure

- To determine the kinetic effects of the enzyme reaction, first determine an appropriate dilution of enzyme extract. Appropriate dilution can be assessed by measuring the rate of reaction given by the diluted enzyme. The rate of reaction of diluted enzyme should be in between 5-10 μm of DOPA converted per minute. For this prepare a serial dilution of enzyme extract.
- Place 9.0 ml of citrate buffer into each of three test tubes and label them 1/10, 1/100 and 1/1000 and pipette 1.0 ml of enzyme extract to make the 1/10 dilution in first test tube (labeled as 1/10) and mix by inversion. Then pipette out 1 ml of the 1/10 dilution into the second tube (labeled as 1/100) and mix by inversion. Pipette 1.0 ml of the 1/100 dilution into the third tube (labeled as 1/1000) and mix by inversion.
- Place all of the dilutions in the ice bath until ready to use. Turn on a spectrophotometer, adjust to 475 nm and with a blank in a tube containing 2.5 ml of citrate buffer and 0.5 ml of enzyme extract. Add 2.5 ml of 8 mM DOPA to each of 4 cuvettes or test tubes. Note that each tube contains 0.0025 x 0.008 moles or 20 μM of DOPA.
- Pipette 0.5 ml of undiluted enzyme extract to one of the tubes containing 8 mM DOPA. Mix by inversion, place into the spectrophotometer and immediately begin timing the reaction. Carefully measure the time required for the conversion of 8 μM of DOPA. Note that since the cuvette will contain a volume of 3.0 ml, the concentration when 8 μM are converted will be 8/3.0 or 2.67 mM dopachrome. Use the data from the standard curve to determine the absorbance equal to 2.67 mM dopachrome. This absorbance value will be the end point for the reaction.
- As the reaction takes place within the cuvettes in the spectrophotometer the absorbance will increase with dopachrome formation. When the absorbance reaches the value above, note the elapsed time from the mixing of the enzyme extract with the 10 μM DOPA.
- Express the time as a decimal rather than minutes, seconds. The time should be between three and five minutes. If the end point is reached before three minutes, repeat this step using the next dilution of enzyme (i.e. the 1/10 after the undiluted, the 1/100 after the 1/10 and the 1/1000 after the 1/100). For the enzyme dilution, which reaches the end point between 3 and 5 minutes, calculate the velocity of reaction.
- Divide the amount of product formed (10 μM) by the time required to reach the end point.

PROTOCOL 5.4

EFFECT OF pH ON ENZYME ACTIVITY

Equipment

10 ml Pipette, Ice bath, Spectrophotometer and cuvettes, Stopwatch

Materials

8 mM DOPA in citrate buffer adjusted to pH values of 3.6, 4.2, 4.8, 5.4, 6.0, 6.6, 7.2 and 7.8.
Enzyme extract

Procedure

- Set up a series of test tubes each containing 2.5 ml of 8 mM DOPA, adjusted to the following pH values: 3.6, 4.2, 4.8, 5.4, 6.0, 6.6, 7.2, and 7.8.
- Begin with the tube containing DOPA at pH 3.6, add 0.5 ml of the diluted enzyme extract which will convert 10 μM of DOPA in 3 to 5 minutes.
- Start timing the reaction, mix by inversion and insert into the spectrophotometer. Note the time for conversion of 10 μM of DOPA.
- Repeat last step for each of the indicated pH values. Calculate the velocity of enzyme reaction (μM/minute) at each pH. Plot pH (X-axis) versus reaction velocity (Y-axis).

PROTOCOL 5.5

EFFECT OF TEMPERATURE ON ENZYME CATALYZED REACTION

Equipment

10 ml Pipette, Ice bath, Spectrophotometer and cuvettes, Stopwatch, Incubators or water baths adjusted to 10, 15, 20, 25, 30, 35 and 40°C,

Materials

Enzyme extract
8 mM DOPA pH 6.6

Procedure

- Set up a series of test tubes each containing 2.5 ml of 8 mM DOPA buffered to a pH 6.6. Place one tube in an ice bath or incubator adjusted to the following temperature; 10, 15, 20, 25, 30, 35 and 40°C.
- Add 0.5 ml of an appropriately diluted enzyme extract (that gives a yield of 10 μM dopachrome in 3-5 minutes) to each of a second series of tubes. Place one each in the corresponding temperature baths. Allow all of the tubes to temperature equilibrate for 5 minutes. Do not mix the tubes.
- Begin with the 10°C tube, and with the spectrophotometer adjusted to 475 nm and properly blanked, pour the enzyme (0.5 ml stored at 10°C) into the tube containing the DOPA and start timing the reaction. Mix thoroughly. Note the time to reach the end point equivalent to the conversion of 10 μM of substrate.
- Repeat last step for each of the listed temperatures, complete the following and plot the data.
- Calculate the velocity of enzyme reaction (μM/minute) at each temperature.
- Plot the graph Temperature (X-axis) versus reaction velocity (Y-axis).

PROTOCOL 5.6

KINETIC ANALYSIS

Equipment

10 ml Pipette, Spectrophotometer and cuvettes, Stopwatch

Materials

8 mM DOPA pH 6.6

Enzyme extract diluted to yield 10 µM of dopachrome in 3 to 5 minutes

Procedure

- Prepare a reaction blank in a clean cuvette to contain 2.5 ml of citrate buffer and 0.5 ml of enzyme extract. Use this blank to adjust spectrophotometer for 100% transmittance.
- Add 2.5 ml of 8 mM DOPA, pH 6.6 to a clean cuvette. Add 0.5 ml of appropriately diluted enzyme extract.
- Shake well and immediately insert the tube into the spectrophotometer. Record the absorbance or transmittance as quickly as possible. Designate this reading as time 0. At 30 second intervals read and record the transmittance until a transmittance value of 10% (or absorbance equal to 1.0) is reached.
- Calculate the amount of dopachrome formed µM by using standard curve.
- Plot time in minutes (X-axis) versus the amount of dopachrome formed (Y-axis).

PROTOCOL 5.7

DETERMINATION OF K_m AND V_{max}

Equipments

10 ml Pipette, Spectrophotometer and cuvettes, Stopwatch.

Materials

Enzyme extract, 8 mM L-DOPA adjusted to pH 6.6

Procedure

- Dilute the DOPA standard (8 mM) to obtain the concentrations of L-DOPA 0.5 mM, 1 mM, 2 mM, 4 mM and 8 mM respectively.
- Repeat kinetic analysis for each of the substrate concentrations listed, substituting the change in concentration where appropriate.
- Plot each set of data and from the data calculate the time required to convert 10 µM of DOPA to dopachrome.
- Calculate the velocity of enzyme reaction (µM/minute) for each substrate concentration and convert that in 1/V. Calculate the 1/[S] with the help of various substrate concentration.

- Plot the rate of DOPA conversion (V) against substrate concentration. That will give a Michaelis-Menten plot. Plot a double reciprocal of the values that is, in between 1/[S] versus 1/V. This plot is Line weaver-Burke plot. Perform a linear regression analysis on the second plot and compute the slope and both Y- and X-intercepts.

Notes

In Michaelis-Menten plot the x intercept is $-1/K_m$ and the negative inverse of it, is the Michaelis-Menten Constant. The y intercept is $1/V_{max}$ and the slope equals to K_m/V_{max}. To repeat the various experiments mentioned above with other enzymes some of the methods to extract and purify the enzymes are discussed below.

PROTOCOL 5.8

KINETIC ANALYSIS OF α- AMYLASE ACTIVITY

Principle

Starchy substances constitute the major part of the human diet for most of the people in the world, as well as many other animals. They are synthesized naturally in a variety of plants. Some plants for examples with high starch content are corn, potato, rice, sorghum, wheat, and cassava. Similar to cellulose, starch molecules are glucose polymers linked together by the alpha-1,4 and alpha-1,6 glucosidic bonds, as opposed to the beta-1,4 glucosidic bonds for cellulose. In order to make use of the carbon and energy stored in starch, the human digestive system, with the help of the enzyme amylases, first breaks down the polymer to smaller assimilable sugars, which are eventually converted to the individual basic glucose units. Since a wide variety of organisms, including humans, can digest starch, alpha-amylase is obviously widely synthesized in nature, as opposed to cellulase. For example, human saliva and pancreatic secretion contain a large amount of alpha-amylase for starch digestion. The specificity of the bond attacked by alpha-amylases depends on the sources of the enzymes. Currently, two major classes of alpha-amylases are commercially produced through microbial fermentation. Based on the points of attack in the glucose polymer chain, they can be classified into two categories, liquefying and saccharifying. Because the bacterial alpha-amylase to be used in this experiment randomly attacks only the alpha-1,4 bonds, it belongs to the liquefying category. The hydrolysis reaction catalyzed by this class of enzymes is usually carried out only to the extent that, for example, the starch is rendered soluble enough to allow easy removal from starch-sized fabrics in the textile industry. The paper industry also uses liquefying amylases on the starch used in paper coating where breakage into the smallest glucose subunits is actually undesirable.

On the other hand, the fungal alpha-amylase belongs to the saccharifying category and attacks the second linkage from the nonreducing terminals (i.e. C-4 end) of the straight segment, resulting in the splitting of two glucose units at a time. Of course, the product is a disaccharide called maltose. The bond breakage is thus more extensive in saccharifying enzymes than in liquefying enzymes. The starch chains are literally chopped into small bits and pieces. Finally, the amyloglucosidase (also called glucoamylase) component of an amylase preparation selectively attacks the last bond on the nonreducing terminals. The type to be used in this experiment can act on both the alpha-1,4 and the alpha-1,6 glucosidic linkages at a relative rate of 1:20, resulting in the splitting of simple glucose units into the solution. Fungal amylase and amyloglucosidase may be used together to convert starch to simple sugars.

The practical applications of this type of enzyme mixture include the production of corn syrup and the conversion of cereal mashes to sugars in brewing. Thus, it is important to specify the source of enzymes when the actions and kinetics of the enzymes are compared. Four types of alpha-amylases from different sources will be employed in this experiment: three of microbial origin and one of human origin. The effects of temperature, pH, substrate concentration, and inhibitor concentration on the kinetics of amylase catalyzed reactions will be studied. Finally, the action of the amylase preparations isolated from microbial sources will be compared to that from human saliva.

Equipment

Erlenmeyer flasks, Beakers, Graduated cylinder, Pipettes (1 ml, 10 ml), Test tubes, Temperature bath, Thermometer, Balance, Syringe, Filter holder and filter paper, Spectrophotometer, Brookfield viscometer

Reagents

Enzymes

Bacterial amylase solution, 3000 SKB units/ml, Fungal amylase powder, 40,000 SKB units/g (concentration of the fungal amylase solution to be used 7.5%), Amylo-glucosidase solution, 75 AG units/ml, human salivary amylase

Corn starch

HCl stopping solution (0.1N HCl)

Iodine reagent stock solution (in aqueous solution, iodine: 5 g/l and KI 50g/l)

Potassium phosphate buffer (KH_2PO_4, $K_2HPO_4.3H_2O$),

$CaCl_2.2H_2O$ (0.1M solution)

Reagents for the analysis of reducing sugars

Procedures

Preparation of 20% starch solution.

- Mix 20 g of soluble potato starch in approximately 50 ml of cold water. While stirring, add the slurry to approximately 900 ml of gently boiling water in a large beaker. Mix well and cool the gelatinized starch solution to room temperature. Add more water to bring the total volume to 1 litre.
- Put a few drops of the starch solution on a glass plate. Add 1 drop of the iodine reagent and see that a deep blue colour is developed. The blue colour indicates the presence of starch in the solution.

Effect of pH

- Prepare 0.1 M pH buffer solutions ranging from pH 4.5 to pH 9 in increments of one pH unit. (Note that phosphate buffer is only good for pH 4.5-9 due to the dissociation constant). Add an equal volume of one of the above buffer solutions to 5.0 ml of the 2% starch solution. The resulting solution should contain 1% of starch in a buffered environment.

- Start the enzymatic digestion process by adding 0.5 ml of the bacterial amylase solution; shake and mix. Let the hydrolysis reaction proceed for exactly 10 minutes at 25°C. Add 0.5 ml of the reacted starch solution to 5 ml of the HCl stopping solution (0.1 N).
- Add 0.5 ml of the above mixture to 5 ml iodine solution to develop color. Shake and mix. The solution should turn deep blue if there is any residual, unconverted starch present in the solution. The solution is brown-red colored for partially degraded starch, while it is clear for totally degraded starch.
- Measure the absorbance with a spectrophotometer at 620 nm.

Effect of temperature

- Take hot water from a hot temperature bath and adjust the temperatures of the temporary water baths in 500 ml beakers so that they range from 30°C to 90°C in increments of 10°C.
- Prepare the starch substrate by diluting 2% starch solution with an equal volume of pH 7 phosphate buffer solution. This results in a working starch concentration of 1%. Add 5 ml of the starch solution to each of the test tubes.
- Allow the temperature of each of the starch solutions to come to equilibrium with that of the water bath.
- Add 0.5 ml of the bacterial amylase solution to each of the thermostated test tubes to start the reaction.
- Stop the reaction after exactly 10 minutes and analyze the starch content by measuring the absorbance at 620 nm spectrophotometrically.

Effect of heat

- Place 0.5 ml of the bacterial amylase solution each of eleven test tubes. Heat-treat the enzyme solution by placing all the test tubes, except one, in a hot (90°C) water bath. The untreated enzyme is used as the control.
- Take out the first test tube after one minute and quickly bring it to room temperature by immersing it in a cold water bath. Remove the second test tube after 2 minutes, the third after 3 minutes, and so on.
- Add 5 ml of the 1% buffered (pH 7) starch solution to each of the test tubes containing the enzyme. Carry out the hydrolysis reaction at room temperature and analyze the sample after exactly 10 minutes. Mix an equal volume of the $CaCl_2$ solution to the enzymes and repeat the same procedures to investigate the heat stabilization of the enzymes in the presence of Ca^{2+} ions.
- This set of studies can be done quickly if the procedures are synchronized. If time permits, try 0.5 ml samples of the amyloglucosidase and 0.5 ml samples of the fungal amylase solution. Compare the sensitivity to heat for these related enzymes.

Effect of substrate concentration

- Add 0.5 ml of the bacterial amylase solution to 50 ml of a 1% starch solution buffered at pH 7.0. Note that less enzyme per ml of substrate is used in this part of the experiment than the previous parts. The objective here is to slow down the reaction so that multiple sampling is possible with reasonable accuracy before all the starch is consumed.

- Take samples periodically to monitor both the decrease in the starch concentration and the increase in the reducing sugars until most of the starch is hydrolyzed. The starch concentration is measured with the same steps outlined above and the sugar concentration with the dinitrosalicylic colorimetric method.
- Continuously monitor the viscosity of the substrate-enzyme mixture with a viscometer. Generate a calibration curve for the viscosity as a function of the starch concentration. Note that this part of the study is fruitful only when the starch solution is extremely thick.

PROTOCOL 5.9

PRODUCTION OF CORN SYRUP USING BACTERIAL AMYLASE

In making industrial sugars, e.g. corn syrup, large gelatinized starch molecules are first chopped into smaller dextrins with the help of bacterial amylase. The liquefaction step is followed by saccharification with either fungal amylase or amyloglucosidase, depending on the end use of the sugar. These sequential enzymatic treatment steps will be simulated in this part of the experiment

Procedure

- Add 0.5 ml of the bacterial amylase solution to 50 ml of the 2% non-buffered starch solution.
- Periodically place a few drops of the reaction mixture on a glass plate.
- Add one drop of the iodine reagent. The colour should finally turn red, indicating the total conversion of starch to dextrin. This liquefaction step should last for approximately 10 minutes.
- When the process of liquefaction is complete, adjust the pH of the starch solution to 4.7 with 1 N HCl.
- Filter the starch solution if it is turbid.
- Separate the solution into two equal parts.
- To the first solution, add 0.5 ml of amyloglucosidase.
- To the second solution add 0.5 ml of fungal amylase solution.
- Measure the sugar concentrations periodically.
- Note that appropriate calibration curves are needed because one is maltose and the other is glucose. Also the initial absorbance at the start of the saccharification process should be measured so that the increase in the sugar concentration can be correctly measured. This saccharification step should last for about 30-60 minutes.
- Taste the two sugar solutions and compare the sweetness.

PROTOCOL 5.10

EVALUATION OF AMINO TRANSFERASES ACTIVITY

The major site of amino acid degradation in mammals is the liver. The α-amino group of many amino acids is transferred to α-keto glutarate to form glutamate, which is then oxidatively deaminated to yield NH_4^+

Aspartate Amino Transferase (Glutamate: Oxaloacetate Amino Transferase).

Principle

Aspartate, a four-carbon amino acid, is directly transaminated into oxaloacetate, a citric acid cycle intermediate. This reversible interconversion is catalyzed by the enzyme, Glutamate oxaloacetate amino transferase (GOT).

$$\text{Aspartate} + \text{2-Oxoglutarate} \rightleftarrows \text{Glutamate} + \text{Oxaloacetate}$$

The oxaloacetic acid gives a brown coloured hydrazone with 2,4-dinitrophenyl hydrazine in alkaline medium, which is measured colorimetrically at 510nm. This constitutes the basis for quantitative estimation of catalytic activity of the enzyme.

Materials

Phosphate buffer, pH 7.4

Anhydrous disodium hydrogen phosphate	11.3 g,
Anhydrous potassium dihydrogen phosphate	2.7 g
Water q.s to	1000 ml

Bring the pH to 7.4, store at 4°C.

Pyruvate standard

Weigh accurately 22.0 mg sodium pyruvate and dissolve in 100 ml distilled water.

Substrate solution

Dissolve 13.3 g D, L-aspartic acid in minimum amount of 1 N sodium hydroxide and adjust the pH 7.4. Add 0.146 g 2-oxoglutarate and dissolve it by adding little more sodium hydroxide solution. Adjust to pH 7.4 and make up to 500 ml with phosphate buffer. Store the substrate solution at –15°C.

2,4-Dinitrophenyl hydrazine solution

Weigh accurately 19.8 mg dinitrophenyl hydrazine and dissolve in 10 ml hydrochloric acid and make up the volume to 100 ml with distilled water. Keep the solution in an amber coloured bottle.

Enzyme extract

Grind the plant tissue in 0.2 M potassium phosphate pH 7.5 in a homogenizer for 2 minutes. Pass it through eight layers of cheesecloth and then centrifuge at 25000g for 15 minutes)

Sodium hydroxide 0.4 N

Procedure

- Warm 0.5 ml substrate solution in a water bath at 37°C for 3 minutes and add 0.2 ml enzyme extract and mix.

- Incubate at 37°C for 1 hour. Then add 0.5 ml dinitrophenyl hydrazine solution and mix.
- Prepare a control by mixing 0.5 ml substrate, 0.5 ml dinitrophenyl hydrazine solution and 0.1 ml enzyme extract. Keep the tubes at room temperature for 20 minutes. Add 5 ml 0.4 N sodium hydroxide, mix and keep for 10 minutes. Measure the absorbance colorimetrically at 510 nm.
- Pipette pyruvate standard 0.05 to 0.20 ml, make up to 0.2 ml then add 0.5 ml substrate and 0.5 ml dinitrophenyl hydrazine solution.
- Similarly, prepare a blank solution by mixing 0.5 ml substrate, 0.2 ml water and 0.5 ml dinitrophenyl hydrazine solution. Then keep the tubes at room temperature for 20 minutes, add 5 ml 0.4 N NaOH, mix and keep for 10 minutes. Measure the absorbance colorimetrically at 510 nm.

Calculation

The difference in absorbance between test and control is due to the pyruvate formed by the enzyme. The pyruvate in standard produces the difference between standard and blank.

Alanine Amino Transferase (Glutamate : Pyruvate Amino Transferase)

Principle

Alanine amino transferase, which is also prevalent in mammalian tissue, catalyzes the transfer of amino group of alanine to α-keto glutarate (2-oxo glutarate).

$$\text{Alanine} + \alpha\text{-ketoglutatate} \longrightarrow \text{Pyruvate} + \text{glutamate}$$

The pyruvate formed after incubation for half an hour is made to react with 2,4-dinitrophenyl hydrazine and measured colorimetrically at 510 nm.

Materials

Substrate Solution

Dissolve 9.0 g alanine in 90 ml water with addition of about 2.5 ml sodium hydroxide (1 N) and adjust to pH 7.4. Then add 0.146 g 2-oxo glutarate and dissolve it by adding a little more sodium hydroxide solution and adjust to pH 7.4, make up the volume to 500 ml with phosphate buffer, store at –15°C.)

Phosphate buffer pH 7.4

Pyruvate standard

2,4-Dinitrophenylhydrazine solution

Sodium hydroxide 0.4 N

Procedure

Use alanine as substrate and follow the steps described for aspartate amino transferase except incubate for 30 minutes instead of 1 hour.

Calculation

Express the enzyme activity as micromoles of pyruvate formed per minute per mg protein.

PROTOCOL 5.11

EVALUATION OF PHOSPHOLIPASE ACTIVITY

These are the enzymes, which hydrolyze phospholipids. Four types of phospholipases having different sites of attack are known.

Phospholipase A

Principle

Phospholipase A acts upon lecithin with the release of lysolecithin which lyses the erythrocytes.

Materials

4% Suspension of saline washed rabbit erythrocytes

Lecithin

Enzyme source (several seeds, yeast, snake venom, etc.)

0.1M Veronal buffer of pH 7.6 is used in which dissolve 01.25 g NaCl (0.22 M), 22 g $CaCl_2$ (20 mM) and 0.037g EDTA

Procedure

- Mix 1 ml of saline washed rabbit erythrocytes suspension (4%) with 1 ml of water and freeze quickly.
- Repeatedly thaw the frozen solid and freeze few times to lyse the erythrocytes.
- Determine the amount of haemoglobin released in the supernatant by centrifuging for 5 minutes at 100g and measuring the absorbance/OD of the supernatant at 560 nm.
- Emulsify 100 mg of lecithin in saline (100 µg/ml) under vigorous shaking.
- Add some enzyme source to 1 ml of erythrocyte suspension and make up the final volume to 2.0 ml with veronal buffer.
- Incubate the mixture at 37°C for 30 minutes.
- Keep the mixture at 4°C for 20 minutes.
- Centrifuge and determine the amount of haemoglobin released in the supernatant by measuring the absorbance/OD at 560 nm and compare to that of completely lysed sample.

Phospholipase D

Principle

The enzyme releases choline by splitting lecithin (phosphatidyl choline), which forms a complex with iodine. Formed complex is measured spectrophotometrically at 365 nm.

Materials

Iodine reagent (as described in official pharmacopoeias)

Enzyme source

Following protocol is followed for the processing of the enzyme.

- Grind and homogenize 100 g fresh cabbage leaves with 75 ml distilled water in a blender.
- Keep it to stand for 1 to 2 hour at 5°C, filter through coarse cloth and centrifuge. The supernatant is a rich source of enzyme.

- Harvest yeast cells by centrifugation and mix the pellet with approximately equal volume of a mixture of carborundum/celite (1:1) mixture. Transfer the resulting dry powder to a mortar kept in ice and grind well till a viscous paste is formed. Extract the paste with citrate-phosphate buffer (0.1 M, pH 5.6, 10 ml/g cells). Decant of the carborundum sediment and centrifuge at 5000 rpm for 10 minutes. The supernatant is a rich source of enzyme.

Substrate egg lecithin (commercially available) 10 mg/ml in ethyl ether.

Procedure

- Pipette 1 ml of ether solution of substrate into a tube and place in warm water bath to remove the solvent. To the residue, add 0.2 ml enzyme source and mix well to form an emulsion. Incubate at 25°C for 90 minutes. Add ether to make up the volume to 5 ml, mix well and keep stoppered for 45 minutes. Centrifuge, discard the ether layer and estimate choline in the aqueous layer spectrophotometrically by the procedure given below.
- To 0.5 ml of a standard solution of choline, add 0.2 ml of iodine reagent, mix well and keep in ice bath for 15 minutes to precipitate out the choline-iodine complex.
- Centrifuge and discard the supernatant and dissolve the precipitate in chloroform (10 ml) and measure the optical density/absorbance of the solution spectrophotometrically at 365 nm. The molar extinction coefficient of choline-iodine complex is 2.7×10^7.
- Prepare a standard curve between absorbance/optical density and concentration. Treat the aqueous phase from the test solution similarly and measure the liberated choline.

PROTOCOL 5.12

DETERMINATION OF ACETYLCHOLINESTERASE ACTIVITY

Principle

Acetylcholine is made to react with hydroxylamine to form the corresponding acylhydroxamic acid, which forms a strongly coloured ferric hydroxamate with ferric salts, and the colour is measured spectrophotometrically at 490 nm. The hydrolyzed acetylcholine per unit time is measured by comparison of the initial concentration in a tube with the final concentration in the experimental tube.

Materials

Blood source

Collect 0.2 ml blood from the test animal in a tube containing 5 ml water. Use the haemolysate for the assay.

Acetylcholine stock solution

3.64% Solution of acetylcholine (200 mM) in distilled water.

Veronal buffer (0.1M pH 8.6)

Dissolve 4.92 g sodium veronal and 3.24 g sodium acetate in 300 ml distilled water, add 3 ml 1N HCl and dilute to 500 ml with distilled water, check the pH.

Sodium hydroxide (10% w/v in distilled water)

Substrate (Acetylcholine solution, 1.33 mM)

Mix 1 ml of acetylcholine stock solution thoroughly in 150 ml veronal buffer.

Hydroxylamine (1N)

7% w/v Hydroxylammonium chloride in distilled water.

Iron solution (0.7M)

Dissolve 2.5 g potassium nitrate in about 10 ml distilled water. Dissolve 33.75 g Fe $(NH_4)(SO_4)_2.12H_2O$ in about 70 ml distilled water with gentle warming. Mix both the solutions and make up the volume to 100 ml with distilled water.

Alkaline hydroxylamine solution

Mix equal volumes of 2.5 N sodium hydroxide and 1 N hydroxylamine solutions.

Citrate Buffer (1 M, pH 1.4)

Dissolve 2.10 g citric acid and 0.8 g NaOH in minimum quantity of distilled water, add 89 ml 1 N HCl and make up the volume to 100 ml with distilled water. Dilute 10 ml of this solution to 100 ml with distilled water. Adjust the pH between 1.2 and 1.4.

Enzyme Source

Grind the fresh sample material (root, leaf or any other part) from plant and extract in 10 mM veronal buffer (pH 8.6) followed by centrifugation at 20,000g for 10 minutes. Grind the pellet containing the enzyme and extract with the above buffer containing 5% ammonium sulphate. Centrifuge the extract at 20,000g for 10 minutes and use the supernatant as the enzyme source.

Procedure

- Pipette out the following into 50 ml volumetric flasks as given below (Table 5.1).

Table 5.1. Volumes of samples and substrates for determination of cholinesterase activity

	Reference (ml)	Test (ml)	Blank (ml)
Sample (enzyme Source)	-	2	-
Substrate solution	25	25	-
Mix well and incubate at 37°C for 30 minutes.			
Alkaline hydroxylamine solution	5	5	5
Sample	2	-	-
Citrate buffer	5	5	5
Ferric solution	10	10	10

- Allow the ferric solution to run slowly down the wall of the flask. Dilute with distilled water to the mark and shake thoroughly. Allow to stand for 20 minutes at room temperature. Filter the solutions and discard the first portion of filtrate.
- Measure the absorbance of the solution spectrophotometrically against blank at 490 nm.

Calculation

The absorbance difference (ΔE) between initial concentration of substrate (reference and final concentration of substrate (test) is used for calculation. The extinction of the dye is 0.961 per μm at 490 nm. Hence the amount of dye formed from the non-hydrolyzed acetyl choline in 50 ml.

C = E x 50/ 0.961 x 1.0 (μM/50 ml).

The acetylcholinesterase activity in whole blood

= E x 50/ 0.961x 1.0 x 1/ 0.08 x 30 x 1000

= E x 21667 (U/litre)

PROTOCOL 5.13

CELLULASES ($C_X\beta_{(1\text{-}4)}$ GLUCONASE) ASSAY

Principle

Glucose, a reducing sugar is produced due to cellulolytic activity, which is colorimetrically, estimated by dinitrosalicylic acid reagent at 540 nm.

Materials

Sodium citrate buffer 0.1 M, pH 5.0

Dinitro salicylic acid reagent

Dissolve 1 g dinitrosalicylic acid, 200 mg crystalline phenol and 50 mg sodium sulphite in 100 ml 1% NaOH and store at 4°C.

Potassium sodium tartrate

40 g in 100 ml of distilled water.

Carboxymethyl cellulose

1% in sodium citrate buffer, 0.1 M, pH 5.0.

Procedure

- Incubate the mixture of 0.45 ml 1% carboxymethyl cellulose solution and 0.05 ml enzyme extract at 55°C for 15 minutes.
- Remove the mixture from the bath.
- Add 0.5 ml dinitrosalicylic acid reagent.
- Heat the mixture in a boiling water bath for 5 minutes.
- Add 1.0 ml potassium sodium tartrate solution.
- Cool to room temperature.
- Make up the volume to 5 ml with distilled water.
- Measure the absorbance at 540 nm.
- Prepare a standard graph with glucose in the concentration range 50-1000 μg/ml.
- Report the enzyme activity as the mg glucose released per minute per mg protein.

PROTOCOL 5.14

EVALUATION OF PAPAIN ACTIVITY

Principle

Papain hydrolyzes benzoyl L-arginine p-nitroanilide (BAPNA) and releases p-nitroaniline which is measured colorimetrically at 410 nm.

Materials

Acetic acid 30% v/v

Enzyme source

0.1 mg/ml Papain in distilled water.

Tris-HCl buffer (50 mM pH 7.5)

Dissolve 0.60 g Tris in 50 ml distilled water. Adjust to pH 7.5 with 0.05 N hydrochloric acid and make up the volume to 100 ml. To the above buffer (100 ml) add 87.80 mg of cysteine hydrochloride (0.005 M) and 74.40 mg of EDTA (0.002 M) and dissolve completely.

Buffered substrate solution

Dissolve 43.5 mg BAPNA in 1 ml of dimethyl sulphoxide and make up the volume to 100 ml with Tris-HCl buffer containing 5 mM cysteine and 2 mM EDTA.

Procedure

- To 0.5 ml papain solution in a test tube add sufficient Tris-HCl buffer to make up the volume to 1.0 ml.
- Add 5 ml of substrate solution and incubate for 25 minutes at 25°C.
- To terminate the enzyme action, add 1 ml acetic acid (30%).
- Measure the absorbance of the released *p*-nitroaniline at 410 nm against a control spectrophotometrically.
- Prepare a standard graph using *p*-nitroaniline.
- Calculate and report the activity per g sample.

  Molar extinction coefficient of *p*-nitroaniline

  (E^{1M}_{1cm}) = 8,800/mole/cm

  1 mM/l = 8.800/1000 = 8.8 Absorbance (A)

  1 μM/l = 8.8/1000 = 0.0088 A

  1 μM/ml = 8.8.

  If the absorbance is 8.8, amount of *p*-nitroaniline = 1 μM/ml

  If X is the absorbance of the sample

$$= \frac{1\ \mu M/ml}{8.8} \times X$$

$$= \frac{X \times \mu M/ml}{8.8}$$

This is for one ml of the sample for 25 minutes.
For 7 ml (volume of the assay mixture) of the sample solution

$$= \frac{X\ \mu M \times 7.0}{8.8 \times 7.0 \times 25}$$

The assay mixture contains 0.5 ml of the enzyme.
Therefore activity of the enzyme in 1 ml

$$= \frac{X\ \mu M \times 7.0}{8.8 \times 0.5 \times 25}$$ (μM of *p*-nitroaniline released per minute)

- Report the activity per g sample.

PROTOCOL 5.15

EVALUATION OF GLUCOSE OXIDASE ACTIVITY

Glucose oxidase catalyses the oxidation of α-D-glucose to D-glucono-1,5-lactone (gluconic acid) with the formation of hydrogen peroxide. The oxygen liberated from hydrogen peroxide by peroxidase reacts with the O-dianisidine and oxidizes it to a red choromophore product. The enzyme can be assayed either colorimetrically or polarographically.

Colorimetric estimation

In colorimetric assay, a coupled peroxidase-o-dianisidine is used. The oxygen liberated from hydrogen peroxide is directly coupled to the dye o-dianisidine, which turns to a brownish red colour which is measured colorimetrically at 460 nm.

Enzyme Source

The moulds like *A. niger, A. oryzae, P. notatum, P. vitale and P. chrysogenum* and red algae like *Iridophycus flaccidum* are the good sources of glucose oxidase. Glucose oxidase has not been found in animal tissues, with the exception of the pharyngeal glands of the honeybee. The enzyme from *Aspergillus* is intracellular whereas that from *penicillium* is extracellular.

Materials

Phosphate buffer (0.1M, pH 6.0)

Coupling enzyme

Aqueous solution of purified horseradish peroxidase containing 60 units/ml

Dye

1% Aqueous solution of o-dianisidine. Add 0.1 ml of this to 12 ml buffer

Substrate

18% Solution of glucose.

Enzyme

Aqueous solution of the crude enzyme in 0.1 M phosphate buffer pH 6.0

Procedure

- Prepare a control by adding 2.6 ml dye buffer solution, 0.3 ml glucose and 0.1 ml peroxidase.
- Prepare a test solution by adding 2.5 ml dye buffer solution, 0.3 ml glucose and 0.1 ml peroxidase.
- Adjust the OD of the test solution to zero against the control at 460 nm. Add 0.1 ml of enzyme to the test solution, mix well. Measure the increase in OD at 460 nm at 30 seconds intervals for 3 to 5 minutes. Plot a graph and calculate the rate.

Polarographic Method

Glucose oxidase causes the conversion of glucose to gluconic acid and the oxygen consumed in this conversion is measured using an oxygen electrode.

Materials

Phosphate buffer 0.1M, pH 6.0
Substrate
  18% Aqueous solution of glucose
Enzyme
  Aqueous solution of crude enzyme in 0.1M phosphate buffer pH 6.0
Azide solution
  0.002% Sodium azide in the buffer

Procedure

- Add 3 ml of well aerated buffer and 0.1 ml of suitably diluted crude extract containing the enzyme in the oxygen electrode cuvette. Add 0.1 ml of glucose solution and record the rates for at least 2 minutes.
- Calculate the enzyme activity from the amount of oxygen consumed per minute, which is equal to the micromoles of oxygen consumed per minute.

PROTOCOL 5.16

SUCROSE SYNTHASE (UDP GLUCOSE: D-FRUCTOSE 2-α-D-GLUCOSYL TRANSFERASE)

It catalyzes the following reversible reaction in plants.

$$\text{UDP- Glucose} + \text{Fructose} \xrightleftharpoons{\text{Sucrose synthase}} \text{Sucrose} + \text{UDP}$$

Principle

The activity of sucrose synthase is estimated by coupling the formation of UDP-glucose to the reduction of NAD^+ in the presence of excess UDP-glucose dehydrogenase and the change in absorbance at 340 nm followed.

Materials

Sucrose 0.5 M (17.11 g/100 ml)
UDP 0.01 M (4 mg/ml)
NAD^+ 0.015 M (9.95 mg/ml)
HEPES-KOH buffer 0.1M, pH 7.5
UDP-glucose dehydrogenase (0.25 mg/ml)
Enzyme extract

> Homogenize 10 g tissue with 20 ml potassium phosphate buffer (10 mM, pH 7.2) containing 1 mM EDTA and 5 mM 2-mercaptoethanol. Filter the homogenate through eight layers of cheesecloth and centrifuge the filtrate at 30,000 rpm for 15 minutes, preferably at 4°C. The supernatant is a rich source of enzyme.

Procedure

Pipette out all reagents as given below (Table 5.2). Set the spectrophotometer to get zero absorbance at 340 nm without adding NAD^+ in the test against blank in a cuvette. Add NAD^+, quickly to the test, mix and record the initial absorbance and set a timer. Record the decrease in absorbance every minute until no further change is observed.

Table 5.2. Volumes of reagents for determination of sucrose synthase activity

Reagent	Assay (ml)	Blank (ml)
HEPES-KOH	0.2	0.3
Sucrose	0.2	0.2
UDP	0.2	0.2
Enzyme extract	0.2	0.2
UDP-glucose dehydrogenase	0.1	0.1
NAD+	0.1	-

Calculation

The change in absorbance at 340 nm is 12.0 for each µM of UDPG per ml. Report the enzyme activity as µM UDPG formed per mg of protein.

PROTOCOL 5.17

LIPASE ENZYME ACTIVITY DETERMINATION

Lipase hydrolyzes triglycerides, releasing free fatty acids and glycerol.

$$\begin{array}{c} CH_2OCOR' \\ | \\ CHOCOR' \\ | \\ CH_2OCOR' \end{array} + H_2O \xrightarrow{Lipase} \begin{array}{c} CH_2OH \\ | \\ CHOH \\ | \\ CH_2OH \end{array} + 3\ R'COOH$$

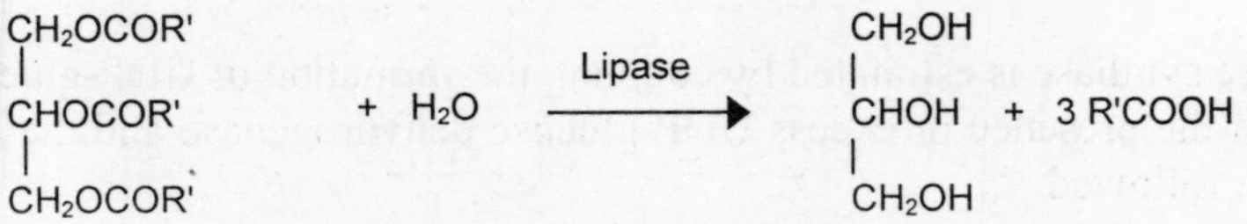

The germinating seeds of groundnut, castor bean and sunflower are good source of lipase.

Principle

The amount of fatty acid released in unit time is measured by the volume of NaOH required to maintain constant pH. The milliequivalent of alkali consumed is taken as a measure of the activity of the enzyme.

Materials

50 mM phosphate buffer (pH 7.0)

0.1N NaOH

Substrate

Neutralize 2 ml of any clear vegetable oil to pH 7.0 if necessary and stir well with 25 ml water in presence of any emulsifying agent (sodium taurochloate, 100 mg) till an emulsion is formed.

Enzyme source

- Germinating oil seeds like castor seeds is a good source. They are pounded in a mortar and pestle. The minced tissue is homogenized with twice the volume of ice-cold acetone. The suspension is filtered and quickly washed with successive portions of acetone, acetone-ether (1:1), ether and then air-dried. The dry powder, called the acetone dry powder can be stored for a long time in a refrigerator. Just before use 1 g of the powder is stirred with 20 ml of ice-cold water (or buffer) for 15 minutes and the residue is removed by centrifugation (15,000 rpm for 10 minutes). The supernatant is used as the enzyme source.
- The pancreatic tissue obtained from a slaughterhouse is also a good source. The tissue is kept in ice during transportation, then cut into very small pieces.

Procedure

- To 20 ml of substrate, add 5 ml of phosphate buffer (pH 7.0).
- Stir the contents slowly at 35°C on a magnetic stirrer cum hot plate. Note the pH of the reaction mixture and adjust it to 7.0.
- Add enzyme extract (0.5 ml), immediately note the pH and set the timer on.
- At frequent intervals (10 minutes) or as the pH drops by about 0.2 unit add 0.1 N NaOH to bring pH to initial value. Continue the titration for 30-60 minutes and note the volume of alkali consumed.

Calculation

The enzyme activity is expressed as the amount of enzyme which releases one milliequivalent of free fatty acid per minute per gram sample.

Note

Cellulose nitrate tube should be filled full otherwise it will collapse during centrifugation.

PROTOCOL 5.18

ISOLATION OF CRYSTALLINE ANIMAL CYTOCHROME C

Principle

Cytochrome c is extracted from muscle at neutral pH after decomposition of cells and particles by a weak acid treatment. The protein is adsorbed on a column loaded with a carboxylic acid cation exchange resin at neutral pH and eluted with neutral buffer of high concentration after washing with a lower concentration. Cytochrome c is oxidized and then further purified by employing a careful fractional elution procedure on a resin column. Some impurity may still present, that is removed by making the solution nearly saturated with ammonium sulphate at weak alkalinity. After dialysis, the preparation is separated into several cytochrome c fractions by chromatography on a resin column and the largest fraction, which contains unmodified cytochrome c, is used for the crystallization. The highly concentrated protein following resin treatment is crystallized in reduced form from nearly saturated ammonium sulphate solution containing ascorbic acid at a alkaline pH.

Starting Material

Beef heart is processed as soon as possible after removal from the animal. The heart should be frozen if the time between removal and processing exceeds 24 hours. Though cytochrome c has been crystallized adopting the present method, or a slightly modified one, from any of the tested animal tissues having a high concentration of cytochrome c, such as beef, pig, horse, human, bonito (*Katsuwonus vagans*) and tuna (*Thunnus alalunga*) hearts, horse thigh and pigeon breast muscle, and beef kidney. Beef heart seems to be the most suitable source. The fishes' heart and pigeon breast muscle are also preferred sources in places where they are easily obtainable.

Procedure

Extraction

Beef heart (or other animal tissue) is made free of fat and ligaments and twice passed through a meat grinder. Two kilograms of the minced muscles are suspended in 1.6 litre of 0.5 N cold acetic acid and kept at 5°C for 1 hour, with stirring (pH 4.3). The suspension is adjusted to pH 6.2-6.5 by addition of about 0.4 litre of 2 N ammonium hydroxide under stirring and placed in a cold room (5-10°C) overnight. The suspension is mixed with 300 g of Celite 545 in the case of pigeon breast muscle or beef kidney (use double of this amount) and squeezed out through a thick cloth in a press. The residue is again suspended in 1 litre of water and squeezed again after 1 hour. The combined extracts are adjusted to pH 6.2-6.5 (indicator paper), filtered through a Buchner funnel with 300 ml of water. The combined extract is a clear brown solution (except with pigeon muscle and beef kidney), volume 4 litres, NH_4^+ concentration 0.2 N, pH 6.2-6.5.

First resin treatment

The combined extracts are passed through a resin bed, which has been prepared by introducing a suspension of 100-200 mesh X E-64 equilibrated with a buffer of pH 7.0 containing 0.1 N ammonium ion (abbreviated 0.1 N NH_4^+ buffer, pH 7.0) into a sintered glass funnel of 7 cm diameter until the bed height becomes 5 cm. This rate of flow is achieved by applying suction. The brown solution passing through is discarded, and the resin bed (upper part is reddish brown from the adsorption of cytochrome c and possibly denatured myoglobin) is washed with about 500 ml of 0.1 N NH_4^+ buffer, pH 7.0. The dark coloured part of the resin is separated after strongly sucking out the washing with a spatula from the colorless part and suspended in 500 ml of 0.05 N NH_4^+ buffer, pH 7.0. The pH of the suspension is adjusted to 7.3-7.6 by the dropwise addition of concentrated ammonium hydroxide and transferred to a 7 cm glass funnel containing about a 1 cm layer of the fresh resin, and the resulting resin layer (upper part, red; lower part, white) is washed with about 2 litre of 0.1 N buffer, pH 7.0 and all the reddish elute is collected (100 ml, NH_4^+ 0.4 N, pH 6.5, purity 60%).

Second resin treatment

The solution is diluted with 3 volumes of water and adjusted to pH 7.0 with ammonia. Then the cytochrome c is completely oxidized with 0.01 M $K_4Fe(CN)_6$ (1 ml). The solution is then made to pass through a resin column (4 x 10 cm, 100-200 mesh, equilibrated with 0.1 N NH_4^+ buffer at pH 7.0) at a rate of 10 ml per minute, and the column is washed with 0.15 N NH_4^+ buffer, pH 7.0, until the red band moves down and cytochrome c just begins to be eluted. This step is carried out at room temperature with pressure applied as needed. Cytochrome c is eluted from the washed column with 0.5 N NH_4^+ buffer, pH 7.0 as before to yield about 30ml of solution approximately 1% with respect to cytochrome c purity 90%.

Ammonium Sulphate Treatment

To the elute collected in a small beaker, 0.7 g of solid ammonium sulphate and 0.02 ml of 30% ammonia are added per ml of the elute (80% saturation). The solution is kept at about 10°C for 2 hours, and passed through a small sintered glass funnel to remove the precipitate with the aid of 0.2 g Hyflow Super-Cel. The filter is washed with 5 ml of 95% saturated ammonium sulphate, pH 8.0, to yield about 35 ml of a solution of Cytochrome c (about 35 ml), NH_4^+ concentration 7 M, pH 8.5, purity nearly 100%.

Chromatography

The combined filtrate and washings are dialyzed in a cellophane bag against 100 volumes of distilled water at 0-5°C overnight. The column is loaded with the resin (200-300 mesh, equilibrated with 0.25 N NH_4^+ buffer, pH 7.0) suspended in buffer into a tube of diameter 2.5 cm and length about 70 cm until the settled resin bed becomes 50 cm high. When the supernatant buffer over the resin bed has just passed down, the dialyzed cytochrome c solution is introduced along the side of tube. Then 0.25 N NH_4^+ buffer is introduced and allowed to pass at the rate of 20-40 ml per hour on a fraction collector at room temperature. The colored solution is collected (belonging to the second fraction) which contains more than 90% of the total cytochrome c and used for crystallization. It is possible to collect the fractions without using the collector by merely observing the band and elute colour. This procedure yields about 200 ml of solution, purity about 100%.

Crystallization

The solution (about 200 ml) is dialyzed against 10 volumes of distilled water in the cold overnight (not more than 24 hours) in order to reduce its cationic concentration to 0.03-0.05 N. The solution is then passed through a column (2 x 2 cm) of the resin (100-200 mesh), held in a sintered glass funnel equilibrated with 0.1 N NH_4^+ buffer, pH 7.0. After the column is washed with 20 ml of 0.1% ammonium sulphate solution pH 8.0 the dark red resin in the upper part of the column is transferred with 0.1% ammonia solution to another column (0.7 cm in diameter). Then 5% ammonium sulphate solution, is slowly passed through the column to elute cytochrome c. A very dark band moves down the column and more than 98% of the pigment adsorbed on the resin is collected in a volume of less than 4 ml (4-8% cytochrome c) in a small centrifugation tube of known weight. After the addition of a drop of octanol, 0.43 g of ammonium sulphate is added per g of the solution. When the salt gets dissolved completely, about 5 g of ascorbic acid and a few drops (1 drop per ml) of 30% ammonia are added and the solution is kept at 10°C for 10 minutes. To the solution, which has been grown light in colour by the reduction of cytochrome c, small quantities of fine powdered ammonium sulphate are added, each portion being dissolved completely by a glass rod until the solution becomes turbid. The solution, tightly stoppered, is allowed to stand at 15-25°C for 1 to 2 days while the cytochrome c crystallizes out as fine needles or in grouped form of needles such as leaflets or rosettes. About 0.02 g of ammonium sulphate is added per millilitre of the suspension and allowed to stand for a few more days. The crystals are collected by centrifugation at 5000g, suspended with a minimum volume of water and recrystallized as above, after the addition of 1 drop of ammonia and 1mg of ascorbic acid. The yield is about 200 mg from 2 kg of the minced muscle. The crystals may be stored as a suspension in saturated ammonium sulphate solution at 0°C or lyophilized after dialysis against 0.08 M NaCl or 0.1 M sodium buffer.

Properties and purity of product

The purity of cytochrome c preparations has been checked by iron content or the ratio of extinction at 280 nm for maximum extinction (this should be altered to 278 nm for maximum extinction) in oxidized form to that at 550 nm in reduced form. The iron content of the present preparation is 0.45% and the extinction ratio (550 nm/ 278 nm) is 1.28 (1.20 and 1.05 with pigeon and fish preparations respectively). Although a few preparations of extinction ratio greater than 1.4 are obtainable from another fraction in the resin chromatography of trichloroacetic acid-treated cytochrome c, it is unlikely that the present crystalline preparation is not a pure one, since the former preparations are thought to be modified. The present preparation is an essentially homogeneous substance that results from ultracentrifugation under several conditions, electrophoresis at weak alkalinity, ion exchange resin chromatography and constancy of the extinction ratio on further recrystallization. Biological activity of the present preparation in the succinic oxidase and the cytochrome oxidase systems is the same as that of the Kieilin and Hartree preparation if based on the extinction at 550 nm in reduced form. However, the cytochrome c described herein is not autoxidizable and is resistant to protease action, in contrast to preparations of cytochrome c, which have been subjected to trichloroacetic acid precipitation.

Method of preparation

In order to get a high yield of crystalline cytochrome c from sources other than beef heart, some steps should be modified slightly. More extensive modifications are necessary for the preparation of the crystals from yeast and wheat germ. The yield of crystalline preparations per unit weight are as follows: pigeon breast muscle >bonito or tuna heart >beef and horse heart > pig or human heart > baker's yeast > wheat germ. There are other reports about the preparation of crystalline Cytochrome c from penguin muscle and beef heart.

PROTOCOL 5.19

DIGESTION OF PROTEINS INTO AMINO ACIDS

Principle

Various species of organisms cannot synthesize or are not efficient in generating all of the twenty amino acids needed to construct the proteins and enzymes essential for their survival. To sustain growth and to maintain metabolic functions, these amino acids must be provided from outside sources. This can be accomplished by the intake of proteins. Humans are a good example of living organisms that ingest proteins as part of their nutritional requirements. Some organisms secrete proteolytic enzymes extracellularly to break down the protein to its component monomeric amino acid units by hydrolyzing peptide bonds at the end of the polymer chain. A series of shorter polypeptides of different lengths are also formed if the broken peptide bonds are not at the end of the polymer chain. Thus, depending on the location of the attack, proteases can be further classified into exopeptidases (attack on the terminal group) and endopeptidases (attack on internal linkages).

In this experiment, an accurate and generally accepted colour method is introduced. In this method, an organic compound called ninhydrin is reacted with the amino acids released during the hydrolysis of the protein. The original unreacted ninhydrin is yellowish in color, but the reacted product of ninhydrin has a deep purple-blue color. For example, the procedure given at the end of this section yields an absorbance of 0.27 for 1 x 10^{-4} M of glutamic acid. Since ninhydrin does not react with the undegraded protein, one can measure the amino acid concentration by following the development of the purple colour by measuring the absorbance of the solution with a spectrophotometer. Because the colour intensity is a measure of the amino acid present, the colour should intensify as more protein is degraded to amino acid over time. The upper limit in colour intensity is reached when all the ninhydrin originally present in the solution has been consumed. Thus, the amount of ninhydrin originally present in the reaction mixture determines the maximum amino acid concentration that can be detected.

Equipments

Beakers (100 ml and 400 ml), Graduated cylinder, Pipettes (1 ml and 10 ml), Temperature bath or Bunsen burner or hot plate), Thermometer, Stirring rod, Funnel and filter paper, Centrifuge, Test tubes, Balance, Blender, Spectrophotometer

Reagents

Amino acid standard (for calibrating spectrophotometer)

Protein source

Cottage cheese or curds (10 g/l)

Protease

Ninhydrin solution

Procedure

- Make a 1% protein solution by dissolving casein in water. Make a saturated protease solution by adding 0.5 g of powder protease to 1 litre of water.

- Spin the solution in a centrifuge to separate the undissolved powder. Keep the supernatant.
- Mix equal volumes of protein solution and protease solution. Note the time at the start of the hydrolysis reaction.
- Withdraw 5 ml of the solution and measure the amino acid concentration of the solution as a function of time by using the ninhydrin colorimetric method. Suggested sampling time interval: 10 minutes for at least one hour.

If time permits, repeat the same procedure for hair.

Notes

Gelatin and albumin may be used in lieu of casein. The hydrolysis rate for different substrates may be studied. Alternatively, add 0.05 g protease directly to 50 ml of the protein mixture. However, one must perform the ninhydrin test on the supernatant obtained either through centrifugation or filtration for each sample.

If reagent grade casein is not available, a 1% mixture can be made by the following steps:

- Add 1 g of protein (cheese) using a blender, liquify the mixture; pour into a 100 ml graduated cylinder or a 100 ml volumetric flask.
- Rinse the blender with about 20 ml of water from a squeezable plastic bottle; pour the rinse into the measurement device and add water to 100 ml.

PROTOCOL 5.20

AMINO ACID ASSAY BY NINHYDRIN COLORIMETRIC METHOD

Principle

The reaction between α-amino acid (NH_2-CHR-COOH) and ninhydrin reagent leads to deep purple blue colour development. The colour development can be explained on following mechanistic steps

$$\alpha\text{-aminoacid} + \text{ninhydrin} \longrightarrow \text{Reduced ninhydrin} + \alpha\text{-iminoacid} + H_2O$$

$$\alpha\text{-aminoacid} + H_2O \longrightarrow \alpha\text{-keto acid} + NH_3$$

$$\alpha\text{-keto acid} + NH_3 \longrightarrow \text{Aldehyde} + CO_2$$

Primarily an oxidative deamination reaction removes two hydrogen atoms from the α-amino acid to yield an α-imino acid simultaneously the original ninhydrin is reduced and loses an oxygen atom with the formation of a water molecule. Then NH group in the α-imino acid rapidly gets hydrolyzed to form an α-keto acid with the production of an ammonia molecule. This α-keto acid further undergoes decarboxylation reaction under a heated condition to form an aldehyde that has one less carbon atom than the original amino acid. A carbon dioxide molecule is also produced here. Overall the reduced ninhydrin and ammonia produce which subsequently develops colour. The overall reaction can be expressed as

$$\alpha\text{-aminoacid} + 2\text{ ninhydrin} \longrightarrow CO_2 + \text{aldehyde} + \text{final complex (blue)} + 3H_2O$$

Ninhydrin, which is a powerful oxidizing agent of yellow colour, turns deep blue purple when reacts with α-amino acid. This deep purple colour is estimated colorimetrically.

Materials

Test tubes, Pipettes, Spectrophotometer

Reagent

Ninhydrin reagent solution

Ninhydrin	0.35g
Ethanol q.s. to	100 ml

Procedure

- Add 1 ml of the ninhydrin solution to 5 ml of sample in a capped test tube. With gentle stirring heat the mixture at 80-100°C for 4-7 minutes.
- After cooling to room temperature in a cold water bath, record the absorbance with a spectrophotometer at 570 nm.

Notes

Ninhydrin is carcinogenic and while handling wear gloves. Isopropanol or a 1:1 mixture of acetone/butanol may be used in place of ethanol in preparing the ninhydrin reagent. Method is not applicable for tertiary and aromatic amines.

PROTOCOL 5.21

DETERMINATION OF TOTAL CARBOHYDRATE CONTENT BY ANTHRONE METHOD

Principle

Carbohydrates are first subjected to hydrolysis using dilute HCl, which converts the polysaccharides to the monosaccharides. These monosaccharides are then dehydrated in hot acidic medium to hydroxymethyl furfural. This compound forms a green colour product with anthrone, which is estimated at 630 nm.

Materials

Test tubes, Spectrophotometer, Water bath, Pipettes

Reagents

2.5 N HCl

Anthrone reagent

Dissolve 200 mg anthrone in 100 ml of ice-cold 95% H_2SO_4. Prepare fresh before use.

Glucose stock solution

Dissolve 100 mg in 100 ml water.

Glucose working standard

10 ml of stock diluted to 100ml with distilled water. Store refrigerated after adding a few drops of toluene.

Procedure

- Weigh 100 mg of the sample into a boiling tube. Hydrolyze by keeping it in a boiling water bath for three hours with 5 ml of 2.5 N HCl and cool to room temperature.
- Neutralize it with solid sodium carbonate until the effervescence ceases. Make up the volume to 200 ml and centrifuge. Collect the supernatant and take 0.5 and 1 ml aliquots for analysis.
- Prepare the standards by taking 0, 0.2, 0.4, 0.6, 0.8 and 1 ml of the working standard. "0" serves as blank. Make up the volume to 1 ml in all the tubes including the sample tubes by adding distilled water.
- Add 5 ml of anthrone reagent. Heat for 8 minutes in boiling water bath.
- Cool rapidly and read the green to dark green colour at 630 nm.
- Plot a standard curve between concentration of standard versus absorbance. Calculate the amount of carbohydrate present in the sample tube by using standard curve.

Note

Before adding ice cold anthrone reagent the contents of the all the test tubes must be cooled.

PROTOCOL 5.22

GLUCOSE ASSAY BY DINITROSALICYLIC ACID COLORIMETRIC METHOD

Principle

This method tests for the presence of free carbonyl group (C=O) present in the reducing sugars. Primarily oxidation of the aldehyde functional group (glucose) and ketone functional group (fructose) takes place and as a result 3,5-dinitrosalicylic acid (DNS) is reduced to 3-amino, 5-nitrosalicylic acid under alkaline conditions.

Materials

Test tubes, Pipettes, Spectrophotometer

Reagents

1% Dinitrosalicylic acid reagent solution

Dinitrosalicylic acid	10 g
Crystalline phenol	2 g
Sodium sulphate	0.5 g
Sodium hydroxide	10 g
Add water q.s. to	1litre

Rochelle salt solution

40% Potassium sodium tartarate solution

Procedure

- Add 3 ml of DNS reagent to 3 ml of glucose sample in a capped test tube.

- Heat the mixture at 90°C for 10 minutes to develop the red brown color.
- Add 1 ml of a 40% potassium sodium tartarate solution to stabilize the colour.
- After cooling to room temperature in a cold water bath, record the absorbance with a spectrophotometer at 510 nm.

Notes

Sodium sulphate which itself is not necessary for the colour reaction, is added in the reagent to absorb the dissolved oxygen as dissolved oxygen can interfere with glucose oxidation.

Phenol in a concentration upto 0.2% intensifies the colour density without affecting the linearity.

Different reducing sugars generally yield different colour intensities so it is advisable to calibrate for each sugar.

PROTOCOL 5.22

ESTIMATION OF AMYLASE IN SALIVA

Principle

The production of blue colour by starch on addition of iodine is not quantitative. Therefore, maltose is estimated using dinitrosalicylic acid.

Procedure

- Prepare a standard graph for maltose as given in Table 5.3. Pipette out different sets of solutions into different tubes following the schedule given below

$$\text{Aldehyde group} \xrightarrow{\text{Oxidation}} \text{Carboxylic acid}$$

$$\text{3,5-dinitrosalicylic acid} \xrightarrow{\text{Reduction}} \text{3-amino, 5-nitrosalicylic acid}$$

Table 5.3. Volumes of reagents for estimation of amylase in saliva

Ingredients	Tube No.*				
	1	2	3	4	5
Phosphate buffer (pH 6.7, 0.1 M)	2.5	2.5	2.5	2.5	2.5
Starch solution	2.5	---	---	2.5	2.5
NaCl, 1%	1.0	1.0	1.0	1.0	1.0
Mix well and keep the tubes for 10 minutes at 37°C					
Water	1.0	1.0	0.5	0.5	0.5
Appropriate diluted saliva	---	---	0.5	0.5	0.5

**Prepare tubes in duplicate*

- After adding the saliva, immediately add 0.5 ml 2 N NaOH to tube 5 to stop the reaction. This is called the 'zero time control'.
- Incubate the rest of the tubes at 37°C for 15 minutes.
- Add 0.5 ml 2 N NaOH to stop the reaction. Add 0.5 ml of dinitrosalicylic acid reagent and mix well. Heat the tubes in a boiling water bath for 5 minutes.
- Cool the tubes to room temperature and measure the OD at 520 nm using tube 1 as blank. This does not contain any enzyme but it is a mixture of enzymes that are being used. Tube 2 is also a control. Any reading in this tube is to be subtracted from the value of reading from tube 4 and 5. Comparing tubes 4 and 5, it is seen that they contain complete mixtures, except that the reaction in tube 5 has been stopped immediately on addition of enzyme. In other words it is the zero time control. Thus the amount of maltose formed in 15 minutes by the amount of saliva added is:

Maltose formed = (OD of tube 4 – OD of tube 3) – (OD of tube 5 – OD of tube 3)

- From the standard graph of maltose, calculate the corresponding amount of maltose formed per ml of saliva.

PROTOCOL 5.24

ISOLATION OF PHOSPHOLIPIDS FROM EGG YOLK

Principle

Many phospholipids are insoluble in acetone and they precipitate out whereas triglycerides, sterols, pigments, etc., are soluble in acetone.

Procedure

- Collect the egg yolk from 6-8 eggs and mix well.
- Add 150 ml of cold acetone and allow to stand for 15 minutes.
- Collect the precipitate by centrifugation and wash 3 to 4 times with cold acetone till the supernatant is clear and colorless.
- Extract the precipitate with 500 ml of chloroform-methanol mixture (2:1 v/v) for 3 to 4 hours at room temperature.
- Evaporate the extract to dryness under a stream of nitrogen.
- Dissolve the residue in a small volume of petroleum ether (20-25 ml) and reprecipitate the phospholipids with the addition of cold acetone (150-200 ml) and collect the precipitate.
- Dry under vacuum and store in dark in a minimum volume of chloroform-methanol system or as solid.

PROTOCOL 5.25

CHROMATOGRAPHY OF PHOSPHOLIPIDS

The individual classes of phospholipids can be separated using silicic acid column. The charges of phospholipids make them adsorbed strongly and hence the use of polar solvents becomes essential. The silicic acid column is prepared in chloroform and the elution is carried out with different concentration of methanol-chloroform mixture. The order of elution of phospholipids will normally be phosphatidic acid, cardiolipin, phosphatidyl ethanolamine, phosphatidyl serine, phosphatidyl inositol and lecithin.

Thin Layer Chromatography of Phospholipids

Chloroform-methanol-acetic acid-water mixture (25:15:4:2 v/v) is the most preferred system for the separation of phospholipids.

Iodine vapour is used as the detecting agent. (Leave a few crystals of iodine in a beaker inside a tightly closed chromatographic jar and it will be full of iodine vapors within a short time.) The lipid spots absorb iodine and will be visible as brown spots on yellow background. These spots however are not stable. Alternately, iodine in chloroform system (1% w/v solution) can also be used as spraying agent.

Paper Chromatography of Phospholipid

The technique is the same as for two-dimensional paper chromatography except that papers are used instead TLC plates. Silicic acid impregnated filter papers are used for the separation of phospholipids.

The solvent systems commonly used to get good results are as follows:

- Chloroform-methanol-28% ammonia 65: 35: 5 v/v
- Di-isobutylketone-pyridine-water 25: 25: 4 v/v
- Di-isobutylketone-acetic acid-water 80: 50: 10 v/v
- Chloroform-methanol-water 65: 25: 4 v/v

Procedure

- Dissolve about 140 g of silicic acid (300-400 mesh) in 500 ml sodium hydroxide solution (147.5 g in 500 ml) with stirring, till the solution is clear and make up the volume 1 litre.
- Cut the Whatman filter No.1 or 3 to size and dip into sodium silicate solution for about 30 seconds. Drain off the excess fluid and keep the papers immersed in 6 N HCl for 30 minutes.
- Wash the papers with tap water to remove traces of acid, and dry in air.
- Develop the chromatogram in diisobutylketone-acetic acid-water solvent system and dry in air. Soak the papers in a tray containing 0.005% aqueous rhodamine B solution for about 2-3 minutes (dye gets absorbed by the lipids).
- Take the paper out and wash under tap water to remove excess dye. Visualize the paper under ultraviolet light while wet.

Note

The phospholipid spots appear as blue or orange fluorescent spots.

PROTOCOL 5.26

ESTIMATION OF SERUM CHOLESTEROL

Preparation of standard curve

- Prepare a standard solution of cholesterol (100 μg/ml) in chloroform or glacial acetic acid.
- Take 40 ml ice cold acetic anhydride in a beaker and to this carefully add 2 ml concentrated H_2SO_4 with gentle stirring and keep the mixture in cold all the time (The mixture should be colorless but if a tinge of blue colour appears, discard it and use a fresh batch of acetic anhydride).
- Pipette out the standard solution into different test tubes in the concentration range from 50 to 500 μg per tube and make the volume up to 1 ml with chloroform (or glacial acetic acid).
- Add 5 ml of the reagent to each of the tubes and the mixture becomes rosy red to blue and greenish blue.
- Leave the tubes covered with a dark cloth for 15 minutes and then measure the OD or absorbance of the solutions at 640 nm (red filter) spectrophotometrically. Draw the standard graph.

Estimation of serum sample

- Collect 0.2 to 0.5 ml of serum in a test tube A. Add 2 ml of Bloor's mixture (ether-ethanol 2:1) to 0.3-0.5 ml of serum in a test tube and mix well and allow it to stand for 10 minutes.
- Centrifuge at 2000 rpm for 10 minutes and transfer the supernatant into a dry flask.
- Extract the residue once more with the same mixture and combine the supernatants.
- Evaporate off the solvent and dissolve the residue in dry chloroform.
- Estimate the amount of cholesterol spectrophotometrically by the Liebermann-Burchard test using suitable aliquots. Prepare the standard graph and determine the amount of cholesterol in the sample. The normal value for human serum lies in the range of 120-180 mg/ml.

SUGGESTED READINGS

Heidcamp, W. H., Cell Biology Laboratory Manual, 1996.

Hwang, M. and Ederer, G. M, *J. Clinical Microbiology*, 1, 114, 1975.

Jayaraman, J., Laboratory Manual in Biochemistry, New Age International Publication, New Delhi, India, 1999.

Jecoby, W. B., Methods in Enzymology, Vol. 22, Academic Press, 1971.

Lehninger, A. L, Biochemistry, Worth Publication, 1975.

Miller, G. L., *Analytical Chemistry*, 31, 426, 1959.

Morell and Copeland, *Plant Physiology*, 78, 1985.

Sadasivam, S. and Manickem, A., Biochemical Methods, 2nd Edition, New Age International Publishers, New Delhi, India, 1997.

Standard SRB Method to Determine Enzyme Activity, *Cereal Chemistry*, 712, 1989.

Strominger, *Methods in Enzymology*, 3, 1957.

Vyas, S. P. and Dixit, V. K, Pharmaceutical Biotechnology, CBS Publishers, New Delhi, India, 1998.

Wang, N. S., Biochemical Engineering Laboratory, ENCH, 1995

CHAPTER 6

Enzyme Linked Immunosorbant Assay (ELISA)

- Introduction
- Direct ELISA
- Indirect ELISA
- Two-site ELISA
- Sandwich (capture) ELISA
- Cellular ELISA

INTRODUCTION

ELISA provides simple, sensitive and quantitative assays to screen large number of samples for the presence of particular antigen and antibody present in relatively high concentration. Quantitation of nanogram quantities of antibodies is difficult to be detected accurately by conventional methods and in such cases ELISA is mandatory, however some times with some modification only.

The performance of any immunoassay is directly dependent on the quality of the antigen used as target or as labeled detector and antibody used as capture or detector. Where antigen sample is crude (impurity of non specific antigens in the sample) the appropriate controls should be used on the basis of similar cross reactions, which can distinguish between specific and non specific interactions.

Selection of Capture Antibody

The important aspect in selection offers tremendous potential as capture antibodies, is that they should have the binding capacity primarily for solid phase and secondarily for specific antigens. The binding capacity should also be high in order to get high sensitivity of assay with substantial reproducibility. The specificity must be detected against epitopes common to all representative antigens.

Monoclonal antibodies

Monoclonal antibodies offer great potential as capture reagents in term of specificity and continuity of supply, as they represent a single antibody lineage in a polyclonal immune response. Use of monoclonal antibodies also eliminated the use of a mixture of antibodies for different epitope specificity. Binding to the base plate (plastic plate) is also a critical parameter in the selection of antibodies. Most polyclonal antibodies bind well to plastics with good retention of activity in comparison to monoclonal antibodies. However, the failure of some monoclonal antibodies may be obviated by altering the pH of coating, chemical coupling to BSA and binding to anti-mouse antibody coated surface.

Conclusively, the selection of most appropriate capture antibody remains largely dependent on its spectrum of reactivity and ability to bind antigen efficiently when immobilized.

Fractionation of serum or ascites

In most of the immunoassays, specific immunoglobulin fraction is preferred rather than whole serum or ascites for coating wells. Use of specific antibodies avoids competitive binding and interference staged by many other proteins present in serum or ascites and hence gives results with good reproducibility.

Storage of antibodies

The storage and handling of antibody is important. Whole serum or ascites are stored in aliquots at –20°C. Purified antibodies can be freeze-dried. The concentration should be determined spectrophotometrically (absorption at 280 nm, for 1 mg/ml concentration OD280 ~ 1.4). The sample is concentrated to 1 mg/ml, most preferably 5 mg/ml, and stored at –20°C in 50% glycerol.

Detector Antibodies

The quality of the detector antibody used for enzyme labeling and the efficacy of conjugation is directly related to assay performance. The requirement of specificity, affinity and purity are often more stringent than for capture reagents. Undesirable cross reactivity with components in the assay must be removed by preabsorption of the unlabeled antibody or by neutralization or by addition of the appropriate material in the conjugate diluent. Anti-species immunoglobulin cross reactivity may be effectively decreased by addition of 1-2% of serum from the offending species.

Most conjugation methods, however carefully performed, result in some polymerization of labeled antibody and presence of free enzyme. Removal of unreacted antibody should be accomplished prior to going for ELISA.

Various Assay Techniques for ELISA

Indirect ELISA

This is the simplest form of ELISA. Antigen is bound passively by incubation to the microtitre plate. This antigen solid phase is then used to bind specific antibodies present in the sample. Unbound material is then removed by washing and bound antibodies are detected using enzyme labeled anti-immunoglobulin (Fig. 6.1). If the enzyme labeled antibody is specific for a particular class of immunoglobulin then the class specificity can also be determined.

Limitation: False negative results due to competitive inhibition and false positive results due to interference by IgM anti-immunoglobulin.

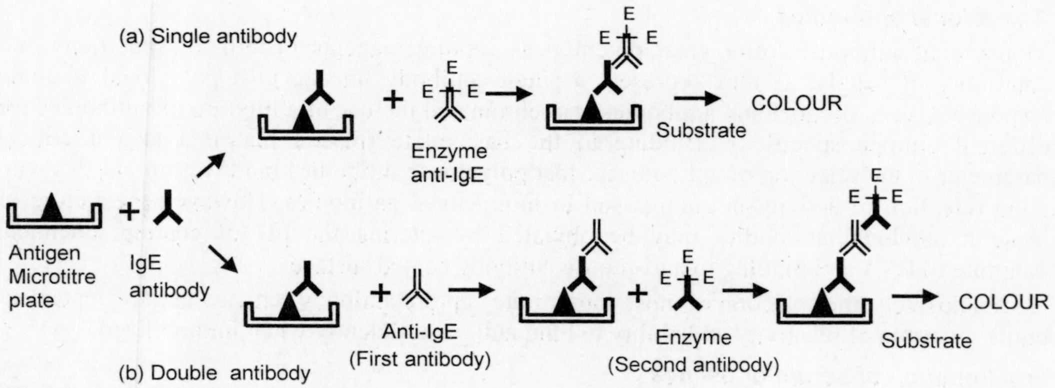

Fig. 6.1. Indirect ELISA. Antibody in the sample binds to antigen in the solid phase and is subsequently detected with (a) an enzyme-labeled antibody or (b) an unlabeled and a second, labeled antibody

Two site ELISA

To determine the concentration of antigen two site ELISA is used. In this assay antibody bound to the microtitre plate/well is used to capture the corresponding antigen in the test samples, the bound antigen is subsequently detected using a second enzyme labeled antibody (Fig. 6.2). This is a rapid, easy method for antigen detection. To avoid the possibility of species cross interaction, monoclonal antibodies having epitope common to different groups can be used.

Class capture assays (sandwich ELISA)

Class capture assays are useful for the sensitive quantitation of clinically relevant antibody from the much larger quantity of antibody of different immunoglobulin class present in the serum. Class capture assays are being used for the detection of specific IgM antibodies to viruses and bacteria and for IgG and IgE antibodies to allergens. In Figure 6.3 class capture assay for IgE antibody is depicted where immunoglobulin of a particular class (e.g. IgE, IgM) is captured by the antibody on the microtitre plate and the presence of antibody activity in the bound immunoglobulin is determined by addition of labeled antigen. Alternatively, antigen can be labeled with the hapten sucas (trinitrophenyl) TNP or with biotin and subsequently detected with enzyme labeled anti-TNP or avidin.

Competitive ELISA

Competitive assays utilize limited concentration of both antigen and antibody so that the amount bound to the solid phase is critical and quantity desorbed or denatured even more so. Competition for binding to antigens can be carried out using an antigen coated microtitre plate (Fig. 6.4) where a fixed level of enzyme labeled antibody competes with varying levels of unlabeled antibody in the sample.

The relative concentration, epitope specificity and affinity of test and reagent antibodies are critical to achieve sensitive, specific and reliable assays for antibody. Sensitivity can be increased if the unlabeled antibody is allowed to bind in a sequential fashion before the labeled reagent is added.

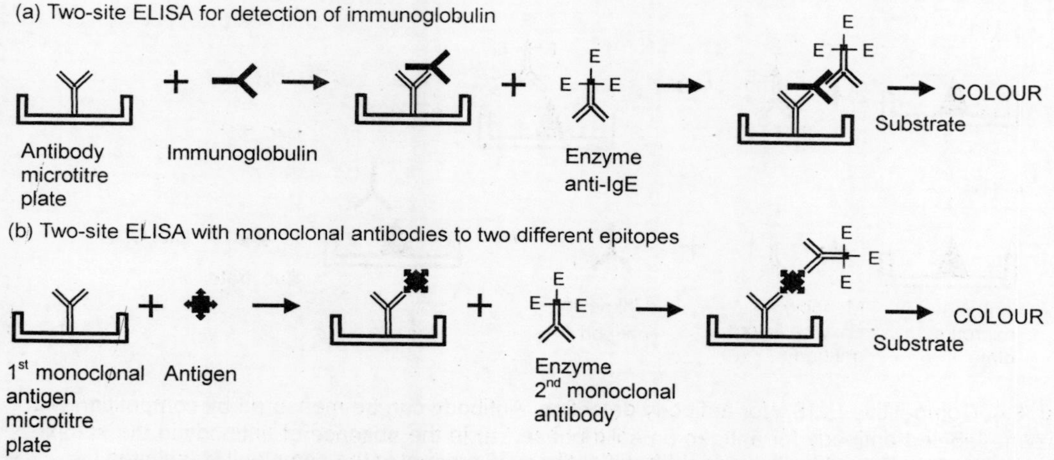

Fig. 6.2. Antibody on the solid phase binds the antigen in the sample, which is subsequently detected using (a) an enzyme-labeled antibody. Alternatively, (b) two monoclonal antibodies that recognize different parts of the antigen can be used.

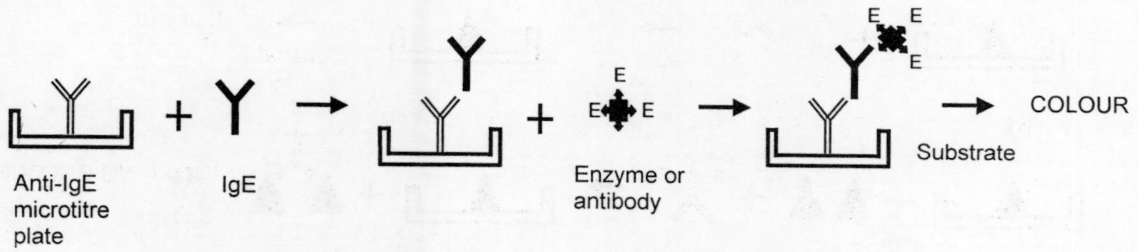

Fig. 6.3. Class capture (sandwich) assay for IgE antibody. Immunoglobulin of a particular class is captured by the antibody on the microtitre plate and the presence of antibody activity in the bound immunoglobulin is determined by association of labeled antigen.

A similar approach can be used to measure antigen (Fig. 6.5). In situations where it is difficult to raise experimental antibodies to the antigen or the objective is to assess the concentration of antigenic determinants recognized by human antibodies, a modification may be used. In this the binding of human antibodies to antigen on the solid phase is inhibited by free unlabeled antigen and resultant activity is measured by adding an enzyme labeled anti-globulin reagent. Such assays have been used to determine the potency of allergen extracts. The presence of antigen in the sample can be determined by competition with labeled antigen for binding to antibody on a solid phase (Fig. 6.6).

Cellular ELISA

Cellular ELISA methodologies are used in the quantitative detection of antibodies from the antibody secreting cells. Cellular ELISAs includes solid phase enzyme linked immunospot assay (ELISPOT) for enumerating antibody secreting cells and ELISA-plaque assay for the detection of single antibody secreting cells. These methods utilize the principle of diffusion-in-gel ELISA (DIG-ELISA). This modification of classical ELISA allows localized antigen antibody reactions to be visualized.

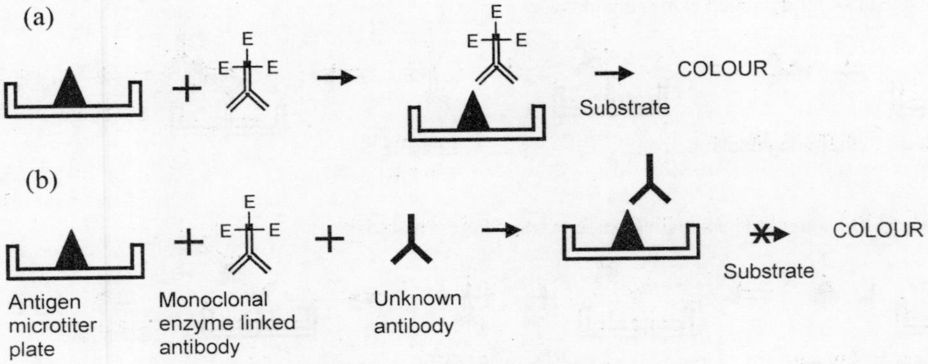

Fig. 6.4. Competitive ELISA for antibody detection. Antibody can be measured by competition with enzyme-labeled antibody for antigen on solid phase. (a) In the absence of antibody in the sample, the enzyme-labeled antibody binds (b) but if antibody is present in the sample, it is inhibited.

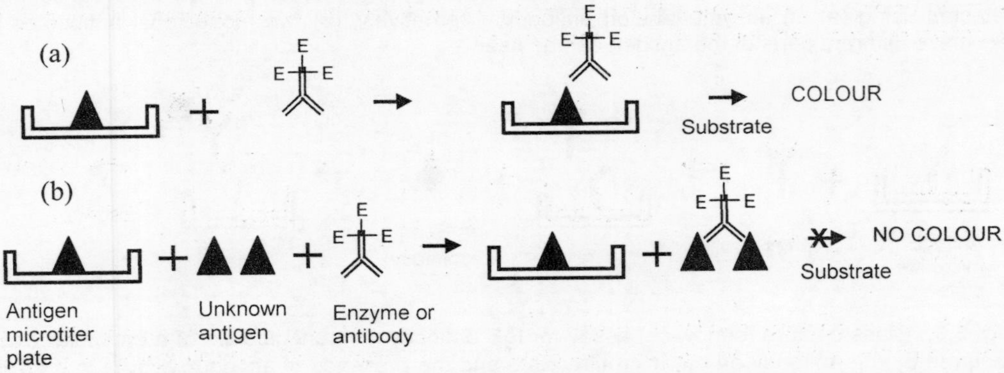

Fig. 6.5. Competitive indirect ELISA for antigen detection. Antigen can be measured by competing with solid phase antigen for binding to enzyme-labeled antibody. (a) In the absence of free antigen in the sample, the enzyme-labeled antibody binds (b) If antigen is present this will be inhibited.

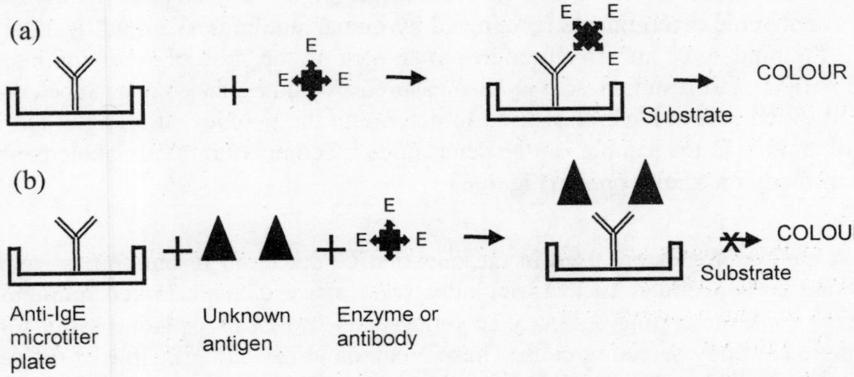

Fig. 6.6. Competitive antigen capture ELISA. Competitive between (a) labeled and (b) unlabeled antigen for binding to antibody on the solid phase can be used for measurement of antigen.

In principle a lymphoid cell suspension containing putative antibody secreting cells is incubated for a few hours in plates that have previously been coated with the pertinent antigen. Following removal of cells, zones or secreted antibody bound to the solid phase are demonstrated by stepwise addition of enzyme-labeled anti-globulin conjugate and agar containing enzyme substrate. Coloured foci or spots appear at the former location of specific antibody secreting cells and can be enumerated with naked eyes or under low magnification. The indicator enzymes used in the assays are horseradish peroxidase and alkaline phosphatase, which can be conjugated with antibody.

PROTOCOL 6.1

DIRECT ELISA

The following is a general procedure for a direct ELISA. The precise conditions should be optimized for a particular assay.

Solution Preparation

Coating solution

Antigen or antibody is diluted in coating solution to immobilize them to the microplate. Commonly used coating solutions are: 50 mM sodium carbonate, pH 9.6; 20 mM Tris-HCl, pH 8.5 or 10 mM PBS, pH 7.2. A protein concentration of 1-10 μg/ml is usually sufficient.

Blocking solution

The blocking agents are BSA, non-fat dry milk, casein, gelatin etc.
Different assay systems may require different blocking agents.

Primary/secondary antibody solution

Primary/secondary antibody should be diluted in 1X blocking solution to prevent non-specific binding. A concentration of 0.1-1.0 μg/ml is usually sufficient.

Wash solution

Typically 0.1 M Phosphate buffered saline or Tris-buffered saline (pH 7.4) with a detergent such as Tween 20 (0.02%-0.05% v/v).

Procedure

Antigen

- Add 100 μl antigen diluted in coating solution to appropriate wells.
- Incubate for1 hour at room temperature.
- Empty plate and tap out residual liquid.

Blocking of Plates

- Add 300 μl blocking solution to each well.
- Incubate for 15 minutes.
- Empty plate and tap out residual liquid.

Adding secondary antibody

- Add 100 µl secondary antibody solution to each well.
- Incubate for 1 hour at room temperature.
- Empty plate and tap out residual liquid.

Washing procedure

- Fill each well with wash solution. Invert plate to empty, tap out residual liquid.
- Repeat 3 to 5 times.
- Give final 5 minutes soak in wash solution. Tap residual liquid from plate.

Substrate reaction

- Dispense 100 µl substrate into each well.
- If desired, after sufficient colour development,
- Add 100 µl of the appropriate stop solution to each well and read plate with a plate reader.

Suggested filters for KPL substrates

2', 2'-Azino-di (3-ethylbenzothiazoline)-6-sulphonate (ABTS)	: 405-410 nm
Orthophenylene diamine (OPD)	: 450 nm non-stopped, 490 nm stopped
Tetraphenylbenzylene hydrochloride (TMB)	: non-stopped 620-650 nm, stopped 450 nm
Nitrophenyl phosphate (NPP)	: 405-410 nm
BluePhos	: 595-650 nm

PROTOCOL 6.2

INDIRECT ELISA

Materials

Antigen
Positive standard
Quality controls
Patients sera
Enzyme-labeled anti-human IgG
Substrate (alkaline phosphatase)
PBS/0.5% animal serum/0.5% Tween 20
Bicarbonate buffer
Nunc Immuno-1 plate (96F)
Spectrophotometer

Procedure

- Coat the plate with antigen at a concentration between 100 µg/ml and 1µg/ml, the optimum having been determined by experimentation. The antigen should be made up in bicarbonate coating buffer. pH 9.6 and incubate with the plate at 100 µl/well overnight at 4°C.

- Wash the plate three times with 300 µl of PBS/0.05% Tween 20.
- Add Positive standards, quality controls and patient's sera at a suitable dilution to the plate (100 µl/well) which is then incubated at 4°C for 2 hours.
- Wash the plate three times with 300 µl of PBS/0.05% Tween 20.
- Add enzyme-conjugated anti-human IgG to the plate at 100 µl/well.
- The optimum concentration is determined by experiment and is usually between 1/100 and 1/500 (typically 5 µg/ml). The incubation time is 1 hour at 4°C.
- Wash plate three times with PBS/0.05% Tween 20 and then once with distilled water.
- Make up substrate in diethanolamine buffer, pH 9.8, as described above.
- Add 100 µl to each well and incubate at 37°C for 1 to 2 hours.
- Stop enzyme reaction by adding 50 µl/well of 3M NaOH.
- Measure absorbance at 405 nm.

PROTOCOL 6.3

TWO-SITE ELISA

Materials

96 well plates
(Phosphate buffer saline)
Tris-buffered saline (TBS)
0.1% Tween 20 in PBS or in TBS
Blocking solution
2% BSA (type V) in PBS. Add 0.02% azide for longer storage.
ELISA buffer
2% BSA in 0.1% Tween 20 in PBS (azide optional)
Enzyme linked antibody horseradish peroxidase
Substrate ABTS
100X (2,2'-azino-bis-(3-ethylbenzothiazoline) sulphonic acid)
Horseradish peroxidase (HRP) buffer
100 mM in Sodium Citrate pH 4.2 (490 mg citric acid + 720 mg sodium citrate dihydrate + 50 ml H_2O, pH 4.2).
Hydrogen peroxide 30% (1000X)

Procedure

Absorption of antigen

- Dilute antigen to 10 µg/ml in PBS.
- Add 100 µl of aqueous solution to each well.
- Leave overnight covered with lid at 4°C.

Blocking

- Wash unbound antigen by inverting the plates and flicking the wells dry.
- Rinse by adding PBS to each well and invert it again (use squirt bottle).
- Rinse twice.
- Add 100 μl of blocking solution to every well.
- Leave 1 hour at room temperature or overnight at 4°C.

Primary antibody

- Add the antibody to be tested.
- Supernatant of cells 25 μl, mix well by pipetting up and down (10 times). Serum, ascites 1:100 and a series of 1:5 dilutions.
- Make dilutions in blocking solution.
- Leave for 1 hour at room temperature or overnight at 4°C.

Secondary antibody

- Wash unbound antibody 4 times with PBS and add 0.1% Tween 20.
- Add 100 μl of enzyme linked antibody to all wells.
- Do the appropriate dilutions in the ELISA buffer. (e.g. HRP is 2000X).
- Leave 1 hour at room temperature or overnight at 4°C.

Substrate

- Dissolve substrate in double distilled water.
- Wash plates 4 times with PBS and add 0.1% Tween 20 (use TBS instead of PBS for alkaline phosphatase).
- Add 100 μl of substrate to every well.
- Match colour development. This could take time from a few seconds to 20 minutes.
- If needed, stop the reaction by adding 50 μl of 4 M NaOH.
- Read absorption in ELISA reader at corresponding wavelength (for horseradish peroxidase system 416 nm, for alkaline phosphatase system 405 nm).

PROTOCOL 6.4

SANDWICH (CAPTURE) ELISA

The general method for a sandwich (capture) ELISA is given below. Moreover, the precise conditions should be optimized for a particular assay.

Solution Preparation

Coating solution

Antigen or antibody is diluted in coating solution to immobilize them to the microplate. Commonly used coating solutions are: 50 mM sodium carbonate, pH 9.6; 20 mM Tris-HCl, pH 8.5; or 10 mM PBS, pH 7.2. A protein concentration of 1-10 μg/ml is usually sufficient.

Blocking solution

Commonly used blocking agents are: BSA, non-fat dry milk, casein, gelatin, etc. Different assay systems may require different blocking agents.

Primary/secondary antibody solution

Primary/secondary antibody should be diluted in 1X blocking solution to help prevent non-specific binding. A concentration of 0.1-1.0 µg/ml is usually sufficient to achieve this.

Antigen solution

Sample antigen should be diluted in 1X blocking solution to prevent non-specific binding. A concentration of 0.1-1.0 µg/ml is usually sufficient.

Wash solution

Typically 0.1 M Phosphate buffered saline or Tris-buffered saline (pH 7.4) with a detergent such as Tween 20 (0.02%-0.05% v/v) are employed.

Apply capture antibody

- Add 100 µl capture antibody diluted in coating solution to appropriate wells.
- Incubate for 1 hour at room temperature.
- Empty the plate and tap out residual liquid.

Block plate

- Add 300 µl blocking solution to each well.
- Incubate for 5 minutes.
- Empty the plate and tap out residual liquid.

Sample antigen reaction

- Add 100 µl diluted antigen to each well.
- Incubate at room temperature for 1 hour to overnight.
- Empty the plate, tap out residual liquid.

Wash procedure

- Fill each well with wash solution.
- Invert plate to empty, tap out residual liquid.
- Repeat the above step 3 to 5 times.

Application of secondary antibody solution

- Add 100 µl diluted secondary antibody to each well.
- Incubate 1 hour at room temperature.
- Empty plate, tap out residual liquid and wash.
- Give final 5 minutes soak with wash solution.
- Tap residual liquid from plate.

Substrate reaction

- Add 100 µl substrate into each well.
- If desired, after sufficient colour development, add 100 µl of the appropriate stop solution to each well.
- Read plate with a plate reader.

Suggested Filters for KPL Substrates

2', 2'-Azino-di (3-ethylbenzothiazoline)-6-sulphonate (ABTS)	: 405-410 nm
Tetraphenylbenzylene hydrochloride (TMB)	: non-stopped 620-650 nm, stopped 450 nm
Orthophenylenediamine (OPD)	: non-stopped 450 nm, stopped 490 nm
P-Nitrophenylphosphate (*p*NPP)	: 405-410 nm
BluePhos	: 595-650 nm

PROTOCOL 6.5

CELLULAR ELISA

Preparation of Formalin Fixed Cell Plates

- Trypsinize confluent flasks.
- Pool and count cells.
- Centrifuge at 1500 rpm for 10 minutes.
- Resuspend to the appropriate concentration in complete medium 4 x 10^5 cells/ml for epithelial cells and 2 x 10^5 cells/ml for fibroblast cells.
- Well to 96 well culture plates.
- Incubate overnight at 37°C.
- Wash plates twice with PBS.
- Add 125 µl/well 10% buffered formalin.
- Fix for 15 minutes at room temperature.
- Wash three times with distilled water.
- Blot dry. Store at 2-8°C.

Reagents

PBS: 1% BSA

PBS: 2% BSA

Carbonate buffer

1.59 g Na_2CO_3

2.93 g $NaHCO_3$

Dissolve in 900 ml distilled water. Adjust pH to 9.6.

Make up the volume to 1 litre with distilled water.

10X Substrate buffer, pH 6.0

36.6 g Citric acid, monohydrate

113.5 g Potassium dibasic phosphate

Dissolve in 900 ml distilled water

Adjust pH to 6.0 and add dilute to make 1 litre.

$0.3\% \ H_2O_2$

Dilute 30% stock peroxide 1 : 100 in distilled water.

Orthophenylenediamine (OPD) stock, 4.0%

4 g OPD in 100 ml distilled water.

Aliquot and store at –20°C. Protect from light.

$4.5 \ N \ H_2SO_4$

12.0 ml Concentrated sulphuric acid

88.0 ml distilled water

working substrate solution

0.5 ml 4.0% OPD

5 ml 30% H_2O_2

1ml 10X Substrate buffer

8.5 ml Distilled water

Procedure

- Wash ELISA plates once with distilled water.
- Add 250 µl/well PBS : 2% BSA.
- Incubate 1 hour at 37°C.
- Wash 3 times with distilled water.
- Add 50 µl/well supernatant, ascites, or controls diluted in PBS : 1% BSA.
- Incubate for 2 hours at 37°C.
- Wash 5 times with distilled water.
- Add 50 µl/well anti-mouse IgG:HRP diluted in PBS : 1% BSA.
- Incubate for 1 hour at 37°C.
- Wash 5 times with distilled water
- Wash once with carbonate buffer.
- Add 50 µl/well working substrate solution
- Incubate for 20 minutes at room temperature.
- Add 25 µl/well 4.5 N sulphuric acid
- Read the absorbance at 490 nm.

Notes

Test all supernatants at 1:5 dilution.

Test ascites at 1:100 dilution.

SUGGESTED READINGS

Carpenter, P. L., Immunology and Serology, Toppan Company Ltd., Tokyo, Japan, 1965.

Crowther, J.R. (1995). Methods in Molecular Biology, Vol. 42-ELISA: Theory and Practice. Humana Press, Totowa, NJ.

Harlow, E. and Lane, D. (1988). Antibodies: A Laboratory Manual. Cold Spring Harbor Laboratory Press, Cold Spring Harbor, NY, 553-612.

Harlow, E. and Lane, D., Antibodies: A Laboratory Manual, Cold Spring Harbor Laboratory Press, New York, 1992.

Kemmemy, D. M. and Challacombe, S. T. (Eds.), ELISA and other Solid Phase Immunoassay: Theoretical and Practical Aspects, John Wiley and Sons, NewYork, USA, 1989.

Perlmann, H. and Perlmann, P. (1994). Cell Biology: A Laboratory Handbook. San Diego, CA, Academic Press, Inc., 322-328.

Talwar, G. P. and Gupta, S. K., A Handbook of Practical and Clinical Immunology, 2nd Edition, CBS Publishers and Distributors, New Delhi, 1992.

CHAPTER 7

Enzyme and Cell Immobilization

- Enzyme immobilization
- Cell immobilization
- Purification of enzymes for immobilization
- Enzyme immobilization in polyacrylamide gel
- Enzyme immobilization in alginate gel
- Enzyme immobilization in gelatin gel
- Immobilization of enzymes in gelatin moulds
- Cell immobilization in agarose
- Cell immobilization with calcium alginate
- Preparation of cell immobilizedcalcium alginate beads
- Immobilization of microbial cells in gelatin
- Yeast cell immobilization on wood chips
- Immobilization of microbial cells by adsorption to solid supports
- Ethanol production by immobilized yeast cell
- Preparation of glucose detector

ENZYME IMMOBILIZATION

Enzymes are biological catalysts that promote the rate of reactions but are not themselves consumed in the reactions in which they participate and they may be used repeatedly for as long as they remain active. However, in most of the industrial, analytical, and clinical processes, enzymes are mixed in a solution with substrates and cannot be economically recovered after the exhaustion of the substrates. This single use is obviously quite wasteful when the cost of enzymes is considered. Thus, there is an incentive to use enzymes in an immobilized or insolubilized form so that they may be retained in a biochemical reactor to catalyze further the subsequent feed. The use of an immobilized enzyme makes it economically feasible to operate an enzymatic process in a continuous mode. Immobilization of an enzyme means that it has been confined or localized so that it can be reused continuously. Immobilization imparts several desirable advantages to an enzyme.

- In cases where processing of some substrate is required with isolated enzyme, they can be used in immobilized form either in the form of beads or immobilized in the reactor bed.

- Enzymes in the immobilized form reportedly retain their activity longer compared to their solution form.
- An immobilized enzyme may be fixed at a location near other enzymes to become a part of participating catalytic sequence, thereby increasing the catalyst efficiency especially in the case of multistep conversions.

The immobilization method greatly influences the property of the resulting biocatalyst. Immobilization causes dramatic change in the rate of enzyme catalyzed reaction, Michaelis-Menten constant, optimum temperature and optimum pH. The major division of methods is between those, which are employed to retain biocatalyst within the support and those, which held biocatalyst on the surface of the support (Fig. 7.1).

On Surface Immobilization

- Adsorption and ionic binding
- Covalent coupling to activated polymers
- Complexation and chelation

Within Support Immobilization

- Copolymerization with multi-functional reagents
- Entrapment by occlusion within cross-linked gels and encapsulation

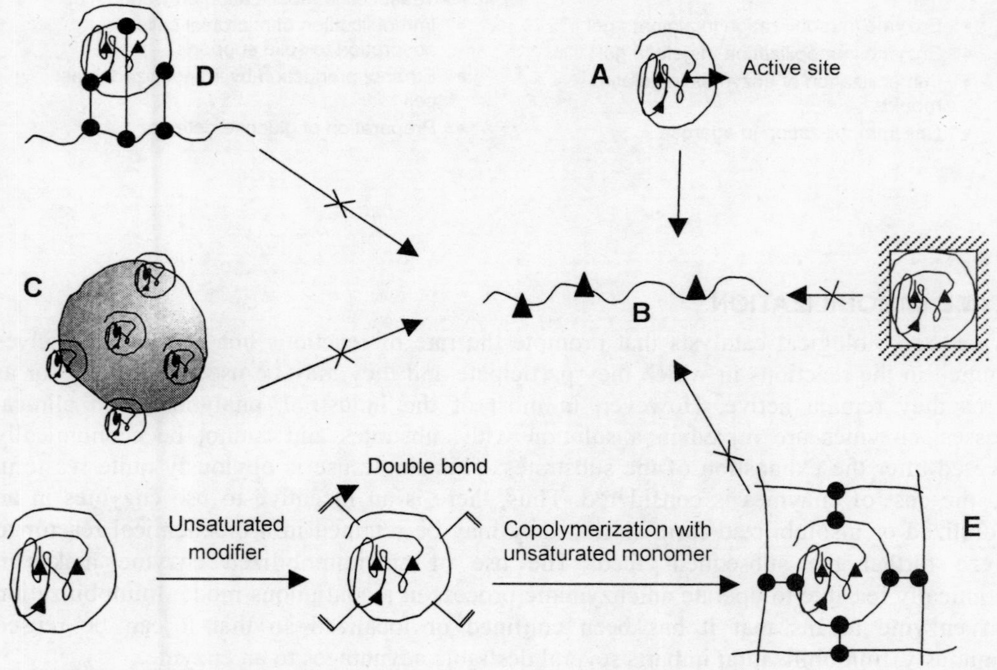

Fig. 7.1. Schematic presentation of possible methods for enzyme stabilization with the use of a carrier (A) native enzyme (B) denatured form of the native enzyme (C) enzyme immobilization by adsorption on a solid support (D) enzyme immobilization on soluble polymer (E), the copolymerization of a modified enzyme with unsaturated monomer into a three-dimensional gel (F) mechanical entrapment of an enzyme into a polymeric gel.

Adsorption and ionic binding

One of the earliest methods of enzyme immobilization is the physical adsorption of the enzyme on to a polymer matrix without involving covalent binding. In this method the adsorbent and enzyme are slowly stirred together for some time. The yields are however low and the enzyme is often partially or totally inactivated. The adsorption of a protein onto a given surface is dependent on ionic strength, pH, temperature, and type of solvent system and enzyme concentration. The most commonly used adsorbents are carbon, alumina, cellulose, clay polystyrene, hydroxyapalite and glass. The binding forces may be ionic, hydrophobic, hydrogen bonds or van der Waal interactions (Table 7.1).

Table 7.1. Interactions and carriers used for enzyme immobilization by adsorption

Interaction	Adsorbents
Physical adsorption	*Activated carbon, Silica gel, Aumina, Starch clay and glass*
	Modified materials: Tannins, Aminohexyl cellulose Concanavalin-A, Sepharose
Ionic binding	Cation exchange
	Carboxymethyl cellulose, Cellulose citrate, P-cellulose Amberlite CG-50, Dowex-50
	Anion exchange
	DEAE-cellulose, TEAE-cellulose, DEAE-sephadex polyaminopolystryene, Amberlite IR-45

The reversible nature of adsorption of enzyme on the support may lead to desorption of the enzyme. The factors responsible for desorption are addition of substrate to the enzyme preparation, fluctuations in pH, temperature and ionic strength. Cellulose is employed to immobilize enzymes in order to achieve high level adsorption of proteins. Table 7.2 lists some therapeutically important enzymes immobilized by adsorption method.

Table 7.2. Some therapeutic enzymes immobilized by physical adsorption

Carrier	Enzyme
Organic Supports	
Concanavalin-A	Arylsulphatase
Gluten	β-amylase
Concanavalin-A-sepharose	Phosphodiesterase
Butyl sepharose	Lipoamide dehydrogenase
Starch	α-Amylase
Activated carbon	Glucose oxidase, α-Amylase, β-Amylase
Inorganic support	
Alumina	Glucose oxidase
Kaolin	Lysozyme
Porous glass	Glucose oxidase
Silica gel	Aspartase
Bentonite	Invertase

Cellulose based ion exchange resins e.g., carboxymethyl cellulose, diethyl aminoethyl (DEAE) cellulose have been extensively used for immobilization of enzymes with higher adsorption capacity (up to 15% w/w protein:cellulose). The ionic binding for enzyme immobilization was first carried out by immobilizing catalase by binding it to the DEAE-cellulose. Ionic binding is influenced by many of the same factors that influence physical adsorption. Most commonly used carriers for ionic binding include polysaccharides and a variety of synthetic polymers having multiple ion exchange groups attached. The ionic binding is usually carried out under relatively mild conditions as compared to covalent coupling and it causes very little or no effect on conformational structure of the enzyme protein (Table 7.3). Another development in immobilization technologies by adsorption has been the use of an effector or activator of an enzyme, attached to a water insoluble polymer to bind that enzyme. Immobilization of the tyrosinase and tryptophanase by adsorption to an insoluble derivative of pyridoxal-5'-phosphate, an activator of these enzymes provides an added advantage that the enzyme is not only specifically adsorbed on to the polymer, but it is activated by the same process.

Table 7.3. Some therapeutic enzymes immobilized by ionic binding

Carrier	Enzyme
Anion Exchangers	
DEAE cellulose	Invertase, Pepsin, L-Asparaginase, Aspartase
DEAE-sephadex	Aminoacylase
Amberlite IR-45	Glucoamylase
Amberlite IRA-410	Invertase
Cation Exchangers	
Carboxymethyl cellulose	Trypsin, α-Chymotrypsin, L-Asparaginase
Cellulose citrate	Trypsin
Amberlite CG-50	Glucose oxidase
Dowex-50	Ribonuclease

Covalent binding to activated polymers

The chemical coupling of enzymes to water insoluble supports and even to water-soluble polymers is the most commonly employed method of enzyme immobilization (Fig. 7.2). By the careful selection of supports with appropriate physical and chemical characteristics, bio-reactors with variety of therapeutic applications can be generated.

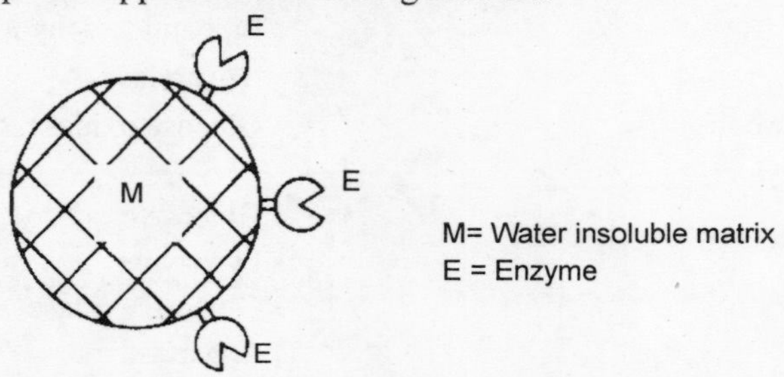

Fig. 7.2. Schematic presentation of immobilization using covalent coupling

Table 7.4 lists several materials, which are employed for covalent enzyme immobilization, and some of their surface functional groups. Other materials, which have been used as support for immobilization of enzymes, include ceramics, glass and other metal oxides. The most important and conventionally used methods of covalent attachment include azo linkage, isocyanates and isothiocynates, carboxymethylazides and carbodiimides coupling.

Table 7.4. Insoluble materials and their surface functional groups useful for covalent enzyme attachment

Natural supports	Synthetic supports
Cellulose (-OH)	Polyacrylamide derivatives
CM-Cellulose (-COOH)	Polystyrene (-NH_2)
Agarose (-OH)	Maleic anhydride copolymer
Dextran (-OH)	Polyethylene glycol
Albumin	

Azo linkage

Any arylamine can be treated with nitrous acid to form a diazonium salt. Diazonium salt reacts with, and couples to many aromatic compounds, particularly phenols such as L-tyrosine, and other abundant constituent of proteins. The most widely used supports include polyamino polystyrene, aryl aminocellulose, arylamine glass and ceramics. Several therapeutic enzymes immobilized by this method are given in Table 7.5.

Table 7.5. Some therapeutic enzymes immobilized by azo linkage carrier

Carrier	Enzyme
Polysaccharide derivative	
m-Aminoanisole cellulose	α-Chymotrypsin, Trypsin
p-Amino benzyl cellulose	α-Amylase, Lysozyme, Trypsin, Chymotrypsin
Amino acid copolymers	
p-Amino-DL-phenylalanine L-leucine	Trypsin, α-Chymotrypsin, Prothrombin Streptokinase, Urease
Polyacrylamide derivatives	Lysozyme, α-Amylase
Styrene resins	
Aminosilane derivatives	Lipase, Diastase
Aminosilanized porous glass	Glucose oxidase, Steroid esterase
Aminosilanized dacron	Acetylcholine esterase, β-Galactosidase Urease, L-Asparaginase

Isocyanates and isothiocyanates

Both alkyl and arylamines can be converted in to isocyanates and isothiocyanates. These active compounds covalently bind with available amine groups. Such groups are common on proteins and are usually provided by the ε-amino group of L-lysine residues of the protein backbone, or by N-terminal α-amino nitrogen atoms. Therapeutically important enzymes, which are immobilized by this method, are given in Table 7.6.

Table 7.6. Enzymes immobilized by amide linkage using isocyanates and isothiocyanates

Carrier	Enzyme
Copolymer of propylene and p-isocyanate styrene	Trypsin
Isothiocyanate derivative of enzacryl amino acid	α-Amylase
Isothiocyanate derivative of aminosilanized hydroxylapalite	Glucose oxidase
Isothiocyanate derivative of aminosilanized porous glass	Glucose oxidase, Trypsin, Papain
Isothiocyanate derivative of aminosilanized silica	Papain
CM-Cellulose isocyanate derivative	ATPase
Sephadex-isocyanate derivative	Trypsin
Polyaminopolystyrene isocyanate derivative	Catalase

Carboxymethylazides

Azides at slightly alkaline pH will react with available amine groups. At acid pH, azide groups become extremely photoactivated coupling agents and could bind to a wide variety of functional and non-functional groups (Table 7.7). Other reactions, which could be used for anchoring enzymes, include cyanogen bromide (CNBr) and dihydroquinoline.

Table 7.7. Some enzymes immobilized by azide linkage using carboxymethylazides

Carrier	Enzyme
Aceto Azide derivative	
CM-Cellulose	Glucoseoxidase
	α-Amylase
	Trypsin
	Bromelain
	Streptokinase
	Urokinase
CNBr-Activated Polysaccharides	
CNBr Activated Cellulose	Xanthine oxidase
	β-D-Glucosidase
	α-Chymotrypsin
	Glucoamylase
CNBr Activated Sephadex	Lactate dehydrogenase
	Glucose 6-Phosphate dehydrogenase
	Carboxy peptidase A
	α-Chymotrypsine
CN-Br Activated Sepharose	Lactate dehydrogenase
	Malate dehydrogenase
	Glucose oxidase

Carbodiimides

Carbodiimides soluble in both aqueous and organic solvents are commonly available. These compounds react with free carboxyl groups forming a pseudourea intermediate addict, which can be coupled with available amines via an amide linkage. Table 7.8 lists some enzymes immobilized by carbodiimide coupling.

Table 7.8. Some enzymes immobilized by carbodiimide coupling

Carrier	Enzyme
AE-Cellulose	Peroxidase
CM-Cellulose	Peroxidase
CM-Sephadex	Pronase
BioGel CM-100	β-Amylase, Trypsin
Copolymer of acrylamide and acrylic acid	β-D-Glucosidase, Trypsin, Urease

Copolymerization with multifunctional reagent

Multifunctional reagents can be used to link enzyme molecules to cellulose or other polymers and to cross-link enzyme molecules to each other. Most commonly used multifunctional reagents are glutaraldehyde and cyanuric chloride. Aldehydes in general and glutaraldehyde in particular have been known to be active against proteins. It is extremely difficult to precipitate an enzyme out of solution using glutaraldehyde; the solution usually gels. In order to produce an insoluble matrix of enzyme and glutaraldehyde it is necessary either to cause the glutaraldehyde to polymerize or to precipitate the enzyme (or adsorb it on to some insoluble surface). The net effect is either to increase the length of the bridging molecule or to decrease the intermolecular distance of the enzyme molecules. Using this approach carboxypeptidase crystals, papain and trypsin have been cross-linked and immobilized. The other multifunctional reagents are N,N′-bisdiazo-benzidine-2,2′-disulphonic acid and 2, 4-dinitro-3, 5-difluorobenzene. These reagents require strong and specific conditions to react with enzyme whereas glutaraldehyde reacts with protein under mild conditions. It is relatively less toxic also. The major problem with this method is that the bifunctional reagents may often preferentially sequester enzyme active site, thus may be rendered inactive.

Entrapment and occlusion

The entrapment of an enzyme molecules can be achieved using one of the following six ways:

- Inclusion within the matrix of a highly crosslinked polymer
- Separation from the bulk phase by a semipermeable membrane
- Dissolution in a distinct non-aqueous phase
- Liposomes
- Reverse micelles
- Resealed erythrocytes

Entrapment within the matrix of highly cross-linked polymer

The most widely used system for enzyme entrapment in a polymer lattice is polyacrylamide gel produced by cross-linking acrylamide in the presence of enzyme. Potassium persulphate is used as a polymerization initiator and β-dimethylamino propionitrile (DMAPN) as an accelerator. The pore size in immobilized enzyme gels remains sufficiently small to retain many enzymes, which have molecular diameter in the range of 200-300 nm.

Separation from the bulk phase by a semipermeable membrane

In this method, the enzyme remains in solution, while a semipermeable membrane physically confines enzyme solution so that the enzyme cannot escape. There is a biological analogy of these techniques. The lysosome within the cell confines hydrolytic enzymes, which would otherwise kill the cell immediately if they were released. In an immobilization method also known as microencapsulation, in which the enzymes are entrapped in small capsules with diameters ranging up to 300 μm. The capsules are surrounded by spherical membranes which have pores permitting small substrates and product molecules to enter and leave the capsule. The pores are too small, however, for enzymes and other large molecules to permeate. There are different methods for the preparation of microcapsules.

Emulsion polymerization method

In this method, a semipermeable membrane is formed by condensation co-polymerization reaction at the interface between an organic phase and a dispersed aqueous phase containing enzyme. By choosing a water insoluble monomer as one of the reactants and a monomer slightly soluble in both phases for the other, the copolymerization occurs only at the interface. Alternatively, an aqueous solution of enzyme dispersed in a solution of PVC or cellulose triacetate may be extruded to form fibres containing droplets of enzymes.

Coacervation phase separation method

The term coacervate is derived from Latin word *acervus*, meaning a heap or aggregation. In coacervation a colloidal dispersion is caused to collapse and separate into a colloidal rich and colloidal poor regions by careful control of temperature, pH, electrolytes addition, or other factors. The coacervate or colloidal rich region forms as droplets, which make the system opaque and sediment to form a separate lower layer. The phase boundary formed is unlike that between immiscible liquids in that the solvent is continuous on both sides of the interface, facilitating free migration of solute between layers.

Interfacial polycondensation

Interfacial polycondensation involves the reaction of various monomers at the interface between two immiscible liquid phases to form a film of polymer that encapsulates the disperse phase (Fig.7.3).

Usually two reactive monomers are employed, one dissolved in the aqueous disperse phase containing a solution or dispersion of core material, and the other dissolved after the emulsification step in the non-aqueous continuous phase. The water-in-oil (w/o) emulsion formed requires the addition of a suitable emulsifying agent as dispersion stabilizer.

Emulsion solvent evaporation

In this method, the polymer is dissolved in a volatile organic solvent and emulsified with the aqueous phase (W_1) containing enzyme to be immobilized. The resulting W_1/O emulsion is again emulsified with another aqueous phase (W_2) containing suitable stabilizer to form a $W_1/O/W_2$ multiple emulsion.

The emulsion is mechanically stirred to evaporate out the organic solvent leaving a thin film of polymer around the phase W_1. Microspheres of poly (L-lactide) glycolide copolymers (PLGA) have been prepared by this method.

Dissolution in a distinct non-aqueous phase

Non-permanent microcapsules can be prepared by emulsifying the aqueous enzyme solution with a surfactant. This liquid-surfactant membrane based capsules can then be added to an aqueous substrate solution. Microcapsules have the potential advantage of a very large surface area (e.g., 2500 cm^2 per ml of enzyme solution) and the possibility of added specificity: the membrane can be made in some cases to admit some substrate selectively while exclude other. Moreover, these methods are applicable to a large variety of enzymes. Various therapeutic enzymes immobilized in microcapsules are given in Table 7.9.

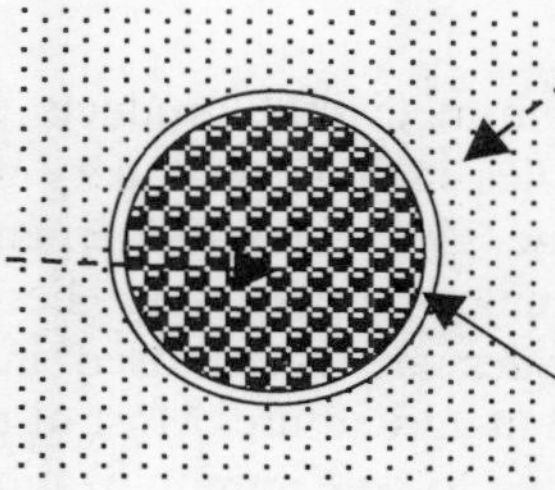

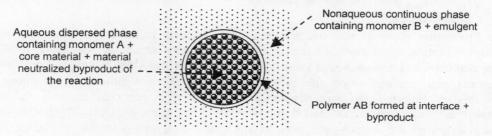

Fig. 7.3. Schematic representation of interfacial polycondensation technique

Table 7.9. Therapeutic enzymes immobilized in microcapsules

Polymer	Enzyme
Agarose	Urokinase
Albumin	L-Asparaginase
Albumin	Urokinase
Collagen	L-Asparaginase
Polydextran	L-Asparaginase
Nylon 6-10	Urease
Nylon 6-10	L-Asparaginase
Poly DL-lactide-co-glycolic acid	L-Asparaginase
Poly DL-lactide-co-glycolic acid	Superoxide dismutase
Poly isobutyl cyanoacrylate	L-Asparaginase and Superoxide dismutase
Poly vinyl pyrrolidone	Lysozyme
Poly acrylamide	L-Asparaginase
Polyhydroxyethylmethacrylate	Urokinase

CELL IMMOBILIZATION

Basically, immobilization of living cells is very similar to that of enzyme immobilization. Various cells have been immobilized, in that noticeable are bacteria, yeasts, fungi, plant tissues, some mammalian tissues and insect tissues. However, true success in cell immobilization is limited to only a few cases. One of the problems is the mass transfer resistance imposed by the fact that the substrate has to diffuse to the reaction site and inhibitory or toxic products must be removed to the environment. Oxygen transfer is often the rate-limiting step in a suspended cell culture, and it is more so in an immobilized cell culture. Oxygenation in an immobilized cell culture is one of the major technical problems that remains to be solved and till date cell immobilization techniques are confined to anaerobic processes in which either obligate anaerobes or only the anaerobic components of the facultative metabolic mechanisms are selectively utilized.

The smaller cell organisms can be easily immobilized with a number of methods :

- Entrapment
- Ion exchange adsorption porous ceramics
- Covalent bonding

Production of medicinal and non-medicinal products is the major part of plant cell immobilization applications. Examples include secondary metabolite production of alkaloid of medicinal and non-medicinal value, glycosides and terpenoids (flavours, and perfumes). In animal cell immobilization the major applicability lies in production of monoclonal antibodies. Immobilized insect tissues are being used in pesticide research and have a potentially large commercial market in agriculture. Most of the principles involved in enzyme immobilization are directly applicable to cell immobilization e.g. covalent bonding, affinity bonding, physical adsorption, and entrapment in synthetic and natural polymer matrices. The most popular and practical immobilization technique deals with cell recycle with an ultrafiltration membrane or a hollow fibre cartridge. The cell recycle devices effectively retain the catalysts in a bioreactor and accomplish the same objective as cell immobilization.

Immobilized cell bioreactor preparation is possible with those cells, whose growth phases and product formation phases are uncoupled. However, cell biomass and primary metabolites are growth associated products, but secondary metabolites such as antibiotics and various enzymes are produced during the stationary phase. The uncoupling of the phases means that productive cells cannot compete with the nonproductive cells in a continuously operated suspension fermenter because the productive cells spend the nutritional and energy resources producing chemicals in quantities far above the amount necessary for their survival, instead of reproducing themselves to propagate further. On the contrary, cell growth in an immobilized cell reactor must be severely limited if gel swelling or breakage is to be avoided. However, once the cells are immobilized, the cell viability must be concomitantly sustained over a long period of time. Thus, immobilization is advantageous for sustaining slowly growing cells, especially plant tissues.

PROTOCOL 7.1

PURIFICATION OF ENZYMES FOR IMMOBILIZATION

Principle

The solubility of protein depends on, among other things, the salt concentration in the solution. At low concentrations, the presence of salt stabilizes the various charged groups on a protein molecule, thus attracting protein into the solution and enhancing the solubility of protein. This is commonly known as *salting-in*. However, as the salt concentration is increased, a point of maximum protein solubility is usually reached. Further increase in the salt concentration implies that there is less and less water available to solubilize protein. Finally, protein starts to precipitate when there are not sufficient water molecules to interact with protein molecules. This phenomenon of protein precipitation in the presence of excess salt is known as salting-out. Many types of salts have been employed to effect protein separation and purification through salting-out. Of these salts, ammonium sulphate has been the most widely used chemical because it has high solubility and is relatively inexpensive.

As the enzymes are proteins, enzyme purification can also be carried out by using same principle, however, some attention must be paid to the consideration of permanent loss of activity due to denaturation under adverse conditions. There are two major salting-out methods:

By increasing salt concentrations

By slow addition of saturated salt solution or powdered salt crystals to the protein mixture to bring up the salt concentration of the mixture. The precipitated protein is collected and categorized according to the concentration of the salt solution at which it is formed. This partial collection of the separated product is called fractionation.

By decreasing salt concentrations

Proteins are first precipitated with a concentrated salt solution. Then a series of cold (near 0°C) ammonium sulphate solution of decreasing concentrations are employed to extract selectively the protein components that are the most soluble at higher ammonium sulphate concentrations. The extracted protein is recrystallized and thus recovered by gradually warming the cold solution to room temperature. This method has the added advantages that the extraction media may be buffered or stabilizing agents be added to retain the maximum enzyme activity. The efficiency of recovery typically ranges from 30 to 90%, depending on the protein.

Equipment

Test tubes, Graduated cylinder, Pipettes, Balance, Centrifuge, Filtration devices

Materials

Protein solution (200 ml, 1% haemoglobin)

Fungal α-amylase (1%)
Protease (1%)
Saturated $(NH_4)_2SO_4$ solution

Add 750 g of ammonium sulphate to 1000 ml of water in a beaker or flask. Simply stir the solution at room temperature with a magnetic stirrer for 15 minutes or until saturation. Gently decant the clear supernatant solution after the undissolved solids settle on the bottom of the flask. (Filtration is not really necessary).

Procedure

Purification of haemoglobin

- Record the absorbance of the haemoglobin solution at the wavelength of 577 nm. This measurement is to be used in the calculation of the recovery of the protein.
- Pipette 4 ml of the haemoglobin solution into a test tube.

- While stirring, add the saturated ammonium sulphate solution drop-wise to the protein solution using a burette until precipitates start to form. It is critical to avoid the spatial nonuniformity in the salt concentration during the addition of the salt solution. Localized concentration hot spots will prematurely initiate the precipitation of other proteins and inadvertently affect the purity of the protein crystals.
- Record the volume of the saturated ammonium sulphate solution needed to cause precipitation. One should keep in mind that protein precipitation is not instantaneous and may require 15 to 20 minutes to equilibrate.
- Centrifuge the mixture at 10,000g for 15 minutes.
- Collect the precipitate by carefully discarding as much supernatant as possible.
- Reconstitute the pelleted haemoglobin by resuspending the precipitate and making the volume to 4 ml with water. For effective recovery of protein, water should be added in small aliquots.
- Measure the absorbance of the reconstituted haemoglobin solution with a spectrophotometer.

Purification of fungal α-amylase

- Instead of haemoglobin solution, use 4 ml of 1% of fungal α-amylase.
- Salt-out the enzyme with a saturated ammonium sulphate solution as described previously.
- Record the volume of the saturated salt solution added.
- Collect the protein precipitates. Avoid the dilution of the enzyme solution too much. Filtration through a syringe filter unit may be conveniently employed if the crystals are not too small and if the collected crystals can be easily washed off the filter paper. Usually the quantitative analysis of the activity of the enzyme collected with the filtration method is not as accurate as the centrifugation method.
- After resuspending the proteins, analyze the enzyme activity.

Purification of protease

- Instead of haemoglobin solution, 4 ml of saturated protease is used. Note that protease may not be totally soluble, and supernatant can be obtained by centrifugation.

Notes

To assure the maximum yield and to avoid unnecessary denaturation of the enzymes, most of the protein purification work is usually carried out at low temperatures, i.e. between 0 and 40°C. However, it is simply far more convenient to work in a regular laboratory room as opposed to a cold room.

The recovery of protein can have significant economical implications. Because a fixed fraction of the original protein stays soluble in the solution, the recovery of protein is often not near 100%. Of course, a yield of over 100% indicates that there may be problems associated with the assay method.

PROTOCOL 7.2

ENZYME IMMOBILIZATION IN POLYACRYLAMIDE GEL

Principle

Three easily available media for enzyme immobilization are polyacrylamide, calcium alginate, and gelatin. All these gels are easy to form and require simple set of equipment. To immobilize the enzyme, enzymes are well mixed with monomers/polymers and cross-linking agents in a solution. The solution is then exposed to polymerization promoters to start the process of gel formation. The solution is poured into a mould to achieve the desired shapes. A gel block may be cut into smaller cubes to increase the surface area. To form spherical beads the unpolymerized solution is forced through a set of nozzles. In such set of preparation adjusting the backpressure applied can easily control size. The resulting beads may be further hardened to enhance structural integrity. In summary, the efficiency of an immobilization process can be measured on following parameters. Most important of all, the percentage of the enzymes initially retained in gel matrices. Secondly, the enzyme activity must be intact during and after immobilization and thirdly, the enzymes must be released by diffusing back into the substrate solution at a later time. Other important parameter is the uniformity of the enzyme dispersion in the gel matrix.

Polyacrylamide is the most widely used matrix for entrapping enzymes. It has the advantage that it is non-ionic. The consequence is that the properties of the enzymes are only minimally modified in the presence of the gel matrix. At the same time, the diffusion of the charged substrate and products is not affected. However, dimethylaminopropionitrile, the polymerization initiator, is highly toxic and must be handled with great care. The requirement to purge the monomer solution with nitrogen is also troublesome, although not totally crippling. This technique is based on the polymerization of acrylamide with N,N'-methylene-bis-acrylamide (Bis) as the cross-linking agent. The degree of cross-linking, thus, can be partly controlled by adjusting the ratio of acrylamide to Bis used.

Equipment

Beakers, Pipettes, Balance, Graduated cylinder, Syringe and needle

Materials

Buffered monomer solution
- 0.1 mM EDTA
- 0.1 M Tris-HCl
- 1.1% N,N'-Methylene-bis-acrylamide and
- 20% Acrylamide
- Adjust the pH to 7.0

Washing solution
- 0.5 M NaCl
- 0.1 mM EDTA
- 0.1M Tris-HCl
- Adjust the pH to 7.0

Dimethylaminopropionitrile (polymerization initiator)

Potassium persulphate solution, 1% (polymerization catalyst)
Nitrogen gas cylinder
Enzyme

Procedure

- Prepare buffered monomer solution by adding 1.1 g of Bis and 20 g of acrylamide to a 100 ml of buffered solution (pH 7.0) of 0.1 mM EDTA and 0.1 M Tris-HCl in a beaker. (The pH of the buffer should be adjusted to match the optimum value of the enzyme to be entrapped).
- To 10 ml of the buffered monomer solution of the above step, add enzyme powders (approximately 0.1 ml of 7.5% fungal amylase or an equivalent concentrated enzyme solution) and mix.
- For 20 minutes, purge the dissolved oxygen in the solution that can interfere with the polymerization process with nitrogen. This step is critical in achieving a high degree of cross-linking. Add 0.1 ml of dimethylaminopropionitrile and mix. Add 1.0 ml of freshly prepared 10% potassium persulphate solution to initiate polymerization.
- Now is the time to pour the solution into a mould if one does not desire the gel to form in the original beaker. Leave the solution undisturbed and approximately 10-30 minutes later gel will form. Hardening can be accelerated by using more dimethylaminopropionitrile.
- Cut the resulting gel into small cubes of approximately 3 mm per side. Alternatively, if smaller pieces are desired, the gel can be forced through a syringe fitted with a fine needle.
- Gently wash the free enzyme off the gel surface in 10 ml of the washing solution. Repeat the washing process for two additional times.

Notes

The above methods of enzyme immobilization by gel entrapment can be directly applied to live cells with minor modifications. For example, dimethylaminopropionitrile used in forming the polyacrylamide gel may not be employed because of its toxicity to viable cells. The monomers of acrylamide are also somewhat toxic to cells. On the other hand, cells can be immobilized with much less degree of cross-linking due to its much larger size.

PROTOCOL 7.3

ENZYME IMMOBILIZATION IN ALGINATE GEL

Principle

Alginate, commercially available as alginic acid sodium salt, commonly called sodium alginate, is a linear polysaccharide normally isolated from many strains of marine brown seaweed and algae, thus the name alginate. The copolymer consists of two uronic acids: D-mannuronic acid (M) and L-guluronic acid (G). Because it is the skeletal component of the algae it has the property of being strong and yet flexible. Alginic acid can be either water soluble or insoluble depending on the type of the associated salt. The salts of sodium, other alkali metals, and ammonia are soluble, whereas the salts of polyvalent cations, e.g., calcium, are water insoluble, with the exception of magnesium. Polyvalent cations bind to the polymer whenever there are two neighbouring guluronic acid residues. Thus, polyvalent cations are responsible for the cross-linking of both different polymer molecules and different parts of the same polymer chain. The process of gelation, simply the exchange of calcium ions for sodium ions, is carried out under relatively mild conditions. Because the method is based on the availability of guluronic acid residues, which will not vary once given a batch of the alginate, the molecular permeability does not depend on the immobilization conditions. Rather, the pore size is controlled by the choice of the starting material.

$$2\ \text{Na(Alginate)} + \text{Ca}^{++} \longrightarrow \text{Ca(Alginate)}_2 + 2\ \text{Na}^{+}$$

The ionically linked gel structure is thermostable over the range of 0-100ºC; therefore heating will not liquefy the gel. However, the gel can be easily redissolved by immersing the alginate gel in a solution containing a high concentration of sodium, potassium, or magnesium. Maintaining a ratio of sodium:calcium smaller or equal to 25:1 will help avoid gel destabilization. In fact, it is recommended to include 3 mM calcium ions in the substrate medium. On the other hand, citrate or phosphate pH buffers cannot be effectively used without destabilizing the alginate gel. Alginate is currently widely used in food, pharmaceutical, textile, and paper products. The properties of alginate utilized in these products are thickening, stabilizing, gel-forming, and film-forming. Alginate polymers isolated from different alginate sources vary in properties. Different algae, or for that matter different part of the same algae, yield alginate of different monomer composition and arrangement. There may be sections of homopolymeric blocks of only one type of monomer (-M-M-M-) (-G-G-G-), or there may be sections of alternating monomers (-M-G-M-G-M-). Different types of alginate are selected for each application on the basis of the molecular weight and the relative composition of mannuronic and guluronic acids. For example, the thickening function (viscosity property) depends mainly on the molecular weight of the polymer; whereas, gelation (affinity for cation) is closely related to the guluronic acid content. Thus, high guluronic acid content results in a stronger gel.

Equipments

Beakers, Graduated cylinder, Balance, Pipettes, Syringe

Materials

Sodium alginate
Sodium salt
Calcium chloride ($CaCl_2$)
Enzyme

Procedure

- Dissolve 30 g of sodium alginate in 1 litre to make a 3% w/v solution.
- Mix approximately 0.015 g of enzyme with 10 ml of 3% w/v sodium alginate solution. The concentration of sodium alginate can be varied between 6-12% w/v depending on the desired hardness.
- The beads are formed by dripping the polymer solution from a height of approximately 20 cm into an excess (100 ml) of stirred 0.2 M $CaCl_2$ solution with a syringe and a needle at room temperature.

- The bead size can be controlled by pump pressure and the needle gauge. A typical hypodermic needle produces beads of 0.5-2 mm in diameter. Other shapes can be obtained by using a mould whose wall is permeable to calcium ions. Leave the beads in the calcium solution to cure for 0.5-3 hours.

Notes

Sodium alginate solution is best prepared by adding the powder to agitated water, rather than vice versa, to avoid the formation of clumps. Prolonged stirring may be necessary to achieve the complete dissolution of sodium alginate. After sodium alginate is completely dissolved, leave the solution undisturbed for 30 minutes to eliminate the air bubbles that can later be entrapped and cause the beads to float.

PROTOCOL 7.4

ENZYME IMMOBILIZATION IN GELATIN GEL

Principle

The main attraction of using gelatin as the immobilization media is that the gel formation process requires only simple equipment and that the reagents are relatively inexpensive and nontoxic. The retention of enzymatic activities for immobilization with a gelatin gel is typically 25-50% of the original free enzyme. Gelatin gel has the advantage that the mass transfer resistance is relatively low compared to other entrapment methods, but the rate of enzyme loss due to leakage is high. The process essentially involves hardening of gel to provide structural strength.

Equipments

Beakers, Graduated cylinder, Pipettes, Constant temperature bath, Freezer

Materials

Gelatin Solution (10% w/v)

Hardening solution

- 20% v/v Formaldehyde
- 50% v/v Ethanol
- 30% v/v Water

Enzyme Extract

Procedure

- Dissolve 10 g gelatin in 100 ml of water to prepare a 10% w/v aqueous solution. Heating the solution gently to facilitate the dissolution process. Adjust the temperature of the gelatin solution to 35-40ºC. The temperature is kept relatively high so that the gelatin solution is not too viscous, but not so high as to cause enzyme denaturation.
- Add approximately 0.015g of the enzyme powder to 10 ml of the gelatin solution. Add 2 ml of the hardening solution to the mixture. Pour the solution into a mould or a small beaker.

- Freeze at –28°C for 4 hours to facilitate the gel formation. If this temperature is not readily available, a regular freezer will also suffice for the purpose of demonstrating the technique.
- When the gel is set, warm the gel to room temperature simply by leaving it on a lab bench. Cut the gel into small cubes of approximately 3 mm per side. Gently wash the gel liberally with deionized water.

PROTOCOL 7.5

IMMOBILIZATION OF ENZYMES IN GELATIN MOULDS

Materials

Essentially the same procedure can be employed for enzymes except that it is preferable to mix gelatin and hardening solution first and within 1 minute to add the appropriate volume of enzyme solution. This has the advantage of reducing the exposure of enzyme to formaldehyde rendering it a more active preparation.

Cylindrical Moulds

A cylindrical mould is constructed of two Plexiglass slabs (1 x 5 x 10 cm) which are held together by two binder clips and have a 9 cm deep hollow (0.8 cm diameter) depression between them. More simply, cylindrical mould can also be constructed from a disposable hypodermic syringe with the needle end of the barrel cut off squarely. Of course, the size of the resulting gelatin cylinder is determined by the sectional area of the syringe and by the position of the plunger, which can be used for removing the hardened gelatin from the syringe barrel.

Spherical beads

The gelatin mixture prepared as described above instead of being poured into a mould, is added dropwise by means of a pipette or syringe to a large volume (at least 10 fold larger) of a tetra-chloroethylene/cyclohexane mixture (1:9 v/v) in a tall beaker or Erlenmeyer flask at –25°C. Beads thus formed are kept overnight under these conditions, then are collected from the solvent mixture (e.g. on a sintered glass filter), abundantly washed with tap water, and stored in a refrigerator.

Flat membrane

Using a flat glass plate having a 10x10 cm square etched with a glass pencil, 10 ml of the gelatin mixture is spread as uniformly as possible between the limits of the square. The glass plate is quickly put into a deep freezer and after at least 4 hours is gradually brought to room temperature. The thin membrane thus formed, once removed from the glass plate, is thoroughly rinsed with tap water and stored in a refrigerator under the same conditions.

Assay of Gelatin Immobilized Biocatalysts

The catalytic activity of gelatin immobilized enzyme or microbial cells is usually measured at 30°C by suspending a number of disks, beads, or other shaped particles in the buffered substrate solution within a miniaturized stirred batch reactor. This consists of a thermostated glass vessel (~70 ml) equipped with a specially designed polyvinyl chloride (PVC) cover with a magnetic stirrer assembly. At fixed time intervals, stirring is interrupted and samples from the supernatant phase are withdrawn and assayed for the reaction product. The total volume of the samples should not exceed 1% of the reaction volume.

A reaction curve is then plotted and the slope is measured at the origin; thus the catalytic activity and the apparent specific activity may be calculated. Towards the end of the activity assay, the immobilized phase is removed from the miniaturized reactor while the sampling of the supernatant phase is continued for at least 1 hour or less depending on the reaction rate. If no further increase in the product concentration is observed, enzyme or cell leakage from the gelatin matrix can be excluded. Then the activity yield can be calculated as the ratio of the activity of the immobilized phase to that of the corresponding free enzyme or cells before being immobilized.

PROTOCOL 7.6

CELL IMMOBILIZATION IN AGAROSE

Principle

Agarose is a linear, neutral polysaccharide isolated from marine red algae. It is basically composed of a repeating agarobios unit consisting of alternating 1,3-linked 3,6-anhydro-L-galactopyranose. This polymer shows hysteresis, which means that it dissolves in water at a higher temperature than the gel forming temperature. The gelling temperature may be influenced by chemical modification of the polymer (introduction of hydroxyethyl groups). The gel formed is noncharged, porous, resistant towards bacterial degradation, and does not require counter ions for stability. Different agarose qualities with gelling temperature down to 15°C are commercially available. Normally agarose preparations with a gelling temperature between 28 and 40°C are employed for the immobilization of microbial and plant cells.

Procedure

- An agarose solution (2.5% w/w, 8 ml) equilibrated at 40°C is mixed with cells (2 g fresh weight plant cells or 2 ml microbial suspension).
- The mixture is dispersed by mechanical stirring in vegetable oil (40 ml) also equilibrated at 40°C. When droplets of appropriate size (0.5-1.0 mm) have been formed, put the mixture on an ice-bath under continuous stirring until the agarose beads have solidified (15°C).
- Culture medium or buffer is added and are allowed to sediment by gravity or gentle centrifugation into the aqueous phase. The oil and most of the aqueous phase is removed by the use of an aspirator and the beads are resuspended in medium or buffer, which is subsequently removed. This procedure is repeated until the bead preparation is free from the organic phase.

Notes

When sterile preparations are required, the agarose solution and the vegetable oil are sterilized at 121°C for 20 minutes. Different agarose preparations are available with gelling temperatures of 15, 30, 36 and 42°C. These temperatures are the dynamic gelling temperatures obtained when a solution is cooled at a constant rate. For the gelling temperature of 36°C one has to equilibrate the agarose solution at 45°C when using it for immobilization.

Depending on the desirable mechanical strength, a final agarose concentration of 1 to 4% (w/v) is chosen depending on the preparation. Chemically modified agarose preparations require a higher polymer concentration than unmodified preparations to achieve certain mechanical stability.

The agarose is usually dissolved in a buffer or culture medium if this is autoclavable. In most of the cases it is not necessary to dissolve the polymer before autoclaving.

Agarose and hydrophobic phases are equilibrated 5-10°C above gelling temperature before the beads are prepared. The dispersion is cooled to at least 10°C below the gelling temperature.

The size of the beads is to some extent dependent on the cell preparation. For microorganisms (e.g., yeast and bacteria) a bead size of 0.1-0.2 mm is suitable, while for large plant cells which usually grow in aggregates a size of 0.5-1.0 mm is more appropriate. Beads down to 1-10 μm can be produced by applying ultrasonication for dispersion.

PROTOCOL 7.7

CELL IMMOBILIZATION WITH CALCIUM ALGINATE

Principle

Calcium alginate is just as widely used as polyacrylamide. Unlike polyacrylamide gels, gelation of calcium alginate does not depend on the formation of more permanent covalent bonds between polymer chains. Rather, polymer molecules are cross-linked by calcium ions. Because of this, calcium alginate beads can be formed in extremely mild conditions, which ensure the integrity of cell in the matrix. However, just as easily as calcium ions can be exchanged for sodium ions, they can also be displaced by other ions. This property can both be advantageous and disadvantageous. If needed, enzymes or microbial cells can be easily recovered by dissolving the gel in a sodium solution.

On the other hand, proper caution must be exercised to ensure that the substrate solution does not contain high concentrations of those ions that can disintegrate the gel. This experiment is to investigate the conversion of glucose to ethanol by entrapped yeast cells in a continuous reactor. Yeast cells are entrapped in calcium alginate gels by using the similar techniques as in enzyme immobilization. Other cell entrapment media that have been previously attempted include polyacrylamide, gelatin, chitosan, and k-carrageenan gels. Due to the constraint in the available equipment to carry out the immobilization procedure aseptically, the experiment will be conducted without autoclaving. The immobilized cell reactor will be employed to convert glucose into ethanol anaerobically. The reasons for choosing this system of microorganism and product are many folds. First, the anaerobic condition will eliminate the need for aeration, which causes many technical problems. Secondly, the lack of oxygen will prevent the uncontrolled growth of aerobic contaminants in an unsterilized fermenter. The presence of high levels of ethanol should also discourage most microorganisms from taking over the fermenter. To reduce further the chance of contamination by bacteria, the pH of the fermenter will be kept low; a value of 4.0 should drastically slow down the growth of most bacteria but only slightly affect the yeast's ethanol producing capacity. The production of ethanol in an immobilized bioreactor is a relatively well studied process. As high as 95% of the theoretical yield of alcohol based on glucose (8.5% ethanol from 14% glucose) has been reported. A high space velocity (the volume of nutrient feed per hour per gel volume), of 0.4-0.5 per hour is commonly used to maximize the ethanol productivity. An ethanol productivity of 20 g/l per hours can be achieved. Both the steady state response and the transient approach to the steady state will be studied in this experiment.

Equipment

Beakers, Graduated cylinder, Balance, Pipettes, Magnetic stirrer, Syringe and needle, Spectrophotometer with flow through cell, pH probe and controller, Microcomputer with data acquisition capabilities.

Materials

Sodium alginate
Calcium chloride
Yeast culture
Ammonium hydroxide
Reagents for glucose analysis
Reagents for ethanol analysis
Growth medium for yeast
 1% yeast extract
 2% peptone
 Autoclave and after autoclaving, add 100 ml of 20% glucose solution to medium.

Procedures

Immobilized cell preparation

Dissolve 9 g of sodium alginate in 300 ml of growth medium, following the same procedure adopted in enzyme immobilization to avoid clump formation. Stir until all sodium alginate is completely dissolved. The final solution contains 3% alginate by weight.

- Thoroughly suspend about 250 g of wet cells in the alginate solution prepared in the previous step. Let air bubbles escape (*see notes*).
- Drip the yeast-alginate mixture from a height of 20 cm into 1000 ml of crosslinking solution. (The cross-linking solution is prepared by adding an additional 0.05 M of $CaCl_2$ to the growth media. The calcium cross-linking solution is agitated on a magnetic stirrer. Gel formation can be achieved at room temperature as soon as the sodium alginate drops come in direct contact with the calcium solution. Relatively small alginate beads are preferred to minimize the mass transfer resistance. A diameter of 0.5-2 mm can be readily achieved with a syringe and a needle. The beads should fully harden in 1-2 hours. Note that the concentration of the $CaCl_2$ is about one fourth of the strength used for enzyme immobilization.
- Wash the beads with a fresh calcium cross-linking solution.

Immobilized cell reactor

A microcomputer will be programmed to take data on the glucose concentration and the rate of NH_4OH addition needed to maintain the pH at 4.0. The off-line samples will be analyzed for the optical density (for free cell concentration), glucose concentration, and ethanol concentration. Furthermore, the liquid and gas flow rate will be measured with a graduated cylinder.

- The reactor operates in a batch manner until no more glucose is utilized. This can be detected with the leveling off in the glucose concentration. Substrate feeding is then commenced at the rate of 0.4/hour.
- Record the substrate flow rate. The approach to the first steady state during the start-up can be followed. Various parameters (nitrogen consumption rate, carbon dioxide evolution rate, glucose concentration, ethanol concentration, and free cell level) at the high steady state are recorded. Decrease the substrate feeding rate to 0.2% per hour. Measure the substrate flow rate and follow the transient approach to the new low steady state.
- Record again the various parameters (nitrogen consumption rate, carbon dioxide evolution rate, glucose concentration, ethanol concentration, and free cell level) for the new steady state.

Immobilized cell reactor construction

- Construct an immobilized cell reactor fitted with a 500 ml Erlenmeyer flask. Place the hardened beads in the flask and seal it with a rubber stopper with appropriate hose connections.
- Make all necessary connections and fill the flask with the growth media (10% glucose) to the working volume of 350 ml.

Notes

Because cell growth can break the bead and is generally considered undesirable beyond what is needed to compensate for the endogenous decay, the cells used for immobilization ideally should have just entered the stationary phase. An equivalent amount of dried cell culture may also be used in lieu of wet cell paste. The actual cell loading may be varied according to the substrate concentration in the feed and the desired product levels. The ratio of wet weight to dry weight is approximately 4 for most cells. If time permits, continue shifting the flow rate and obtain more information on steady states. Continue operating the bioreactor until noticeable deterioration in the performance is detected due to gel swelling, cell death, or severe contamination.

PROTOCOL 7.8

PREPARATION OF CELL IMMOBILIZED CALCIUM ALGINATE BEADS

Preparation of Sodium Alginate Solution

Sodium alginate is freely soluble in distilled or deionized water at room temperature (25°C). To avoid the formation of lumps a high shear mixer is employed. The concentration of sodium alginate employed can be varied from 0.5% w/v to 8% w/v or higher if lower viscosity types of alginate are used. If some additional solute such as sucrose (as osmoticum), has to be included in sodium alginate solution, dry mixing of it with the alginate enhances the dissolution of the latter.

Dispersion of Cells in Sodium Alginate Solution

Cells to be entrapped are first centrifuged to convert them in the form of a paste or cream of material concentrate. For the entrapment of yeast cells it is satisfactory to stir 5 g of cell paste into 15 ml of 1% w/v sodium alginate using a pastle mortar or magnetic stirrer operated very gently. However, for the entrapment of bacteria it is most satisfactory to suspend cells at a concentration of 20% w/v fresh in a 5% w/v sodium alginate aqueous solution.

Bead Formation

The suspension of cells in sodium alginate is passed drop wise into a solution of a calcium salt (0.1 M) that may contain an osmoticum such as sucrose, glucose, or sorbitol. On a laboratory scale syringe with an outlet diameter of about 1 mm can be used. On a larger scale a single channel peristaltic pump with tube diameter about 1 mm may be used. The beads should be left in the calcium bath for at least 20 minutes and preferably for 1 hour to allow gelation of the beads to occur.

PROTOCOL 7.9

IMMOBILIZATION OF MICROBIAL CELLS IN GELATIN

Equipment

Cylindrical moulds, Desiccator, Refrigerator

Materials

Deionized water
Ethanol
Silica Gel
Gelatin
Formaldehyde
Microbial Cells

Procedure

- Microbial cells are suspended in deionized water and dispersed in a 10% w/v gelatin-aqueous solution at 35-40°C to give a final cell to gelatin ratio of 1:10 on a dry weight basis.
- To 9.5 ml of this dispersion, 0.5 ml of a hardening solution consisting of 20% w/v formaldehyde in 50% v/v ethanol is added. The mixture is poured into a cylindrical mould (0.8 cm diameter) and kept in a deep freezer (about –25°C).
- After at least gelatin cylinder obtained is thoroughly rinsed with tap water, kept over night in a large volume of deionized water at refrigerator temperature (4-5°C), and then cut into

thin disks (0.2-04 cm). The gel disks can be stored refrigerated for months without any appreciable loss of enzyme activity (e.g., yeast cell invertase), either wet in deionized water containing a proper preservative or dry in a desiccator over silica gel.

PROTOCOL 7.10

YEAST CELL IMMOBILIZATION ON WOOD CHIPS

Culture Conditions

Strain *Saccharomyces cerevisiae* is used for the study. The culture is maintained on malt extract-yeast extract-glucose-peptone slants. Prior to experimental use, cells are grown aerobically for 24 hours in an environmental incubator maintained at 30°C in 250 ml Erlenmeyer flasks each containing 100 ml of yeast medium containing 10 g/l glucose, 5 g/l peptone, 3 g/l yeast extract and 3 g/l malt extract. The pH of the yeast medium is adjusted to about 5.0 prior to sterilization in a Barnstead autoclave at 121°C. The concentration of cells is increased to 5-15 g dry weight cells per litre by batch centrifugation. The concentration of suspended cells may be measured either by turbidimetry or by a gravimetric method. The turbidimetric method involves measurement of the optical density with a spectrophotometer while the gravimetric method involves filtration with Millipore filter (pore size 4.5×10^{-7} m).

Column Design and Support

The packed bed reactor used for the immobilization studies consisted of a jacketed glass column 80 cm in height and 4.7 cm internal diameter during immobilization, a concentrated cell suspension (5 to 15 g/l) is circulated from a surge tank through the packing of wood chips in an upflow mode of operation. The surge tank is equipped with a temperature indicator controller by which means the contents are maintained at the desired test temperature. The column reactor, together with the support material and connecting tubes, is presterilized in an autoclave at 121°C for 30 minutes. The cell suspension in the surge tank was pumped with a precalibrated Sigma motor pump at a constant flow rate through a latex tubing 6.35 mm in diameter to the bottom of the packed column and upward through the column. The effluent from the top of the packing is then recycled to the surge tank. Cell loading is determined as follows. The column is packed with the support particles of known dimension and together with the connecting tubings, are sterilized at 121°C for 30 minutes. After allowing the packed column to cool to room temperature, immobilization of the column for a period of 10-12 hours at a superficial velocity of about 1.7×10^{-4} m/second. The column is then washed by the passage of 0.1% w/v glucose solution through the column in order to remove the nonadsorbed cells from the column. The optical density of the effluent is then monitored to determine when nonadsorbed cells become eluted from the column. The liquid flow velocity is then increased to 1.0×10^{-2} m/second in order to strip off any adsorbed cells held by the support. This velocity is maintained until the determined dry weight of the support is completely loaded with cells.

The above procedure may be repeated for various support particles sizes and for different pH values and temperature.

Factors Influencing the Adsorption of Yeast Cells

Initial culture concentration

A major factor influencing the quality of cells adsorbed onto the support particles is the initial cell concentration used during the immobilization process. This factor may be related, to surface area presented by the support particles. The immobilization is generally more successful when relatively high initial cell concentrations are employed.

Support size and time

A finite time is required to establish the adsorption process. The effect of particle size is related to the specific surface area available for adsorption. The smaller the particles size, the greater would be the specific surface area.

PROTOCOL 7.11

IMMOBILIZATION OF MICROBIAL CELLS BY ADSORPTION TO SOLID SUPPORTS

Culture Conditions

Saccharomyces uvarum cells from a strain used in the brewing industry could be cultivated in a liquid Sabouraud medium at 30°C and without stirring in Erlenmeyer flasks. The cells are harvested either in active growth phase or 48 hours after all activity is ceased by centrifugation at 4°C for 10 minutes at 3000g. They are then washed thrice resuspending in a buffer solution.

Supports

Porous Brick (Used for the preparation of bacterial filters, this support is in the form of cylindrical pellets, 1 mm in diameter and 2 to 3 mm in length. Pore size is between 0.5 and 6 μm, with an average value of 4.5 μm) and porous silica (In the form of beads between 100 and 200 μm in diameter. Supports with pore diameters of 7 to 550 nm for respective specific areas of 445 to 6 m^2/g are available.)

Procedure

The *S. uvarum* cells are suspended in 100 ml of buffer solution (pH 3.0) [sodium citrate phosphate 0.1 M (pH 5.0), sodium phosphate 0.1 M (pH 8.0), sodium pyrophosphate 0.1 M] and percolated through a bed consisted either of 15 g of silica or 16 g of brick in a glass column 20 cm long and 1.5 cm in diameter. The cell suspension is recirculated at 25°C by a pump and samples are periodically taken. Determination of the number of the residual cells in the solution allows the number of cells retained on the support to be calculated at any given moment.

This calculation is performed using a Coulter Counter device allowing the numeration of the particles suspended in the liquid. A Coulter Channelyser type C1000, used in conjunction with this counter, gives the size distribution of the particles counted. Myuneration was performed using a 70 μm orifice probe using 0.25 ml of suspension for 80 ml of electrolyte solution (NaCl, 0.9%) filter twice in a 0.22 μm millipore membrane. The apparatus is calibrated using a monodisperse suspension (2.01 μm) distributed by using coultronics.

PROTOCOL 7.12

ETHANOL PRODUCTION BY IMMOBILIZED YEAST CELL

Principle

Fermentation using the substrates has shown excellent fermentation rates and reactor stability. Other potential advantages include a relatively high productivity, a much lower effluent cell yield compared to free suspension culture and a lower susceptibility to process upsets. The high productivity obtained suggested that capital cost for the reactors may be reduced.

For the fermentation studies a two stage packed bed bioreactor, 6 cm in diameter and 2.15 m in height, was used as a cost-effective means of fermenting glucose and molasses substrates to ethanol. For initial glucose concentration in the range 22-26%, ethanol productivity in the range 2.1-2.8% per hour and affluent ethanol concentrations of 8-11.8%, respectively, were obtained at 30°C. Similar ethanol productivity was obtained with molasses substrate for effluent ethanol concentrations of 5-8.3%. The ethanol productivity obtained with the surface immobilized yeast cell bioreactor are either comparable to or higher than those previously reported for adsorbed cell systems and generally are higher (20-80%) than productivity reported for entrapped cell systems.

The potential of packed bed bioreactor designs comparable to the performance reported for stirred tank fermenters employed cell recycling. However, the packed bed bioreactor system possesses several economic and operational advantages compared to a stirred tank. With cell recycle the former is much less subject to process upsets and requires less complex piping and control systems and less power input.

Procedure

Follow the similar procedure as given in alcohol production by using yeast cells (refer protocol 4.4). Use immobilized and non immobilized yeast cells and compare the productivity rate.

PROTOCOL 7.13

PREPARATION OF GLUCOSE DETECTOR

Principle

Doctors commonly use highly specific test strips, for detection of glucose in urine or in blood. All of these tests utilize the enzyme glucose oxidase and peroxidase, immobilized on a paper pad (test strips). The pad is covered with a thin cellulose membrane, which is permeable only to small molecules such as glucose. In the presence of oxygen and glucose, the products of the enzyme activity react with a chemical to produce a colour change. The intensity of the colour developed indicates the glucose concentration (Fig. 7.4).

The principles behind these diagnostics can be demonstrated, using potassium iodide as the chromogen (colour change reagent). Different sugars can be used to indicate the specificity of the reaction catalyzed by glucose oxidase. Chemical reaction steps of glucose detector strips are as follows :

- Glucose oxidase acts specifically on glucose to give hydrogen peroxide and gluconic acid

$$\beta\text{-D- glucose} + \text{Oxygen} + \text{Water} \longrightarrow \text{Hydrogen peroxide} + \delta\text{-Gluconolactone}$$

$$\delta\text{-Gluconolactone} \downarrow \text{Gluconic acid}$$

- Horseradish peroxidase then catalyzes the reaction of hydrogen peroxide with potassium iodide. The colourless iodide is oxidized to brown iodine

$$\text{Hydrogen peroxide} + \text{Potassium iodide} \longrightarrow \text{Iodine} + \text{water}$$

Materials

Thick filter paper or blotting paper
2% potassium iodide solution
Glucose oxidase / Horseradish peroxidase mixture
Fermcozyme 952 DM
Glucose solution
Fructose solution
Sucrose solution

Procedure

- Cut out a small square of filter paper, roughly 10 x 10 mm.
- Place a drop of potassium iodide solution on the paper.
- Allow it to dry slightly.
- Add a drop of the enzyme mixture to the paper.
- Add a drop of a sugar solution to the paper.
- Note the colour change.
- Compare the colour with the standard to find out glucose concentration in the sample.

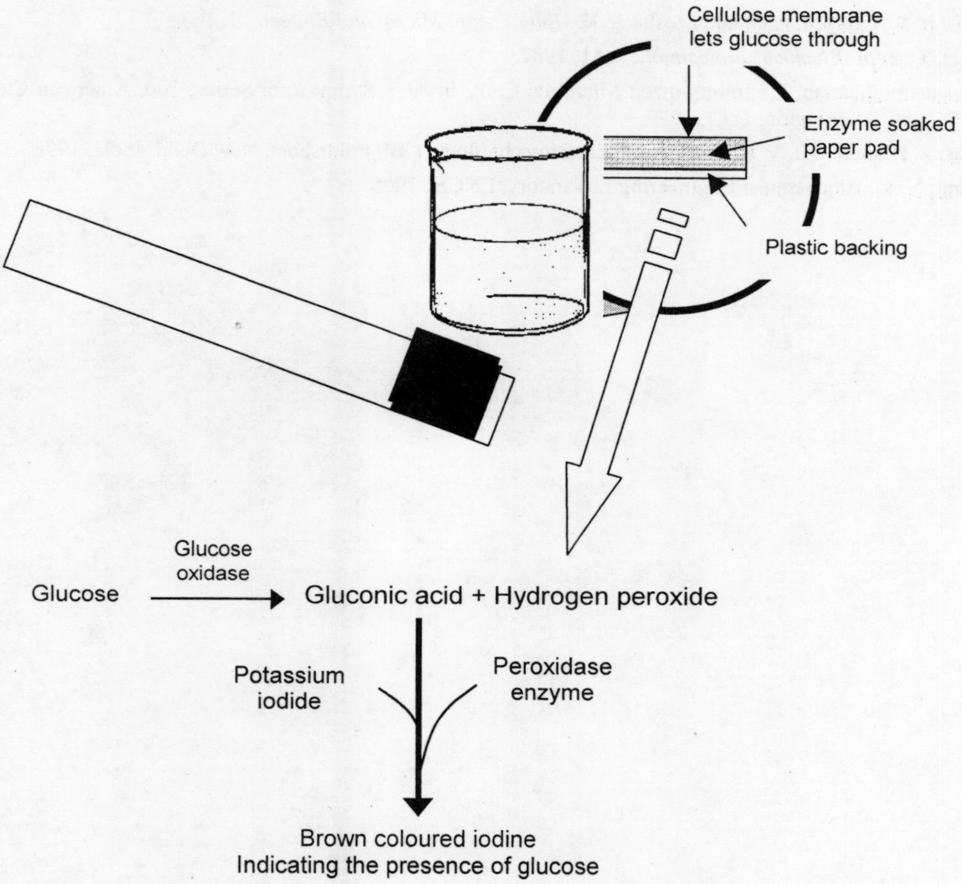

Fig. 7.4. Schematic diagram showing glucose detector and the basic reaction

SUGGESTED READINGS

Alteris, E. D., Parascandola, P., Salvadore, S. and Sardi, V., *J. Chem. Tech. Biotech*, 35B, 60, 1985.

Hagashima, M., Azuma, M. and Haguchi, S., *Annual New York Academy Science*, 413, 457, 1983.

Jayaraman, J., Laboratory Manual in Biochemistry, New Age International Publication, New Delhi, India, 1999.

Lee, J. M. and Woodward, J., *Biotech. Bioeng.*, 25, 2411, 1983.

Lehninger A. L., Nelson, D. L. and Cox, M., Principles of Biochemistry, 2nd Edition, CBS Publishers and Distributors, New Delhi, India, 1993.

M. D. Trevan and S. Grover, *Trans. Biochem. Soc.*, 7, 28, 1979.

Mattison, B., Immobilized Cells and Organelles, Vol. 1 and 2, CRS Press, 1983.

Nagashima, M., Azuma, M., and Noguchi, S., *Ann. N.Y. Acad. Sci.*, 413, 457, 1983.

Ohlson, S., Larsson, P. O. and Mosbach, K., *Eur. J. App. Micro. and Biotech.*, 7, 103.

Vaija, J., *Appl. Biochem. Biotechnol.*, 7, 51, 1982.

Venkatsubramanian, K., Immobilized Microbial Cells, in ACS Symposium Series, 106, American Chemical Society, Washington, D.C., 1979.

Vyas, S. P. and Dixit, V. K, Pharmaceutical Biotechnology, CBS Publishers, New Delhi, India, 1998.

Wang, N. S., Biochemical Engineering Laboratory, ENCH, 1995.

CHAPTER 8

DNA and RNA Isolation

INTRODUCTION

Deoxyribonucleic acid (DNA), genetic material of cell and a very long, thread like macromolecule, is a double helix consisting of antiparallel strands. Each strand of polynucleotide chain consists of purine deoxyribonucleotides of adenine and guanine bases, and the pyrimidine deoxyribonucleotides of cytosine and thymine bases. Uracil is found instead of thymine in Ribonucleic acid (RNA). In DNA, pentose sugar is 2-deoxyribose, whereas in ribonucleic acid, pentose sugar is ribose (Fig. 8.1). A base is linked to sugar is called nucleoside; when a phosphate group is added as the base-sugar-phosphate it is called a nucleotide. The nitrogenous bases are linked to the 1′-carbon atom of deoxyribose residues. They are located perpendicular to the long axis. The two polynucleotide strands in which the nucleotide units linked by 5′-3′ phosphodiester bonds (Fig. 8.2 and 8.3) are joined together by hydrogen bonds between purine and pyrimidine bases. Guanine is linked to cytosine through three hydrogen bonds, and adenine is linked with thymine by two hydrogen bonds. The bases sequence of one strand is complementary to bases sequence of another strand.

In the eukaryotic cells, DNA is found in the nucleus as well as in mitochondria and chloroplast. Chromosomal DNA exists in two forms, heterochromatin and euchromatin. The DNA in heterochromatin is genetically inert as it is tightly coiled whereas euchromatin is more loosely organized and is believed to be the functional genetic material. These are distinguished by their differential ability to accept basic stains. Heterochromatin stains more intensely than euchromatin. DNA fibers can be extracted from wide variety of cultured cells and virus particles. However, the amount of DNA recovered is often limiting, especially with viruses, so that it is necessary to incorporate radioactive atoms into structure of the macromolecule to provide the means for the detection. DNA can be labeled with radioactive ^{14}C, ^{3}H or ^{32}P.

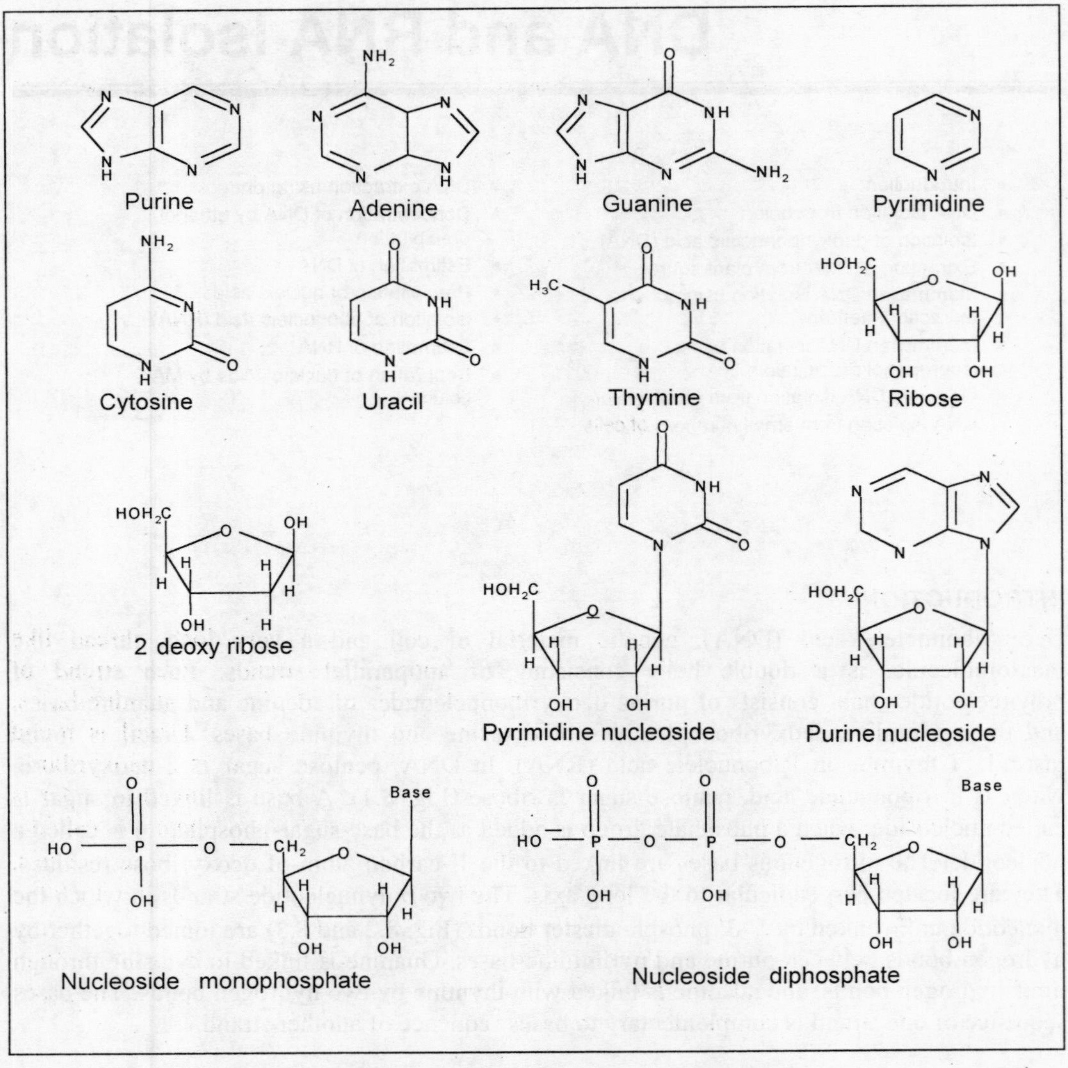

Fig. 8.1. Structure of purine and pyrimidine bases

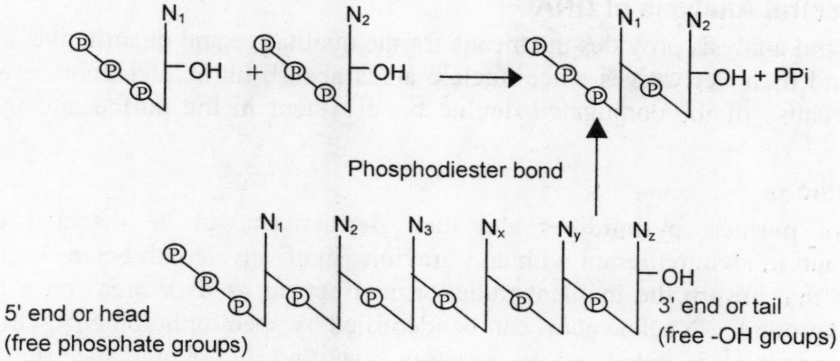

Fig. 8.2. The schematic presentation of nucleic acid assembly

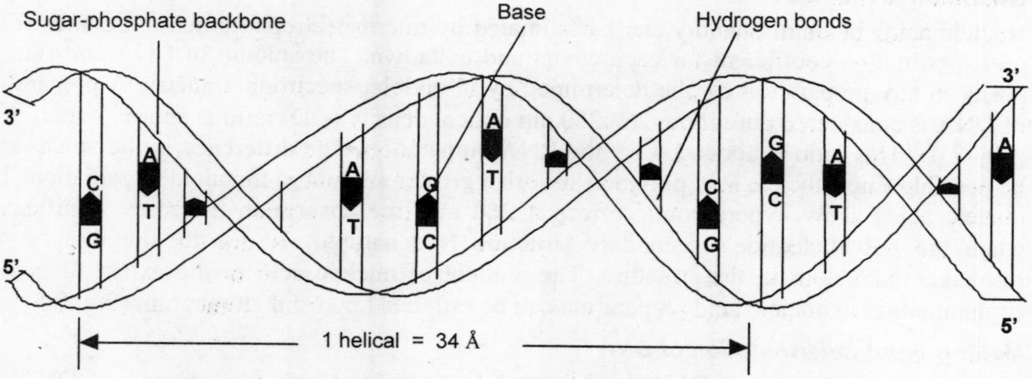

Fig. 8.3. Structure of DNA

Ribonucleic acids are single stranded polynucleotide chains in which nucleotides are linked together through 5′-3′ phosphodiester bonds. Although they are much shorter than DNAs, they are much more abundant in most cells. There are three major classes of RNA namely messenger RNA (mRNA), ribosomal RNA (rRNA) and transfer RNA (tRNA). mRNAs are the information carrying intermediates in protein synthesis, while tRNA and rRNA are part of the protein synthesizing machinery. Ribonucleic acid occurs as ribonucleoprotein in intact cells. RNA molecules can be separated by using different methods like zonal centrifugation method in sucrose gradient, separation in agarose-acrylamide composite gel, affinity column chromatography and phenol method. These methods exploit different physicochemical properties of RNA molecules for selective and successive isolation.

Electron Microscopy of DNA

Electron microscopy can visualize DNA molecules if a basic protein is adsorbed to increase the fibre thickness and the nucleic acid is converted from three dimensional to two dimensional form for complete structure to be located on a single plane. DNA molecules may be spreaded on an artificially prepared protein monolayer on the surface of an aqueous salt solution to accomplish either of prerequisite conditions.

Ultraviolet Spectral Analysis of DNA

Ultraviolet spectral analysis provides the means for the qualitative and quantitative analysis of nucleic acids and their derivatives since nucleic acids absorb ultraviolet light between 220 and 300 nm because of the conjugated double bond system in the purine and pyrimidine bases.

Qualitative methods

The location of purines, pyrimidines and their derivatives can be detected on paper chromatogram and ionophoretogram with an ultraviolet light wavelength between 250 to 290 nm compounds that absorb the incident radiation and appear as dark areas on a light-blue fluorescent background. Nucleic acids can be identified by spectrophotometry. The aqueous solution of compounds is subjected to spectral scan and individual spectrum of each compound can be obtained, which varies characteristically with pH.

Quantitative methods

Nucleic acids in small quantity can be estimated by microspectrophotometric methods if the molar extinction coefficient for each compound is known. The amount of DNA and state of purity in any preparation can be determined by ultraviolet spectrophotometry. A preparation of DNA is considered pure if the 260:280 nm optical density (OD) ratio is approximately 1.85 (Fig. 8.4). This ratio is about 2.0 for the RNA preparation. The difference in the values may be possible since nucleic acid polymers absorb a greater amount of the incident radiation. The nucleic acids show hyperchromic effect at 260 nm (the absorption increases significantly when the polynucleotide's secondary structure is denatured) is due to alteration in the resonance behaviour in the structure. The amount of nucleic acid or the extent of protein contamination in nucleic acid preparation can be estimated by using nomogram (Fig. 8.5).

Melting-point determination of DNA

The bihelical structure of DNA is disrupted by heat in which two strands of DNA are completely separated as hydrogen bonds are broken and the temperature at which the helix is ruptured is referred to as helix-to-coil transition temperature. The melting point is defined as the temperature at the midpoint of the reaction. The separated single DNA strands absorb 40 percent more ultraviolet light at 260 nm than rigid bihelical molecules. This increase in absorption (hyperchromic shift) is used to construct and analyze DNA melting profiles spectrophotometrically.

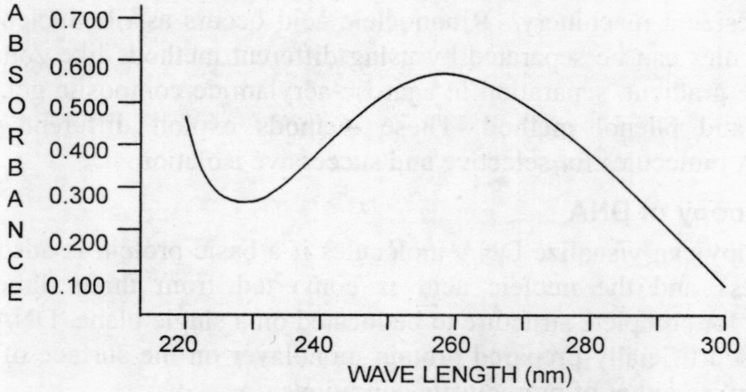

Fig. 8.4. Spectral analysis of purified DNA

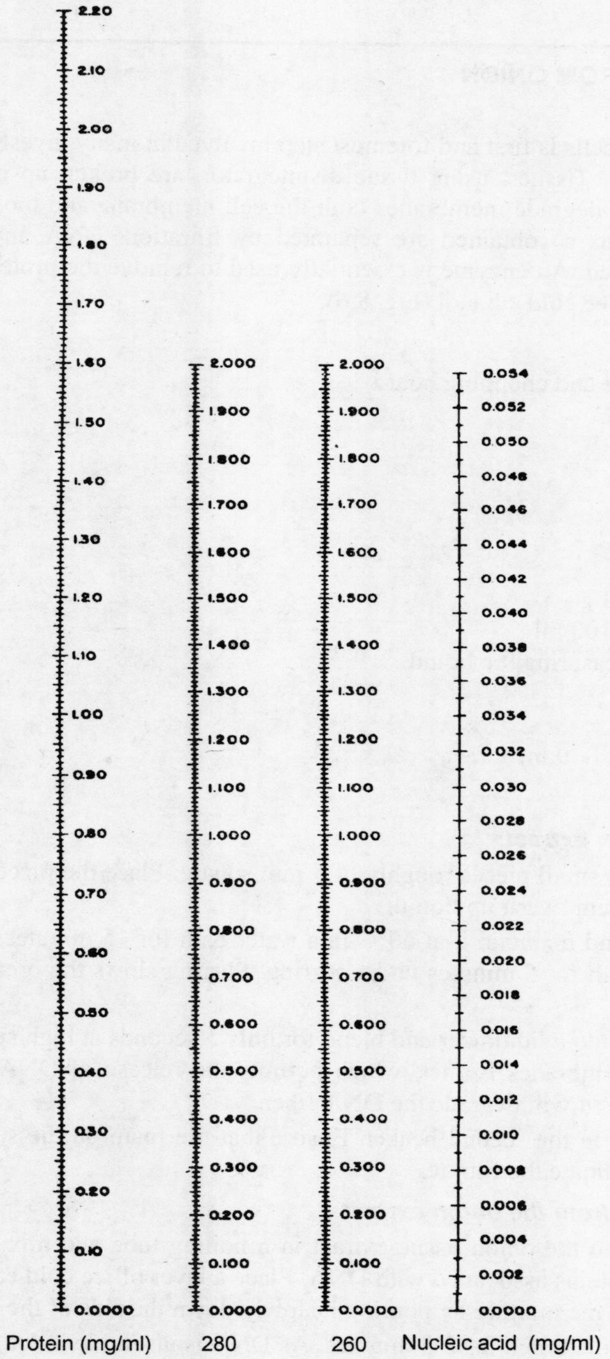

Fig. 8.5. Nomogram to estimate protein contamination in a liquid sample of nucleic acid.

PROTOCOL 8.1

DNA ISOLATION FROM ONION

DNA isolation from cells is first and foremost step involved in many investigations especially in molecular biology. Tissues, using tissue disintegrator, are broken up mechanically, then detergent is added to degrade membranes both the cell membrane and those surrounding the nuclei. Cell fragments so obtained are separated by filtration. DNA and soluble proteins remained, are collected. An enzyme is essentially used to remove the proteins, then the DNA is precipitated using ice cold ethanol (Fig. 8.6).

Materials

Sharp vegetable knife and chopping board
Water bath set at 60°C
Ice
Thermometer
Coffee filter paper
Onion, 100 g
Wash up liquid
  Sodium chloride, 3 g
  Distilled water to 100 ml
10 ml Syringe for measuring the liquid
Onion extract, 6 ml
Protease enzyme
95% Ethanol (Ice cold), 9 ml

Procedure

Preparation of onion extract

- Cut the onion into small pieces roughly of 5 mm square. Place the pieces in a beaker, then pour on the detergent/ wash up liquid.
- Stir the mixture and maintain it at 60°C in a water bath for 15 minutes. Mixture is cooled in an ice water bath for 5 minutes under stirring. Stirring slows the breakdown of DNA at high temperature.
- Pour the mixture into a liquidizer and blend for only 5 seconds at high speed to degrade the cell walls and membranes further, which permits the release of DNA. Take care not to blend for longer as it will degrade the DNA fiber.
- Filter the mixture in the second beaker. Ensure that the foam on the surface of the liquid should not contaminate the filtrate.

Separation of DNA from the onion extract

- Add the enzyme to the onion tissue extract in a boiling tube and mix well. This enzyme will digest the proteins associated with DNA. Place a layer of ice cold ethanol on top of the onion extract/enzyme mixture by pouring it slowly down the side of the boiling tube.
- Leave the tube undisturbed for 2-3 minutes. As DNA is insoluble in ice cold ethanol, it can only digest other compounds in the mixture leaving DNA as a precipitate.

- Gently rotate the glass rod in the liquid, at the interface of the alcohol and detergent mixture. Care should be taken not to mix the layer so that fragile DNA broken up.
- The white web of mucus like DNA can be drawn from the tube with the help of a Pasteur pipette, which is resuspended in 4% sodium chloride solution.

Further possible extensions include:

- Stain the DNA using acetoorcein and examine under a microscope.
- Assess the acidic nature of the DNA using universal indicator solution.
- Extract DNA from animal tissues (e. g. cod roe, liver, calf thymus) or microorganisms by treating in a similar way.

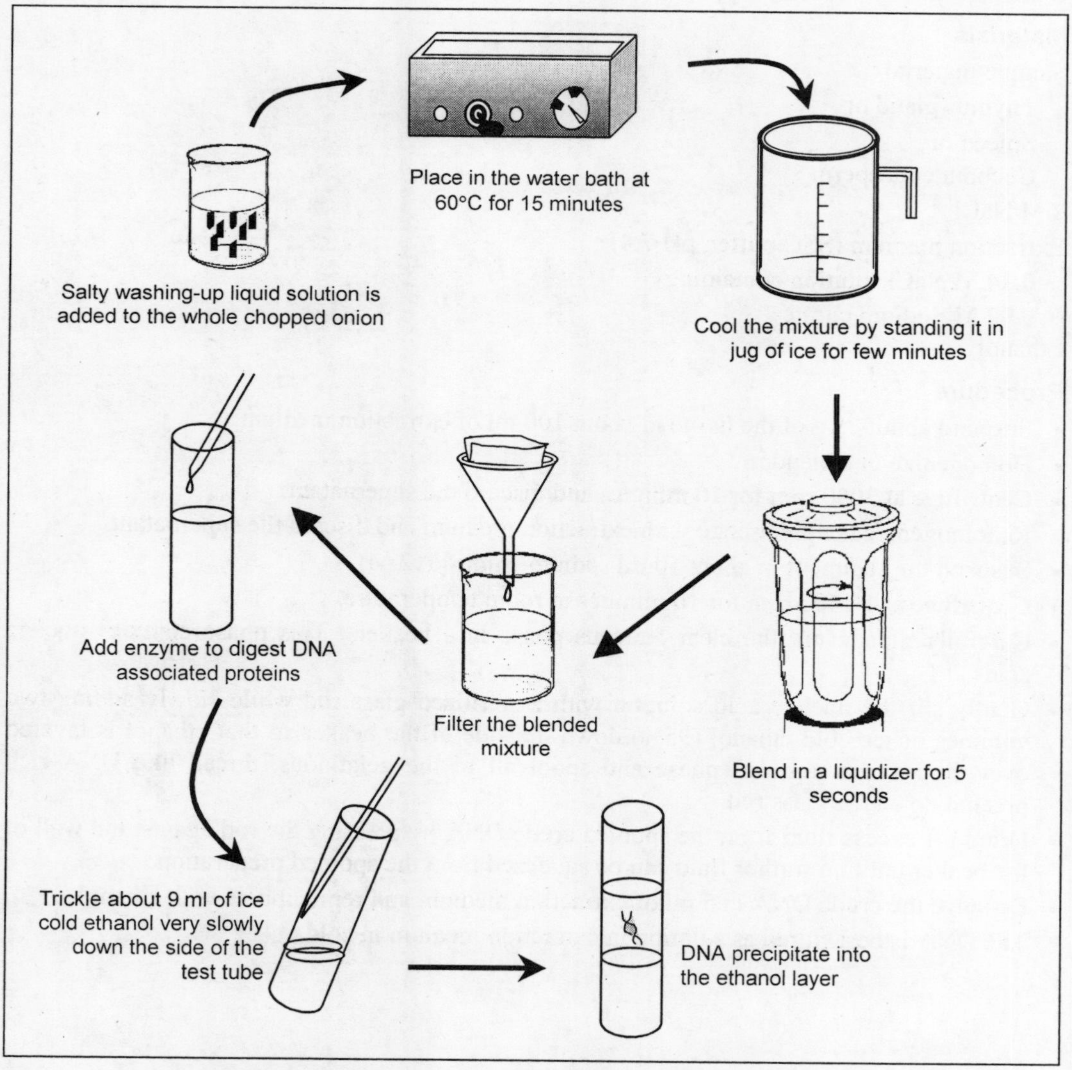

Fig. 8.6. Schematic diagram showing isolation of DNA from onion

PROTOCOL 8.2

ISOLATION OF DEOXYRIBONUCLEIC ACID (DNA)

Thymus gland, spleen and coconut endosperm, apart from being soft tissues, contain relatively large amount of nucleic acid material. These materials are a good source for DNA isolation experiments. The addition of detergent in the minced tissue causes the rupturance of cell membrane and dissolves the lipid and protein of the cells.

To isolate the DNA, cell wall and nuclear membrane are ruptured, deproteinized and DNA is precipitated after adding ethanol.

Materials

Sample material

Thymus gland or

Spleen or

Coconut endosperm

2 M NaCl

Extraction medium (SSC buffer, pH 7.4)

0.14 M NaCl solution containing

0.02 M Sodium citrate

Ethanol

Procedure

- Suspend about 25 g of the tissue in about 100 ml of extraction medium.
- Homogenize in a blender.
- Centrifuge at 3000 rpm for 10 minutes and discard the supernatant.
- Rehomogenize the precipitate with extraction medium and discard the supernatant.
- Suspend the sediment in about 50 ml sodium chloride (2 M).
- Centrifuge at 10,000 rpm for 10 minutes at room temperature.
- Carefully pipette out the clear aqueous phase in a beaker. This phase contains nucleic acids.
- Gently stir the nucleic acid solution with a sterilized glass rod while slowly adding two volumes of ice-cold ethanol (95%) down the side of the beaker so that ethanol is layered over the viscous aqueous phase and spool all of the gelatinous, thread like DNA rich precipitate on the glass rod.
- Drain off excess fluid from the spooled crude DNA by pressing the rod against the wall of the beaker until no further fluid can be squeezed from the spooled preparation.
- Dissolve the crude DNA in 5 ml of extraction medium and reprecipitate with ethanol.
- The DNA is best stored as solution in extraction medium in cold.

PROTOCOL 8.3

EXTRACTION OF DNA FROM PLANT SOURCE

Plant DNA can be extracted by a number of methods, which depend upon the starting tissues, homogenization conditions, etc.

Materials

Fresh plant tissue
Liquid nitrogen
5 M potassium acetate
3 M sodium acetate
Extraction Buffer (TES buffer)

100 mM Tris-HCl (pH 7.8)	6.06 g
10 mM Disodium EDTA	9.30 g
500 mM NaCl	14.61 g
Water q.s.to	500 ml.

Suspension buffer

50 mM Tris-HCl (pH 8.0)	0.61 g
10 mM Disodium EDTA	0.37 g
Water q.s. to	100 ml

TE Buffer

10 mM Tris-HCl (pH 7.5)	0.12 g
10 mM Disodium EDTA	0.37 g
Water q.s. to	100 ml.

Procedure

- Grind 10 g of plant tissue (frozen in liquid nitrogen) to a fine powder.
- Add 150 ml extraction buffer in small aliquots and grind thoroughly.
- Transfer the homogenate to a flask. Add 10 ml of 20% sodium dodecylsulphate (SDS) and mix thoroughly for 15 minutes using a magnetic stirrer.
- Incubate the contents at 65°C for 10 minutes.
- Add 100 ml potassium acetate solution, mix and incubate at 0°C for 30 minutes to precipitate polysaccharides and proteins.
- Centrifuge at 25,000g for 15 minutes and remove the precipitate.
- Add six tenth volume (of supernatant) of isopropanol and keep at 20°C for 30 minutes to precipitate DNA.
- Centrifuge again at 20,000g for 15 minutes to pellet DNA.
- Discard the supernatant and drain off any liquid. Redissolve DNA pellet in suspension buffer (3 ml). Add 3.6 ml isopropanol and 360 ml 3 M sodium acetate solution and keep at –20°C for 1 hour. Centrifuge again for 15 minutes (20,000g), wash with ice-cold ethanol (80%) and dry in vacuum.
- Redissolve the DNA pellet in a suitable volume (1-5 ml) of TE buffer.
- Estimate the DNA content and check purity by UV spectrophotometry.

PROTOCOL 8.4

MAMMALIAN DNA ISOLATION USING PHENOL EXTRACTION METHOD

This procedure avoids use of phenol and chloroform by high salt concentrations to remove proteins. It is rapid, safe and inexpensive. This procedure is for DNA extraction from white blood cells (one or two tubes of blood). Average yields are similar to that obtained with the phenol-chloroform extraction procedure (50-200 μg), with quality of DNA excellent. The procedure may be scaled up to handle larger samples.

Reagents

Buffer A

0.32 M sucrose	109.5 g
10 mM Tris-HCl, pH 7.6	10 ml
5 mM $MgCl_2$	5 ml
Deionized water q.s. to	1 litre
1% Triton X-100	

Sterilize above solution by autoclaving, then add 10 ml Triton X-100.

Buffer B

25 mM EDTA pH 8.0	50 ml
75 mM NaCl	40 ml
Deionized water q.s. to	1 litre

Sterilize by autoclaving.

Saturated NaCl solution

Dissolve 35 g of NaCl in a total volume of 100 ml (deionized water). If the solution has no precipitate, add 2 g NaCl and mix. Repeat until no more NaCl goes into solution. Filter and sterilize.

Procedure

- Take 1-2 tubes of blood. Add 9 volumes buffer A, mix well and hold on ice for 2 minutes.
- Centrifuge at 1500 rpm at 4°C for 15 minutes. Nuclei pellet will be formed.
- Resuspend the nuclei pellet in 5 ml buffer B and transfer to a 15 ml polypropylene centrifuge tube. Add 500 μl of 10% sodium dodecylsulphate (10% SDS) and 55 μl proteinase K (10 mg/ml stock). Incubate at 37°C overnight on a low-speed rocker or orbital shaker.
- After 24 hours add 1.4 ml saturated NaCl solution (approximately 6 M) to each tube. Shake vigorously for 15 seconds.
- Spin the tubes at 2500 rpm in the Beckman low speed centrifuge for 15 minutes.
- Transfer the supernatant to another 15 ml polypropylene tube, leaving behind the precipitated protein pellet. Add exactly two volumes of absolute ethanol and invert the tube several times until the DNA precipitate is visible.
- Remove the DNA strands with a plastic spatula or pipette tip and transfer to an Eppendorff tube containing 100-200 μl TE.
- Allow the DNA to dissolve at 37°C before quantitation.

PROTOCOL 8.5

MAMMALIAN DNA ISOLATION USING ISOPROPANOL PRECIPITATION

Reagents

Lysis buffer

100 mM Tris HCl (pH 8.5)	5 ml
0.5 M EDTA	0.5ml
10% SDS	1ml
5 M NaCl	2 ml
Proteinase K (20 mg/ml)	0.25 ml

Make up to 50 ml with double distilled water.

Procedure

Lysis

The lysis buffer (usually 0.5 ml) is added to the tissue or cell (for a 75 ml flask, add 5 ml directly to the cell). Digestion is complete within several hours at 37°C (for cells, 2-3 hours) or 55°C (for tissues) with agitation.

Isopropanol precipitation

One volume of isopropanol is added to the lysate and the samples are mixed or swirled until precipitation is complete (about 10-20 minutes, until viscosity completely gone).

Recovery of precipitate

The DNA is recovered by lifting the aggregated precipitate from the solution using a disposable yellow tip. Excess liquid is dabbed off and the DNA is dispersed in a prelabeled Eppendorff tube, (depending on the size of the precipitate) containing 20 to 500 μl to 10 mM Tris-HCl, 0.1 mM EDTA (pH 7.5). Complete dissolution of the DNA requires several hours of agitation at 37°C or 55°C (may need overnight). It is important that the DNA is completely dissolved to ensure the reproducible removal of aliquots for analysis.

PROTOCOL 8.6

GENOMIC DNA ISOLATION FROM MOUSE LIVER

Unlike plasmid DNA, genomic DNA is vulnerable to mechanical shearing forces such as vigorous shaking or vortexing, and pipetting through a narrow pipette tip. So for each of the following steps, pay attention to the degree of shaking required for the mixing during phenol/chloroform extraction and precipitation of DNA.

Procedure

- Dissect mice to get liver. Weigh 0.5 to 1 g of mouse liver.
- In a large plastic weighing boat, mince the liver into tiny chunks using a razor blade.

- Add liquid nitrogen (about 25 ml) to a mortar, and place pestle back into mortar. After the liquid nitrogen is about half gone, add another 10 ml nitrogen. Immediately scrape the mouse liver chunks into the liquid nitrogen and let it freeze until the liquid nitrogen is nearly gone. Grind the liver to a powder or as nearly to a powder as possible and add 5 ml digest buffer and allow to thaw. When the slush has started to thaw into liquid, stir so that the extraction buffer gets mixed well.
- When totally thawed, pour slurry into a 15 ml graduated disposable falcon tube. Scrape any remaining part of it into the tube using a spatula while pouring. Mix and incubate them in an oven at 50°C for overnight.
- Add an equal volume of phenol/chloroform to the 15 ml tube containing liver homogenate, cap the tube securely and mix by hand with a medium through up and down motion with the wrist. The idea here is to mix at least hard enough to form a sol (homogeneous mixture) between the DNA phase and the phenol/chloroform phase (step A).
- Place in high-speed centrifuge (adjacent lab) and centrifuge at 4500 rpm for 5 minutes. Remove upper aqueous layer using a plastic disposable pipette and transfer to a new 15 ml tube (step B).
- Repeat steps A and B.
- Adjust the volume to 4 ml (of DNA solution) by either adding TE or removing DNA solution. Add 2 ml of 7.5 M ammonium acetate, gently mix by inversion. Slowly add 8 ml of 100% ethanol by layering it over the DNA solution with a disposable pipette. Precipitate the DNA by slowly inverting the tube and rocking it back and forth. A thread like DNA appears as a result of through mixing after about 3 minutes or so.
- Centrifuge in a big centrifuge at 3000 rpm for 2 minutes. Discard the supernatant and wash the pellet by adding about 5 ml of 70% ethanol directly from the bottle. Invert the tube and centrifuge at 3000g for 2 minutes. Slowly discard ethanol and remove the last traces with a Pasteur pipette. Resuspend the pellet in 500 μl of TE. Try gently rolling the tube to redissolve. If this does not work, use a 1 ml pipette with the tip trimmed off a little to widen the bore of the tip. Transfer to a labeled 1.5 ml centrifugation tube and place on ice.

PROTOCOL 8.7

DNA ISOLATION FROM SMALL NUMBERS OF CELLS

Procedure

Preparation of Cells

- Centrifuge cell suspension for 5 minutes at 1200 rpm, 4°C and keep on ice.
- Remove supernatant from each sample and resuspend pellets in 1 ml of ice-cold Tris-buffered saline (50 mM Tris, 150 mM NaCl, pH 8.0) and keep on ice.
- Centrifuge the cells again (5 minutes, 1200 rpm, 4°C) and resuspend them in 1 ml (or another required volume) of ice-cold Tris-buffered saline and keep on ice.
- Count the cells.

- Transfer the required number of cells from which DNA should be isolated into Eppendorff tubes (optimum is 2 x 10^5 but 1 x 10^5 and even 5 x 10^4 occasionally give good results).
- Recentrifuge the Eppendorff tubes (5 minutes, 1200 rpm, 4°C) and remove the supernatant using an automatic pipette, without disturbing the pellets.
- Centrifuge the tubes for 15 seconds (14000 rpm, 4°C) to clear the walls.
- After returning the tubes to ice, all remaining supernatant should be carefully removed. Cells should then be frozen rapidly in liquid nitrogen.

Proteinase K Digestion

- Transfer samples to ice. Add 10 µl of ice-cold buffer A and centrifuge for 15 seconds (14000 rpm, 4°C) and incubate for 1minute at 50°C.
- Add 10 µl of buffer A containing 2% agarose and 0.5 mg/ml freshly prepared proteinase K at 50°C. If necessary, centrifuge the tube for 15 seconds, 14000 rpm at room temperature.
- Incubate the cells for 2 hours at 50°C (do not overheat as proteinase K is inactivated above 50°C).

Removal of Detergent and Other Small Molecules

- Centrifuge each sample for 15 seconds, at 14,000 rpm and 4°C. Allow to solidify on ice.
- Add 500 µl of sterile 10 mM TE buffer at 4°C.
- Incubate the samples at 4°C with changing buffer after 1 hour, 18 hours and 24 hours.

RNase and Restriction Enzyme Digestion

- Restriction enzyme digestion can be carried out in the presence of LGT agarose. Melt the samples by heating at 65°C for 5 minutes and cool to 37°C.
- Samples are digested in a final volume of 35 µl. To each sample add 6 µl distilled water, 3.5 µl BSA (10 mg/ml), 3.5 µl restriction buffer, 1 µl RNase (10 mg/ml) and restriction enzyme (units depend on type of experiment as well as on enzyme itself). Water, BSA, buffer and RNase should be added as a mixture to avoid long handling of samples.
- Centrifuge samples for 5 seconds (14,000 rpm, room temperature).
- Digest for 18 hours at 37°C.

PROTOCOL 8.8

DNA EXTRACTION USING PHENOL

Phenol extraction is a common technique used to purify a DNA sample. Conventionally, an equal volume of TE-saturated phenol is added to an aqueous DNA sample in a microcentrifuge tube. The mixture is vigorously vortexed, and then centrifuged to facilitate phase separation. The upper, aqueous layer is carefully removed to a new tube, avoiding the phenol interface and then is subjected to ether extractions twice to remove residual phenol. An equal volume of water-saturated ether is added to the tube, the mixture is vortexed, and the tube is centrifuged to allow phase separation. The upper ether layer is removed and discarded, including phenol droplets at the interface. The extraction is repeated and the DNA is concentrated by ethanol precipitation.

Procedure

- Add an equal volume of TE-saturated phenol to the DNA sample contained in a 1.5 ml microcentrifuge tube and vortex for 15-30 seconds.
- Centrifuge the sample for 5 minutes at room temperature to separate the phases.
- Remove about 90% of the upper aqueous layer to a clean tube, carefully avoiding proteins at the aqueous:phenol interface. At this stage the aqueous phase can be extracted a second time with an equal volume of 1:1 TE-saturated phenol:chloroform, centrifuged and removed to a clean tube as above but this additional extraction is not necessary if care is taken during the first phenol extraction.
- Add an equal volume of water-saturated ether, vortex briefly, and centrifuge for 3 minutes at room temperature. Remove and discard the upper ether layer, taking care to remove phenol droplets at the ether:aqueous interface. Repeat the ether extraction.
- Ethanol precipitates the DNA by adding 2.5-3 volumes of ethanol-acetate, as discussed below.

PROTOCOL 8.9

CONCENTRATION OF DNA BY ETHANOL PRECIPITATION

Typically, 2.5-3 volumes of an ethanol/acetate solution are added to the DNA sample in a microcentrifuge tube, which is placed in an ice-water bath for at least 10 minutes. Frequently, this precipitation is performed by incubation at –20°C overnight. To recover the precipitated DNA, the tube is centrifuged, the supernatant discarded, and the DNA pellet is rinsed with more dilute ethanol solution. Centrifuge again, the supernatant is discarded, and the DNA pellet is dried under vacuum.

Procedure

- Add 2.5-3 volumes of 95% ethanol/0.12 M sodium acetate to the DNA sample contained in a 1.5 ml microcentrifuge tube, invert to mix, and
- Incubate in an ice-water bath for at least 10 minutes. At this stage, the sample can be placed at –20°C overnight.
- Centrifuge at 12,000 rpm in a microcentrifuge (Fisher) for 15 minutes at 4°C.
- Decant the supernatant, and drain inverted on a paper towel.
- Add 80% ethanol, incubate at room temperature for 5-10 minutes and centrifuge again for 5 minutes, decant and drain the tube as above.
- Place the tube in a Savant Speed-Vac and dry the DNA pellet for about 5-10 minutes, or until dry.
- Always dissolve dried DNA in 10 mM Tris-HCl, pH 7.6-8.0, 0.1 mM EDTA (termed 10:0.1 TE buffer).

- It is advisable to aliquot the DNA purified in large scale isolations (i.e. 100 µg or more) into several small (0.5 ml) microcentrifuge tubes for frozen storage because repeated freezing and thawing may adversely affect the DNA structure.

Isobutanol concentration of DNA

DNA samples may be concentrated by extraction with isobutanol. Add slightly more than one volume of isobutanol, vortex vigorously and centrifuge to separate the phases. Discard the isobutanol (upper) phase, and extract once with water-saturated diethyl ether to remove last traces of isobutanol. The nucleic acid may be then precipitated by addition of ethanol as described above.

PROTOCOL 8.10

ESTIMATON OF DNA

Deoxyribonucleic acid can be estimated by a number of methods based on the physical or chemical property of the nucleic acid. The deoxyribose in DNA, in presence of acid forms hydroxylevulinylaldehyde, which reacts with diphenylamine to give blue colour, which is estimated colorimetrically at 595 nm.

Materials

Standard DNA solution, 100 µg/ml

Standard Saline citrate (SSC buffer)

0.15 M NaCl.

0.015 M Sodium citrate.

Diphenylamine reagent

Mix 1 g diphenylamine, 100 ml acetic acid and 2.75 ml concentrated sulphuric acid. This reagent is stable for six months at 2°C.

Procedure

- Prepare a standard solution of DNA (100 µg/ml) and a solution of isolated DNA in saline citrate.
- Set up different tubes with increasing concentration of standard DNA and a separate blank. Make up the volume to 3 ml with water.
- Add 6 ml diphenylamine reagent to each tube.
- Mix well and heat the tubes in a boiling water bath for 10 minutes and then cool the tubes.
- Measure the absorbance or optical density at 595 nm against the blank.
- Draw a standard graph between absorbance or optical density (ordinate) versus concentration of DNA and determine the concentration of isolated DNA dissolved in saline citrate solution.

Note

The method is commonly used for samples containing 50-500 µg DNA.

PROTOCOL 8.11

PRECIPITATION OF NUCLEIC ACIDS

Most nucleic acids may be precipitated by addition of monovalent cations and two to three volumes of cold 95% ethanol, followed by incubation at 0 to –70°C. The DNA or RNA then may be pelleted by centrifugation at 10 to 13,000g for 15 minutes at 4°C. A subsequent wash with 70% ethanol, followed by brief centrifugation, removes residual salt and moisture.

Procedure

- Add one-tenth volume (of nucleic acid solution) of 3 M sodium acetate, pH 5.2 to the nucleic acid solution.
- Add two volumes of cold 95% ethanol.
- Place at –70°C for at least 30 minutes, or at –20°C overnight.
- Alternatively procedure given below may be followed for nucleic acid precipitation.
- Add 95 ml of 100% ethanol with 4 ml of 3 M sodium acetate (pH 4.8) and 1ml of sterile water.
- Mix by inversion and store at –20°C.
- Add 2.5 volumes of cold ethanol/acetate solution to the nucleic acid solution to be precipitated.
- Place at –70°C for at least 30 minutes or at –20°C for two hours to overnight.

Note

5 M ammonium acetate (pH 7.4), NaCl and LiCl may be used as substitute to sodium acetate. DNA may also be precipitated by addition of 0.6 volumes of isopropanol.

Oligonucleotides Precipitation

Procedure

- Add one tenth volume of 3 M sodium acetate, pH 6.5 and three volumes of cold 95% ethanol.
- Place at –70°C for at least one hour.

RNA Precipitation

Procedure

- Add one tenth volume of 1 M sodium acetate, pH 4.5 and 2.5 volumes of cold 95% ethanol.
- Large volume samples can be precipitated by keeping at –20°C overnight.
- Small volume samples may be precipitated by placing in powdered dry ice or dry ice-ethanol bath for 5 to 10 minutes.

PROTOCOL 8.12

ISOLATION OF RIBONUCLEIC ACID (RNA)

The ribonucleoprotein complex is dissociated into RNA and protein, deproteinized by phenol and the free RNA left in aqueous solution is precipitated in the cold after adding alcohol.

Materials

Yeast tablets

Phenol

Potassium acetate, (20% w/v; pH 5)

Ethanol

Ether

Centrifuge

Mechanical stirrer.

All glassware should be dried at 120°C overnight. There should not be any contamination with any nuclease.

Procedure

- Powder the active yeast tablets and suspend in 120 ml warm water (37°C) and stir for 15 minutes.
- Add freshly redistilled phenol (about 150 ml) and stir for about 30 minutes.
- Centrifuge the resulting mixture at 3000 rpm for 10 minutes (preferably in cold) to separate the layers. The lower (phenol) phase contains DNA among other things and the upper aqueous phase contains RNA and polysaccharides, etc.
- Transfer the upper aqueous phase into a separate flask and filter through a funnel packed with glass wool.
- Measure the volume of the filtrate and add potassium acetate solution so that the final volume is 2% w/v (1 ml potassium acetate to 9 ml filtrate).
- Add twice the volume of ethanol and leave the flask at –20°C for RNA precipitation.
- Collect the precipitate of RNA by centrifugation at 2000g for 10 minutes.
- Wash the pellet (RNA) with 70% ethanol, ethanol: ether (1:1) and finally with ether.
- Dry the pellet gently in vacuum.

This preparation may contain polysaccharides also.

Notes

All the glassware and solutions should be sterile.

Any contaminating DNA will appear just like cotton wool during ethanol addition.

Chloroform : phenol (1:1) mixture is an effective deproteinizing agent.

PROTOCOL 8.13

ESTIMATION OF RNA

Ribonucleic acid (RNA) releases ribose, a pentose on acid hydrolysis. Colorimetric procedures suitable for pentose determination have been used for estimation of RNA. These include reactions with orcinol, aniline, fluoroglucinol etc. The reaction between ribose and orcinol has been widely used (Bial's test).

Principle

The ribose gets converted to furfural, in the presence of hot acid. Orcinol reacts with furfural to give a green colour in the presence of ferric chloride, which is measured colorimetrically at 660 nm. Purine nucleotides are generally more reactive than pyrimidine nucleotides.

Materials

Standard RNA solution, pure yeast RNA, xylose or adenylic acid.

Sample RNA solution.

Orcinol acid reagent

Add 1 ml of a 10% (w/v) of ferric chloride ($FeCl_3.6H_2O$) to 200 ml concentrated HCl.

6% w/v Orcinol solution

Dissolve 6 g orcinol in 100 ml ethanol (95%) and keep it in cold.

Tris-acetate buffer

10 mM Tris-acetate, 1 mM EDTA, Adjust the pH 7.2.

Procedure

- Prepare a standard RNA solution (100 μg/ml) in ice cold Tris-acetate buffer or any suitable buffer (pH 7.2).
- Prepare the solution of isolated RNA in the above buffer to get an approximate concentration of 100 μg/ml.
- Set up different tubes with increasing concentration of standard RNA and make up the volume to 3 ml with water.
- Prepare a blank containing 3 ml of water. Add 6 ml orcinol acid reagent to each of the tubes.
- Add 0.4 ml solution of orcinol in alcohol (6% w/v) to each tube.
- Shake the tubes to mix the contents and then keep the tubes in boiling water bath for 15-20 minutes.
- Cool the tubes to room temperature and measure the absorbance at 660 nm against the blank.
- Draw a standard curve between absorbance and concentration of standard RNA and determine the amount in the isolated RNA solution using the graph.

Notes

If the concentration of the sample is high, n-butanol can be used to dilute it.

PROTOCOL 8.14

SEPARATION OF NUCLEIC ACIDS BY MAK COLUMN

Nucleic acids can be separated with fair accuracy by ion-exchange chromatography. The protein albumin after methylation, to protect the negative charge on the molecule, is used as the column material. Thus only the positive charge groups are exposed. Kieselguhr is used as support for this methylated albumin and hence the column is called Methylated Albumin Kieselguhr (MAK) column.

Materials

Nucleic acid sample
Glass column of 2 cm diameter
Albumin
Kieselguhr
0.1 M NaCl, pH 7.0
0.4 M NaCl, pH 7.0

Preparation of Methylated Albumin Kieselguhr

- Suspend 20 g of Kieselguhr in 100 ml of 0.1 M NaCl (pH 7.0) in a beaker and boil the suspension slowly to expel air.
- Cool and add 5 ml of esterified albumin solution (1%) and stir well. Wash the material thoroughly with 0.4 M NaCl (pH 7.0) solution.
- The material suspended in 0.4 M NaCl can be stored in cold for a longer period.

Preparation of MAK Column

- Pack one end of a glass column with a small amount of glass wool.
- Boil and cool a suspension of 6 g Kieselguhr in 40 ml of 0.1 M NaCl and pour it down the tube to form the first layer. Add 10 ml of MAK suspension to form the second layer.
- Add a boiled and cooled suspension of 1 g Kieselguhr in 10 ml of 0.4 M NaCl.
- Wash the column repeatedly with 0.4 M NaCl and should be kept wet with this solution.

Procedure

- Load the column with 0.5 mg nucleic acid sample in 0.4 M saline (adjusted to pH 6.7).
- Elute the column with 0.4 M and going upto 2 M sodium chloride solution.
- Collect the eluent in 5 ml fractions and measure the OD/absorbance of each of the elutes spectrophotometrically at 260 nm.
- Plot a graph between the number of fractions (X-axis) and OD at 260 nm (Y-axis).
- After measuring the OD, estimate for the presence of both RNA and DNA in various fractions.

SUGGESTED READINGS

Jayaraman, J., Laboratory Manual in Biochemistry, New Age International Publication, New Delhi, India, 1999.

Kuchler, R. J., Biochemical Methods in Cell Culture and Virology, Dowden, Huchinson and Ross, Inc., Strausberg, USA, 1977.

Miller, A. S., Dykes, D. D., and Polesky, H. F., *Nucleic Acids Research*, 16, 1215, 1988.

Marmur, J., *J. Molecular Biology*, 3, 208, 1961.

Sadasivam, S. and Manickem, A., Biochemical Methods, 2nd Edition, New Age International Publishers, New Delhi, India, 1997.

CHAPTER 9

Cloning and Molecular Analysis of Genes

- Introduction
- Isolation of plasmids
- Purification of plasmid DNA
- Large-scale isolation of cosmid and plasmid DNA
- Miniprep double-stranded DNA isolation
- Midiprep double-stranded DNA isolation
- Plasmid DNA isolation (from large culture)
- Plasmid miniprep I by Birnboim method
- Plasmid miniprep II by Boiling method
- 96 well double-stranded template isolation
- Cultivation of lambda (λ) phage
- Isolation of lambda DNA
- Isolation of lambda DNA by quick method
- Single-stranded M13 DNA isolation using phenol
- Biomek-automated modified-eperon isolation procedure for single-stranded M13 DNA
- Isolation of *Aspergillus* DNA
- Isolation of *Aspergillus* DNA by Quiagen method
- Genomic DNA isolation from blood
- Restriction digestion
- Agarose gel electrophoresis
- Bacterial cell maintenance
- Notes on restriction/modification bacterial strains
- DNA transfection by protoplast fusion
- Fragment purification on Sephacryl S-500 spin columns
- PCR amplification of DNA
- Kinase end-labeling of DNA
- Elution of DNA fragments from agarose
- Fusion of protoplast to adherent mammalian cells
- Delivery of liposome-encapsulated RNA to cells expressing influenza virus haemagglutinin
- Resistant bacterial system for DNA transformation
- DNA transformation of bacteria red colony
- Solubilization of Inclusion bodies
- Solubilization of recombinant proteins from inclusion bodies reagents
- Assays for gene transfer
- DNA transfection in retrovirus stocks
- Titration and analysis of recombinant retrovirus stocks
- Assay for gene transfer and expression by PCR based techniques

INTRODUCTION

Gene is invariably in all descriptions defined as a segment of DNA responsible for producing an RNA molecule or template containing an information, which decodes itself as a polypeptide chain. It includes regions preceding (leader) and following the coding regions (trailer) as well as intervening sequences (introns) between individual coding segments (exons). A gene has two main regions:

- Regulatory region
- Transcription region unit

After the development of tool that can manipulate genes or DNA molecules the immense possibilities are visible for the transformation of animal and plant breeding and of a variety of chemical and industrial process. The whole concept based on biochemical manipulation of genes and subsequent applicability in various fields is termed as genetic engineering. The various methodologies e.g. cutting and joining of genes (gene manipulation), amplification, modification and cloning, the separation and sequencing of genes and subsequent generation of protein molecules *in vitro* are the basic tools for genetic engineering.

Gene manipulation involves essentially the breakage of DNA into fragments using restriction endonuclease and then selection of gene of interest and their subsequent joining to other DNA molecule, which has high replication potency bringing about recombination. The gene of interest is termed as target or foreign DNA whereas, high replication part of DNA is termed as vehicle or vector DNA. Thus assembled DNA is termed as recombinant DNA or r-DNA. To generate several identical copies of r-DNA, it is inserted into some host cells usually of bacterial origin. The generated identical copies are called cloned gene and this particular phenomenon is termed as gene cloning. These cloned copies are separated and sequenced and eventually can be studied for the structure and function of protein generated because of manipulated gene sequence. As a whole a complete information of a particular gene can be obtained. General steps of cloning of DNA are outlined in Figure 9.1.

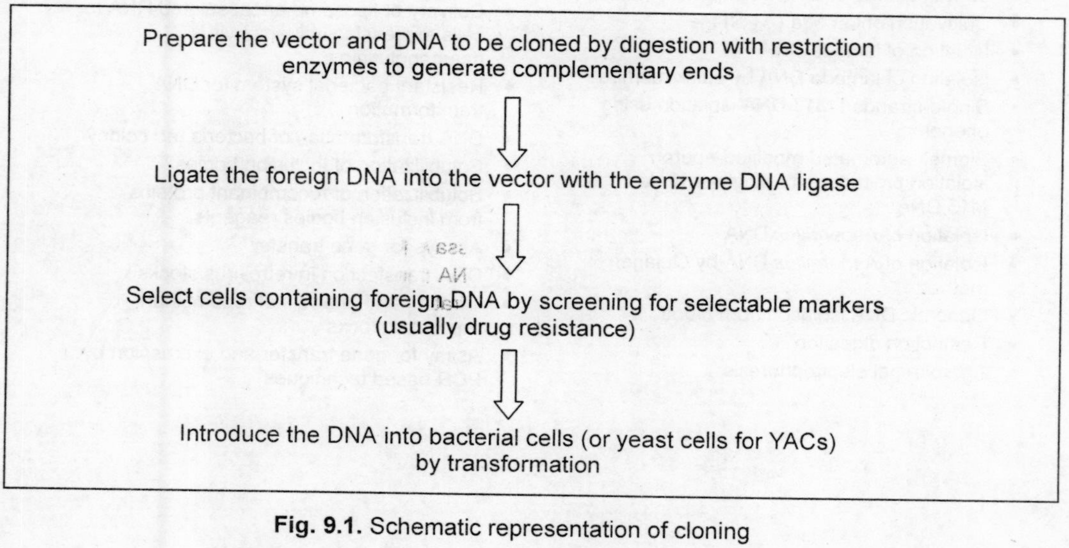

Fig. 9.1. Schematic representation of cloning

Restriction Endonucleases

The most widely recognizable enzymes that are used in molecular genetics are restriction enzymes. These enzymes are part of the restriction-modification system that bacterial species use to prevent foreign organisms from overtaking their cells. Presumably, each species has one or more of these systems. These systems consist of a restriction enzyme that cleaves DNA at a specific sequence and a methylase that protects the host DNA from being cleaved.

Restriction endonuclease enzymes recognize specific nucleotide sequences in double stranded DNA, that are usually four, five or six nucleotides long and then cut both strands of the DNA at specific locations. There are basically three ways in which the DNA can be cut

- A staggered cut to leave a cohesive end with 5' overhang.
- A staggered cut to leave a cohesive end with 3' overhang.
- A cut in the same place on both strands to leave a blunt end.

Cohesive ends allow any two DNA fragments produced by the same restriction enzyme to form complementary base pair. Various restriction endonuclease enzymes with their source and specific cut site are listed in Table 9.1.

Table 9.1. List of restriction endonuclease enzyme with their source and specific cut site

Restriction endonuclease enzyme	Source	Specific cut site
Acc I	*Acinetobacter calcoaceticus*	GA*A(C)T (G)AC CAT(G)A(C)*TG
Alu I	*Arthrobacter luteus*	AG*CT TC*GA
ApaL I	*Acetobacter pasteurianus*	G*TGCAC CACGT*G
Ava I	*Anabaena variabilis*	5'…C*PyCGPuG…3' 3'…G PuGCPyC…5'
BamH I	*Bacillus amyloliquefaciens*	G*GATCC CCTAG*G
Bcl I	*Bacillus caldolyticus*	T*GATCA ACTAG*T
Bgl I	*Bacillus globigii*	GCCNNNN*NGGC CGGN*NNNNCCG
Bgl II	*Bacillus globigii*	A*GATCT TCTAG*A
BstE II	*Bacillus stearothermophilus ET*	G*GTNACC CCANTG*G
Cla I	*Caryophanon latum*	A*TCGAT TAGC*TA
Dra I	*Deinococcus radiophilus*	TTT*AAA AAA*TTT

continued.....

Table 9.1. Continued.

EcoR I	*Escherichia coli*	G*AATTC CTTAA*G
EcoR V	*Escherichia coli*	GAT*ATC CTA*TAG
Hae III	*Haemophilus aegyptius*	GG*CC CC*GG
Hha I	*Haemophilus haemolyticus*	GCG*C C*GCG
Hinf I	*Haemophilus influenzae Rf*	G*ANTC CTNA*G
Hinc II	*Haemophilus influenzae*	GT(T/C)*(A/C)AC CA(A/G)*(T/C)TG
Hind III	*Haemophilus influezae Rd.*	A*AGCT T TTCGA*A
Hpa I	*Haemophilus parainfluenzae*	GTT*AAC CAA*TTG
Hpa II	*Haemophilus parainfluenzae*	C*CGG GGC*C
Kpn I	*Klebsiella pneumoniae*	GGTAC*C C*CATGG
Mbo I	*Moraxella bovis*	*GATC CTAG*
Mlu I	*Micrococcus luteus*	A*CGCGT TGCGC*A
Msp I	Moraxell species	C*CGG GGC*C
Nco I	*Nocardia corallina*	C*CATGG GGTAC*C
Not I	*Nocardia otidiscaviarum*	GC*GGCCGC CGCCGG*CG
Nhe I	*Neisseria nucosa heidelbergensis*	G*CTAGC CGATC*G
Nru I	*Nocarkia rubra*	TCG*CGA AGC*GCT
Pst I	*Providencia stuartii*	CTGCA*G G*ACGTC
Pvu I	*Proteus vulgaris*	CGAT*CG GC*TAGC
Pvu II	*Proteus vulgaris*	CAG*CTG GTC*TAC

continued.....

Table 9.1. Continued.

Sac I	*Streptomyces achromogenes*	GAGCT*C C*TCGAG
Sal I	*Streptomyces albus G*	G*TCGAC CAGCT*G
Sau3A I	*Staphylococcus aureus 3Al*	*GATC CTAG*
Sfi I	*Streptomyces fimbriatus*	GGCCNNNN*NGGCC CCGGN*NNNNCCGG
Sma I	*Serratia marcescens*	CCC*GGG GGG*CCC
Spe I	*Sphaerotilus species*	A*CTAGT TGATC*A
Ssp I	*Sphaerotilus species*	A*ATATT TGATC*A
Stu I	*Sphaerotilus species*	AGG*CCT TCC*GGA
Taq I	*Thermus aquaticus YTI*	T*CGA AGC*T
Xba I	*Xanthomonas badrii*	T*CTAGA AGATC*T
Xho I	*Xanthomonas holcicola*	C*TCGAG GAGCT*C
Xma I	*Xanthomonas malvacearum*	C*CCGGG GGGCC*C

* *represents the specific cut site recognized by the restriction enzyme*

Other Enzymes Used in DNA Cloning

Use of enzyme in molecular cloning of DNA depends upon their substrate specificity. Most polymerase strongly prefers DNA template to synthesize DNA *in vitro* (DNA dependent DNA polymerase). However they can also synthesize DNA using RNA as a template (RNA dependent DNA polymerase). Most frequently used DNA dependent DNA polymerase are *E. coli* DNA polymerase I (holozymes), the large fragment of *E coli* DNA polymerase I (Klenow fragment), the DNA encoded by Bacteriophages T4 and T7, modified bacteriophage T4 DNA polymerase (Sequenase^{TM}) and thermostable DNA polymerase (Taq DNA polymerase and Ampli Taq^{TM}). Reverse transcriptase is the example of RNA dependent polymerase which can use both DNA and/or RNA as a template for the synthesis therefore it can be used for the synthesis of double stranded DNA. Terminal transferase (Terminal deoxynucleotidyl transferase) is a special type of DNA polymerase which does not copy a template but adds nucleotide only to the termini of existing DNA molecule. This enzyme is used for adding a tail to the cDNA and the vector DNA for cloning by homopolymer tailing. DNA ligase enzyme is used for the joining of two pieces of DNA fragments, as it forms a phosphodiester bond in between the free 3' OH group of one piece and free 5' PO_4 group of other piece.

DNA polymerase I (Holoenzymes)

DNA ploymerase I consists of a single polypeptide chain that can function as a 5'-3' DNA polymerase, a 5'-3' exonuclease and a 3'-5' exonuclease activity. It can act on the DNA with various ways according to its substrate specificity

- It shows 5'-3' DNA polymerase activity when substrate is single stranded DNA template with a DNA primer bearing a 3'-hydroxyl group.

5'.... pC pC pG OH3'
3'....Gp Gp Cp Tp Ap Tp Cp Gp Ap ....5'

↓ Mg^{++}, dATP, dTTP, dGTP, dCTP; *E. coli* DNA polymerase I

5'....pC pC pG pA pT pA pG pC pT.....3'
3'....Gp Gp Cp Tp Ap Tp Cp Gp Ap ....5'

- It shows 5'-3' exonuclease activity when substrate is double stranded DNA or RNA: DNA hybrid. It degrades double stranded DNA from the 5' termini and also degrades RNA component of RNA: DNA hybrid.

5'.... pC pG pC pA pT pC pT.....3'
3' GpCp Gp Cp Gp Tp Ap Gp Ap.....5'

↓ Mg^{++}; *E. coli* DNA polymerase I

5' pC pA pT pC pT.....3'
3' GpCp Gp Cp Gp Tp Ap Gp Ap.....5'
+ 5'pC+ 5'PG + 5'pC pG

- It shows 3'-5' exonuclease when substrate is double stranded or single stranded DNA containing 3' hydroxyl termini. Exonuclease activity on double stranded DNA is blocked by 5'-3' DNA polymerase activity and is inhibited by dNMPs with 5' phosphate.

5'... pC pG pC pA pT pC pT 3'
3'....Gp Cp Gp 5'

↓ Mg^{++}; *E. coli* DNA polymerase

5'... pC pG pC OH 3'
3'....Gp Cp Gp 5'
+ 5' pA + 5' pC + 5' pT

- It also shows exchange (replacement) reaction when only one dNTP is present, the 3'-5' exonuclease activity will degrade double stranded DNA from the 3' hydroxyl terminus until a base is exposed that is complementary to the dNTP. A continuous series of synthesis and exchange reactions will then occur at that position.

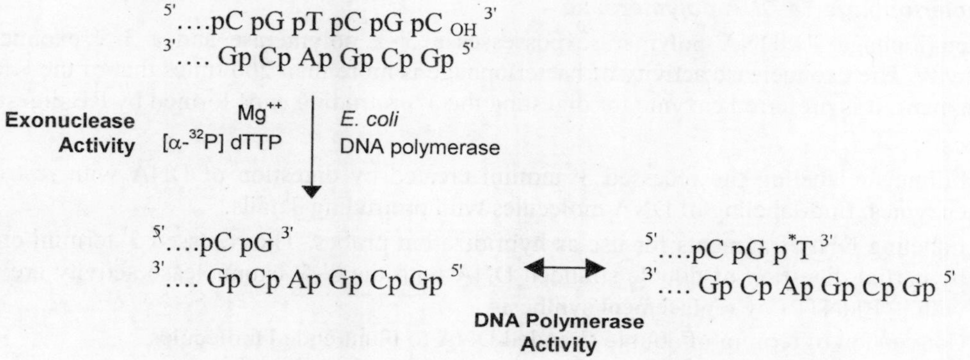

Uses

- Labeling of DNA by nick translation
- The holoenzyme is used for the synthesis of the second strand of cDNA in cDNA cloning as 5'-3' exonuclease of *E.coli* DNA polymerase I degrades oligonucleotides that may serve as primers for the synthesis of the second strand of cDNA.
- It is also used for the end labeling of DNA molecules with protruding 3' tails, which is accomplished in two stages. In first stage 3'-5' exonuclease activity removes protruding 3' tails from the DNA and creates a blunt 3' terminus. Then in the presence of high concentrations of one radiolabeled precursor, exonucleolytic degradation is balanced by incorporation of dNTPs at the 3' terminus. This reaction, which consists of cycles of removal and replacement of the 3' terminal nucleotides from recessed or blunt ended DNA is sometimes called an exchange or replacement reaction.

Large fragment of DNA polymerase I (Klenow fragment)

This enzyme is produced by cleavage of intact DNA polymerase I. It possess 3'-5' exonuclease activity and DNA polymerase activity. For cloning purposes it is more useful than the holoenzyme of *E. coli* DNA polymerase as it does not possess the 5'-3' exonuclease activity. 5'-3' exonuclease activity is responsible for the degradation of 5' terminus of primers that are bound to DNA template and also removes 5' terminus phosphates which are to be used as substrates for ligation.

Use of Klenow fragments

- Filling or labeling the recessed 3' termini created by digestion of DNA with restriction enzymes.
- End- labeling of DNA molecules with protruding 3' tails.
- Labeling DNA fragments for use as hybridization probes. The recessed 3' termini created by partial digestion of double stranded DNA with the 3'-5' exonuclease activity are filled with [^{32}P]dNTPs by replacement synthesis.

- Synthesis of the second strand of cDNA in cDNA cloning.
- Synthesis of double stranded DNA from single stranded templates during *in vitro* mutagenesis.
- Sequencing of DNA using the Sanger's dideoxy mediated chain termination method.

Bacteriophage T4 DNA polymerease

Bacteriophage T4 DNA polymerase possesses a 5'-3' polymerase and a 3-5' exonuclease activity. The exonuclease activity of bacteriophage is more than 200 times that of the Klenow fragment. It is preferred enzyme for digesting the 3' protruding ends formed by RE digestion.

Uses

- Filling or labeling the recessed 3' termini created by digestion of DNA with restriction enzymes. End-labeling of DNA molecules with protruding 3' tails.
- Labeling DNA fragments for use as hybridization probes. The recessed 3' termini created by partial digestion of double stranded DNA with the 3'-5' exonuclease activity are filled with [^{32}P]dNTPs by replacement synthesis.
- Conversion of termini of double stranded DNA to blunt ended molecules.
- Polishing the ends of cDNA after its synthesis.

Taq DNA polymerase and AmpliTaq™

Taq DNA polymerase is a thermostable DNA dependent DNA polymerase. These enzymes have a 5'-3' polymerization-dependent exonuclease activity. 5'-3' DNA polymerase acts on single stranded template primer with 3' hydroxyl. The enzyme is most active in between 75-80°C. Taq DNA polymerase is used for DNA sequencing and to amplify specific sequences that flank the region of interest. The first oligonucleotide is complementary to sequences of one strand of the template upstream of the region of interest, and the second is complementary to the other downstream from the region.

The enzyme is useful in the amplification of the cDNA or genomic DNA (10^6 times) of specific sequence.

Reverse transcriptase (RNA dependent DNA polymerase)

This enzyme lacks the 3'-5' exonuclease activity on DNA but having activity of 5'-3' polymerase for RNA or DNA template with an RNA or DNA primer bearing a 3' hydroxyl group. It is also having RNase H activity (5'-3' and 3'-5' exoribonuclease) activity.

- It is used chiefly to transcribe mRNA into double stranded cDNA that can be inserted into prokaryotic vectors.
- Labeling the termini of DNA fragments with protruding 5' termini.
- In sequencing of DNA by the dideoxy chain termination method.

Terminal transferase (terminal deoxynucleodidyl transferase)

Enzyme catalyzes the addition of dNTPs to the 3'- hydroxyl termini of DNA molecules in the presence of divalent cations.

$$\text{Single stranded DNA } DNA_{OH} \xrightarrow[\text{Terminal transferase}]{\substack{Mn^{++} \text{ or } Mg^{++} \\ \text{dATP, dTTP, dGTP, dCTP}}} DNA\text{-}({}_{p}dN)_n + nPPi$$

DNA ligase

The enzyme use to joins two pieces of DNA, are called DNA ligase. The ligases used more often in cloning are encoded by bacteriophage T4, although there is a less versatile enzyme available from uninfected *E. coli.*

Bacteriophage T4 DNA ligase

It catalyzes the formation of phosphodiester bonds between adjacent 3' hydroxyl and 5' phosphate termini in DNA.

Uses

- It joins double stranded DNA molecules when compatible cohesive termini are present on the strands, which are to be ligated. In addition, the enzyme is active on nicked DNA and on RNA substrate.

5'….pApCpGOH pApApTpTpCpGpT…..3'
3'…..TpGpCpTpTpApAp HOGpCpAp….5'

Mg++, ATP — Bacteriophage T4 DNA ligase

5'….pA pC pG pA pA pT pT pC pG pT…..3'
3'…..Tp Gp Cp Tp Tp Ap Ap Gp Cp Ap….5'

- Joining blunt ended double stranded DNA molecules to one another or to synthetic linker. For such ligation a high concentration of blunt ended, double stranded DNA containing 5' phosphate and 3' hydroxyl termini.

5'….pC pG pA OH pC pG pT pA…3'
3'….Gp Cp Tp HO Gp Cp Ap Tp….5'

Mg++, ATP — Bacteriophage T4 DNA ligase

5'….pC pG pA pC pG pT pA…3'
3'….Gp Cp Tp Gp Cp Ap Tp….5'

E. coli DNA ligase

E. coli DNA ligase catalyzes the formation of phosphodiester bonds in double stranded DNA containing complementary protruding 5' or 3' termini. The reaction is catalyzed by NAD^+. This enzyme is used for the ligation of cohesive ends, however blunt ends can also be ligated in the presence of PEG or ficoll which also act as volume extenders.

5'….pApCpGOH pApApTpTpCpGpT…..3'
3'…..TpGpCpTpTpApAp HOGpCpAp….5'

Mg^{++} / ATP — *E. coli* DNA ligase

5'….pA pC pG pA pA pT pT pC pG pT…..3'
3'…..Tp Gp Cp Tp Tp Ap Ap Gp Cp Ap….5'

cDNA Cloning

The cloning that has been described here is suitable for any random piece of DNA. But since the goal of many cloning experiments is to obtain a sequence of DNA that directs the production of a specific protein, any procedure that optimizes cloning will be beneficial. One such technique is cDNA cloning. The principle behind this technique is that an mRNA population isolated from a specific developmental stage should contain mRNAs specific for any protein expressed during that stage. Thus, if the mRNA can be isolated, the gene can be studied. mRNA cannot be cloned directly, but a DNA a copy of the mRNA can be cloned (cDNA). This conversion is accomplished by the action of reverse transcriptase and DNA polymerase (Fig. 9.2). The reverse transcriptase makes a single-stranded DNA copy of the mRNA. The second DNA strand is generated by DNA polymerase and the double- stranded product is introduced into an appropriate plasmid or lambda vector.

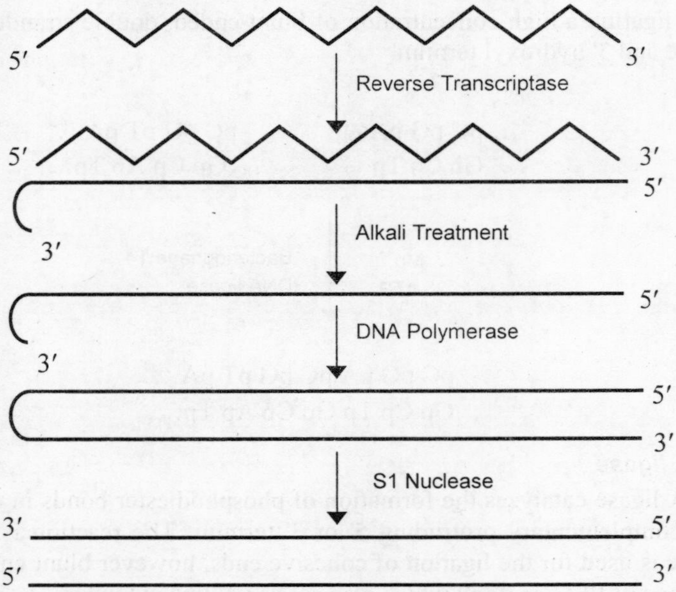

Fig. 9.2. Synthesis of double stranded DNA from mRNA

Cloning Vectors

The molecular analysis of DNA has been made possible by the cloning of DNA. The two molecules that are essentially required for cloning are the DNA to be cloned and a cloning vector.

Selection of a cloning vector is mainly based on three features

- Sequences that permit the propagation of itself in bacteria (or in yeast for YACs)
- A cloning site to insert foreign DNA; the most versatile vectors which contain a site that can be cut by many restriction enzymes
- A method of selecting for bacteria (or yeast for YACs) containing a vector with foreign DNA; usually accomplished by selectable markers for drug resistance

Types of Cloning Vectors

Plasmids

An extrachromosomal circular DNA molecule that autonomously replicate inside the bacterial cells. Usually, it has a cloning limit of 100 to 10,000 base pairs or 0.1-10 kilobases (kb). Plasmid DNA carries few genes, e.g. resistance to antibiotics, heavy metals and bacteriocins and toxins, which are conferred to bacterial host cells and serve as a marker gene(s). Plasmids may be self-transmissible or non-self-transmissible.

Non self-transmissible plasmids pass from one cell to another during conjugation aided by other plasmids present in the cell, such as pSC101 and ColE1.

Self-transmissible plasmids can be easily transmitted to many bacterial cells. Examples are RK2 and RK4 as self-transmissible plasmids. Some commonly used plasmid vectors are given in Table 9.2. A commonly used plasmid pBR322 is shown in Figure 9.3. In a number of plasmids a small synthetic oligonucleotide is added which makes the cloning site recognizable to number of restriction enzymes in a continuous manner. This site is called multiple cloning site (MCS) or a polylinker region. The pUC series of vectors are the good example of such plasmids. The polylinker regions of the typical pUC plasmids are shown in Figure 9.4.

Table 9.2. List of commonly used plasmid vectors

Plasmid	Copy number
pBR322 and its derivative	15-20
pUC vectors	500-700
pACYC and its derivatives	10-12
pSC101 and its derivatives	~5
Col E1	15-20

Phages

These vectors are the derivatives of bacteriophage lambda, which contain a linear DNA molecule, whose region can be replaced with foreign DNA without disrupting its life cycle. Usually, it has a cloning limit of 8-20 kilobases. For replication, any of the two pathways are followed by phages. The selection of the replication path of the phages depends on phenotype of host and MOI. In lytic mode of growth the circular viral DNA replicates manyfold, a large number of bacteriophage gene products are synthesized, progeny bacteriophage particles are assembled and the cell eventually lyses, releasing many new infectious virus particles.

In lysogenic mode of growth, the infectious phage genome becomes integrated into the bacterial host DNA by site specific recombination and subsequently replicated and transmitted to progeny bacteria like any other chromosomal gene (During lysogeny only one bacteriophage gene is expressed, the CI gene, which codes for repressor gene). Map of bacteriophage vector is shown in Figure 9.5.

Cosmids

A cosmid is an extrachromosomal circular DNA molecule that combines features of plasmids and phage. It has a cloning limit of 35-50 kilobases. Cosmids are artificially constructed vector with an extracircular DNA molecule that has combined features of plasmids and phages, these are also referred as the phagemids.

The origin of replication on cosmid takes place from a plasmid and the cohesive sites from λ phage. Cosmids can infect bacteria just like a phage and can be propagated as plasmids. To clone in cosmids, segments of foreign DNA are isolated and ligated to linearized vector DNA *in vitro*. This segment of DNA is flanked by cosmid molecules and the two cos sites are arranged in the same orientation. During *in vitro* packaging reaction the *cos* sites are cleaved by *ter* function of the bacteriophage λ gene proteins and the DNA between the two cosmids is packaged into mature bacteriophage λ particles.

During infection of *E. coli* by such bacteriophage particles, the linear recombinant DNA is injected into the cells, where it circularizes. Because the resulting circular molecule contains a complete copy of plasmid vectors, it replicates as a plasmid and confers drug resistance upon its bacterial host. Using media with appropriate antibiotic recombinant cosmid containing bacteria can easily be separated out.

Bacterial artificial chromosomes (BAC)

Based on bacterial mini-F plasmids. Cloning limit: 75-300 kb.

Yeast artificial chromosomes (YAC)

An artificial chromosome that contains telomeres, origin of replication, a yeast centromere, and a selectable marker for identification in yeast cells. Cloning limit: 100-1000 kb.

Cloning Strategies

After obtaining suitable gene fragment (either the cDNA molecule or the genomic fragment) these are ligated with vector DNA. Various strategies to accomplish such ligation are :

Homopolymer tailing

In homopolymer tailing, 20-40 nucleotides are added at the 3'end of both the strands of the insert in the presence of deoxynucleotide (TdT). Then complementary nucleotides are added to linearized vector. Subsequently, DNA is annealed by providing appropriate buffer conditions, which result in the formation of the open circular recombinant molecule. This molecule is then used for the transformation of the host cells.

Commonly used technique of cloning is G:C tailing at PstI site. This can be achieved by using restriction endonuclease PstI and adding a tail of poly G to it, which also reconstituted the PstI site (Fig. 9.6).

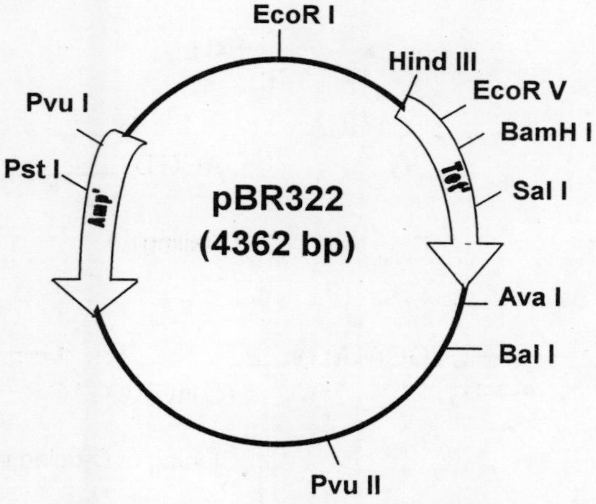

Fig. 9.3. Restriction map of plasmid vector pBR322

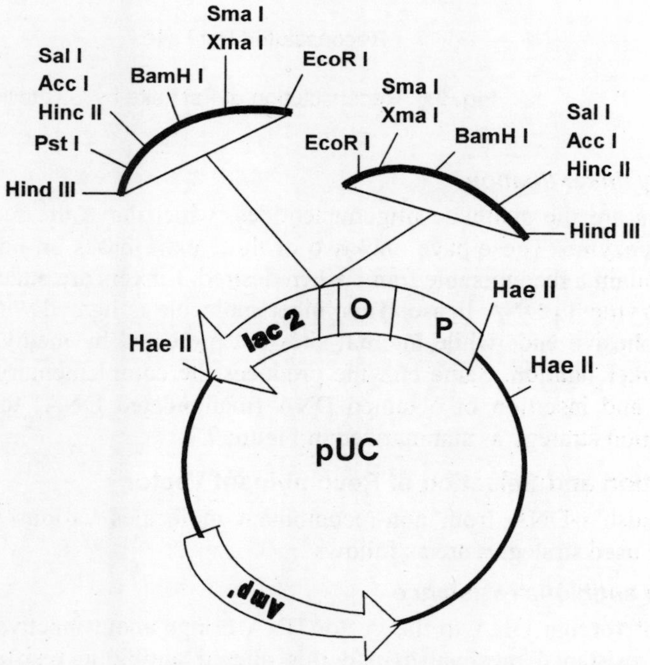

Fig. 9.4. Restriction map of plasmid vector pUC

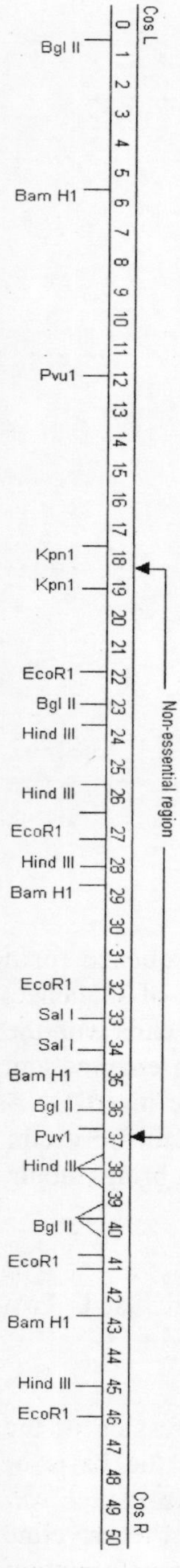

Fig. 9.5. Restriction map of bacteriophage λ

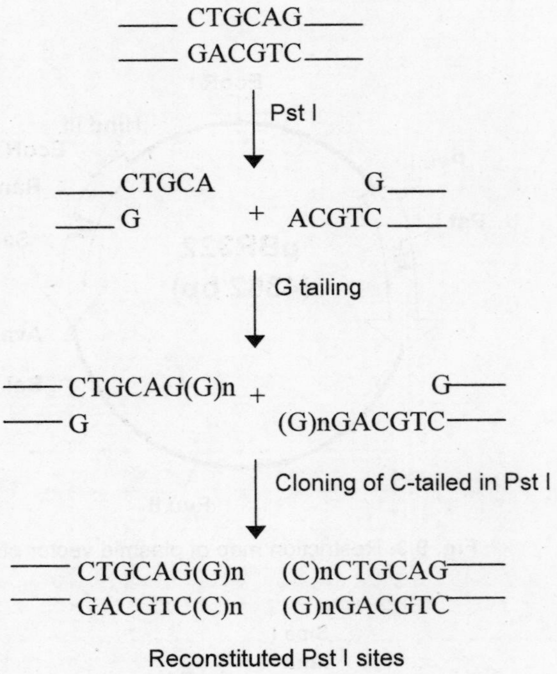

Fig. 9.6. Reconstitution of Pst I site by G:C tailing

Cloning by linker ligation

The linkers are the synthetic oligonucleotides, which have the recognition sequence for a particular enzyme. These have one, two or three extra bases on both the sides of sequence, which maintain a recognizable frame when desired. Linkers are attached to both ends with the help of enzyme T_4 DNA ligase. This linker molecule is ligated with restriction enzyme and produce cohesive ends while internal sites are protected by methylation of the insert DNA prior to linker ligation. Same enzyme produces the complementary sequences to the vector molecules and insertion of obtained DNA (manipulated DNA) to the vector brings about recombination strategy as summarized in Figure 9.7.

Identification and Selection of Recombinant Vector

To distinguish r-DNA from non-recombinant molecules various strategies are used. Two commonly used strategies are as follows :

By altered antibiotic resistance

Insertion of foreign DNA to the vector DNA brings about inactivation or repression of the antibiotic resistance mechanism and this altered antibiotic resistance makes the basis of recombinant DNA selection. For example insertion of foreign DNA fragment in PstI, *E.coli* site of pBR 322 inactivates ampicillin resistance mechanism and does not affect tetracycline resistance. For the detection of recombinant plasmids tetracycline resistance transformation can be scored for ampicillin resistance.

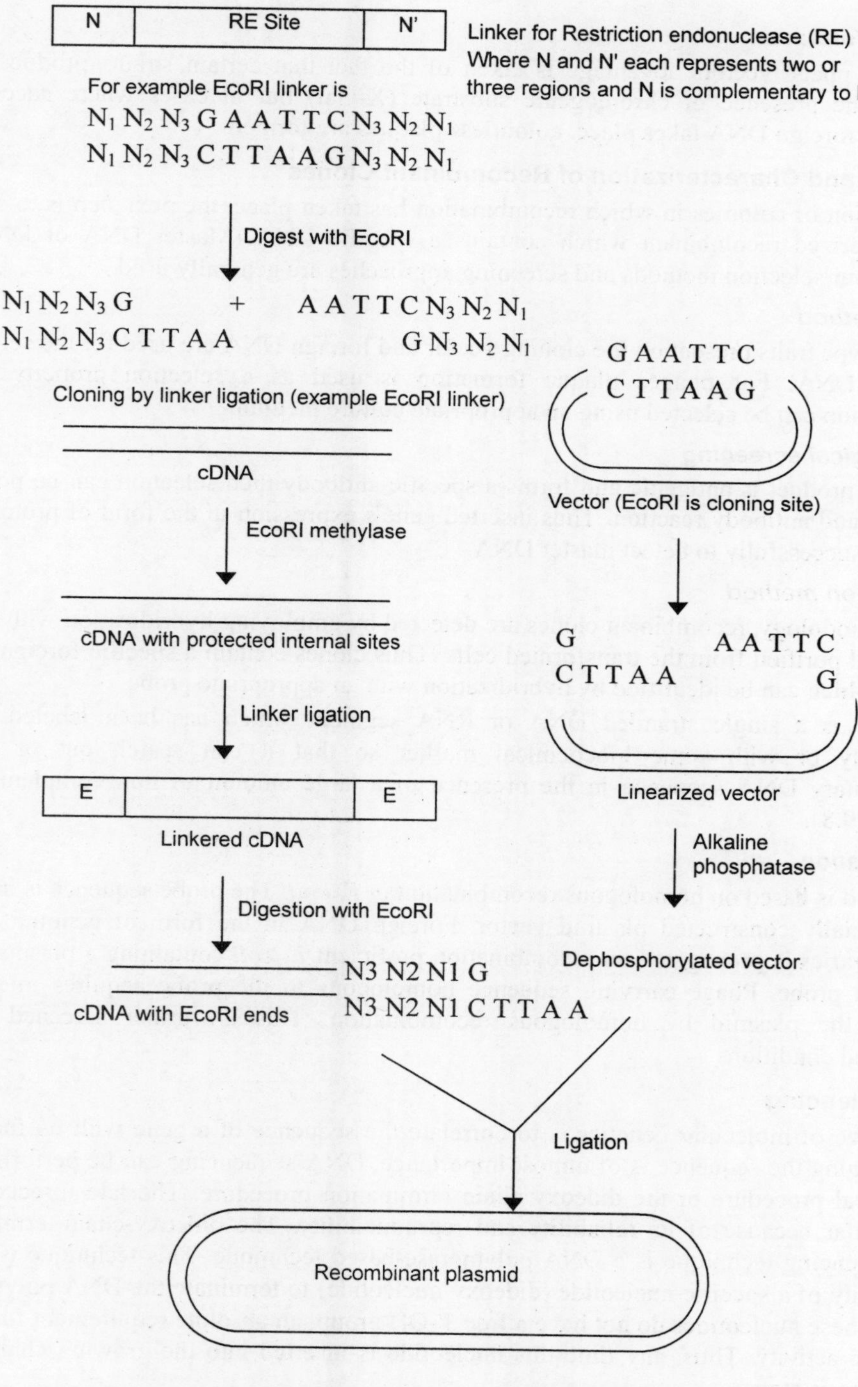

Fig. 9.7. Cloning by linker ligation

By plaque formation

In cases of phage vectors advantage is taken of the fact that certain strains produce blue plaque in the presence of chromogenic substrate (X-Gal) but in cases where successful insertion of foreign DNA takes place, colourless plaques are formed.

Screening and Characterization of Recombinant Clones

After isolation of colonies in which recombination has taken place, the next step is to screen the characterized recombinant which contains a specific DNA (Master DNA or DNA of interest). Four selection methods and screening approaches are generally used.

Genetic method

The phenotype traits present on the cloning vector and foreign DNA are used for the selection of master DNA. For phages plaque formation is used as a selection property. Thus transformation can be selected using an appropriate culture medium.

Immunological screening

If the gene product is antigenic and forms a specific antibody then selection can be possible by antigen and antibody reaction. Thus inserted gene's expression in the form of protein can be utilized successfully to detect master DNA.

Hybridization method

In this methodology, recombinant clones are detected by employing hybridization with DNA, isolated and purified from the transformed cells. Thus clones contain a specific foreign DNA sequence which can be identified by hybridization with an appropriate probe.

A probe is a single stranded DNA or RNA segment which has been labeled either radioactively or with some biochemical marker so that it can search out or locate complementary DNA sequence in the presence of a large amount of non complementary DNA (Fig. 9.8).

Recombination

This method is based on homologous recombination in *E. coli.* The probe sequence is inserted into a specially constructed plasmid vector. Foreign DNA in the form of genomic phase lambda libraries is propagated on recombination proficient *E. coli* containing a plasmid with an inserted probe. Phage carrying sequence homologous to the probe acquires integrated copies of the plasmid by homologous recombination. This is further screened under appropriated conditions.

DNA Sequencing

An objective of molecular genetics is to correlate the sequence of a gene with its function. Thus obtaining the sequence is of utmost importance. DNA sequencing can be performed by the chemical procedure or the dideoxy chain termination procedure. The later procedure is more popular because of its reliability and reproducibility. The dideoxy-chain-termination DNA sequencing technique is a DNA polymerase-based technique. This technique is based on the ability of a specific nucleotide (dideoxy nucleotide) to terminate the DNA polymerase reaction. These nucleotides do not have a free 3'-OH group, an absolute requirement for DNA polymerase activity. Thus, any time this nucleotide is inserted into the growing chain and DNA synthesis stops.

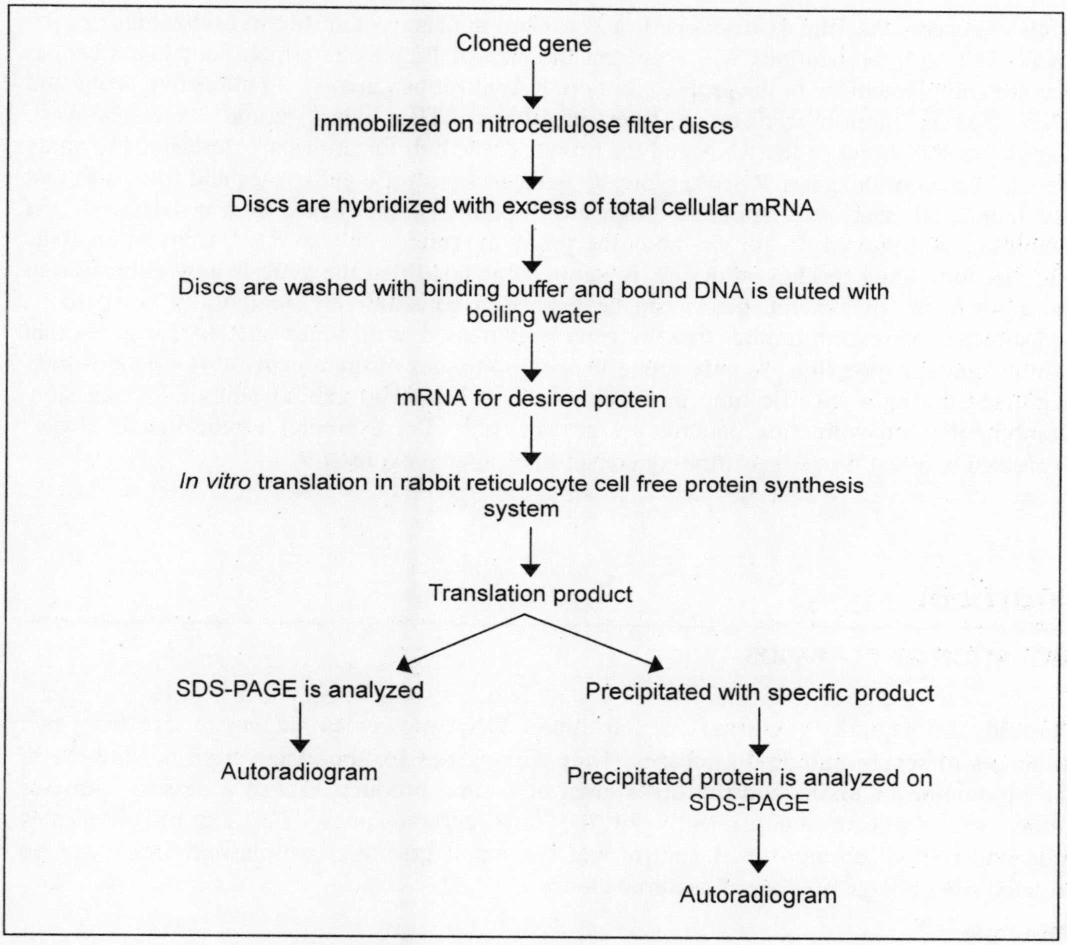

Fig. 9.8. Schematic showing hybrid selection

Technically, four polymerase reactions are performed, each containing the four nucleotides dATP, dTTP, dCTP and dGTP. In addition the reactions contain a limited amount of the one of the four dideoxybases so that all possible terminations can occur. After the reactions are finished, the products from the four reactions are separated side-by-side on a polyacrylamide gel. Each of the fragments within a lane ends with the base corresponding to the dideoxy nucleotide used in the reaction. Thus by reading the four lanes from the bottom of the gel to the top, the sequence of the DNA can be obtained.

Southern and northern hybridization analysis

The hybridization or binding of a clone to DNA or RNA provides important information regarding the structure and the expression of the gene. Southern hybridizations involve the binding of a radioactive probe to a DNA molecule that is immobilized on a nitrocellulose membrane filter. After a series of washes, the filter is used to expose a piece of X-ray film.

After exposure, the film is developed, and a band appears where the hybridization occurs. Each of these hybridizations will represent the size of fragments, which contain sequences that are complementary to the probe. Northern hybridizations involve a radioactive probe and RNA that is immobilized on a filter membrane. The hybridization occurs between complementary bases in the RNA and the probe. These hybridizations are performed to study the expression of the gene. RNA is typically isolated from different tissues and from different developmental stages of species. After electrophoresis, the RNA is transferred to the membrane and probed. If, for example, the probe hybridizes only to RNA from heart tissue after the individual reaches adult age, it can be concluded that the gene is only expressed in the adult heart. In general, genes can be expressed constitutively, temporally or spatially. Constitutive expression implies that the gene is expressed at all times. mRNA for genes that exhibit spatial expression are only found in specific tissues of the organism. If a gene is only expressed during a specific time in development, it is said to exhibit temporal expression. Combinations of expression patterns are also possible. For example, a gene that is always expressed in a leaf tissue, is exhibiting constitutive, spatial expression.

PROTOCOL 9.1

ISOLATION OF PLASMIDS

Plasmids are naturally occurring circular duplex DNA molecules ranging in size from two kilobases to several hundred kilobases. They carry genes for the inactivation of antibiotics, the production of toxins and the breakdown of natural products. These accessory chromosomes can replicate independently of the host chromosomes. The plasmid replicates independently of chromosomal control and the small quantities of plasmid DNA can be isolated from a large number of bacterial clones.

Principle

The bacterial cells are cultured, harvested and gently lysed with lysozyme treatment followed by the use of the detergent sodium dodecyl sulphate. This weakens and ruptures the cell wall releasing high molecular weight DNA that is removed by high-speed centrifugation. The plasmid DNA is left in the cleared lysate, which is then deprotenized and treated with ethanol to precipitate the nucleic acids. The plasmids are then purified by equilibrium density centrifugation in cesium chloride.

Materials

Bacterial strain carrying the plasmid (e.g. *E. coli,* JA221 carrying pBR 328).

Lysozyme solution 5 mg/ml in 0.25 M Tris-HCl (pH 8.0).

Phenol-chloroform mixture (1:1 v/v).

Saline sodium citrate solution

0.15M NaCl	0.88 g
0.015M, Sodium citrate	0.44 g

Water q.s. to	100 ml	
Dilute it ten times.		
Luria Broth (LB)		
Yeast extract	5 g	
NaCl	10 g	
Tryptone	10 g	
Water q.s. to	1 litre	
0.25 EDTA solution		
Ethidium bromide		
5 mg/ml in 0.1 M saline sodium citrate solution.		
TE + Sucrose (pH 8.0)		
0.05 M Tris (hydroxymethyl) aminomethane		0.61 g
25% (w/v) sucrose		25 g
Water q.s. to		100 ml
TES Buffer (pH 8.0)		
30 mM Tris (hydroxymethyl) aminomethane		0.36 g
5 mM disodium EDTA		0.19 g
50 mM NaCl		0.28 g
Water		100 ml

Procedure

- Grow the bacterial strain carrying the plasmid in 250 ml LB broth containing antibiotic (ampicillin) at 37°C with shaking and vigorous aeration to stationary phase.
- Centrifuge at 5000 rpm in a refrigerated centrifuge at 4°C for 10 minutes to harvest the cells.
- Resuspend the cells in TES buffer and centrifuge at 6000 rpm for 10 minutes. Repeat this step.
- Resuspend the cells in a small volume of TE in sucrose buffer.
- Make up the volume to 3.75 ml with TE in sucrose buffer and transfer to a precooled 100 ml flask.
- Add 0.75 ml of lysozyme solution and 1.25 ml of 0.25 M EDTA (pH 8.0) solution and shake the contents on ice for 10 minutes. Add 0.75 ml of sodium dodecyl sulphate solution and mix the contents uniformly.
- Incubate without shaking at 37°C in a water bath until the suspension is clear (cell lysis, 10-60 minutes). Cool on ice. Centrifuge the lysate at 40,000 rpm (in an ultracentrifuge) for 1 hour at 20°C. This will clear the lysate and the supernatant will contain most of the plasmids with RNA and proteins as contaminants. High molecular weight chromosomal DNA is removed in the pellet.
- Decant the supernatant into a measuring cylinder, note the volume and transfer into a 100 ml flask. Add 0.1 volume supernatant 2.0 M Tris-base (pH unadjusted). Add an equal volume of phenol:chloroform. Shake gently for 4 minutes at room temperature and centrifuge at 5000 rpm for 10 minutes to separate the aqueous and organic phases.

- Transfer the aqueous phase using Pasteur pipette, without disturbing the protein precipitate at the interface. Repeat previous step.
- Remove the aqueous phase and note its volume. Add 0.25 times the volume of 4.5M potassium acetate to give a 0.9 M solution to precipitate DNA completely.
- Add two volumes of chilled ethanol and place at –20°C for 1 hour to precipitate DNA completely.
- Centrifuge the contents at 10,000 rpm for 10 minutes at 0°C to pellet the DNA. Decant the supernatant and drain off any liquid completely. Dry gently in a vacuum desiccator.
- Dissolve the precipitate in 0.4 ml 0.1M saline sodium chloride solution and pipette 20 ml for testing by electrophoresis.
- Make up the volume of the remaining solution to 3.6 ml with 0.1 saline sodium citrate solution.

PROTOCOL 9.2

PURIFICATION OF PLASMID DNA

Equilibrium centrifugation in CsCl-ethidium bromide gradients has been the method of choice to prepare large amount of plasmid DNA. For some purposes it is essential to have DNA preparation that are free from contaminating RNA. Although the weight of such contaminants in bromide gradients is small, the number of RNA molecules can be relatively large and can contribute significantly to the total number of 5' termini in a restriction digest. RNA can be removed from plasmid preparations by the following two methods :

Purification by Cesium Chloride Centrifugation

Procedure

- Dissolve 3.9 g cesium chloride in the preparation completely and add 0.4 ml ethidium bromide.
- Centrifuge at 1,40,000 rpm for 40 hour at –20°C in a swing-out rotor.
- The DNA-ethidium bromide complex fluorescence under long wave ultraviolet light. The top band consists of linear plasmids and fragments of nuclear DNA while the more intense lower band is formed by circular plasmids.
- Draw out the plasmid band using a sterile syringe (fitted with a long needle) and the top DNA band using a Pasteur pipette.
- Extract plasmic fraction three times using two volumes each of isopropyl alcohol to remove ethidium bromide.
- Cesium chloride and ethidium bromide are removed by exhaustive dialysis for 16 hours against several changes of 0.1 M saline sodium chloride solution.
- Transfer the plasmid solution to sterile tubes and measure the absorbance spectrophotometrically at 260 and 280 nm. The A260 should be nearly double of A280 for a good preparation.

- Calculate the concentration of plasmid DNA using the relationship that if A260 is 1.0 then equivalent concentration of DNA is 50 µg/ml. The preparation can be stored for several weeks at –20°C.

Chromatography through Bio-gel A-150m or Sepharose CL-4B

Procedure

- Add 0.1 volume of 3 M sodium acetate (pH 5.2) and precipitate the nucleic acids with 2 volumes of ethanol for 30 minutes at 4°C.
- Recover the nucleic acids by centrifugation at higher than 10,000g for 15 minutes at 4°C. Drain off as much of the supernatant as possible and then store the open tube on the bench to allow the last traces of ethanol to evaporate.
- Dissolve the pellet in TE buffer (pH 8.0) at a concentration of at least 100 µg/ml.
- Add DNase-free pancreatic RNase to a final concentration of 10 µg/ml. Incubate the mixture for 1 hour at room temperature.
- Extract the solution once with an equal volume of phenol equilibrated in TE buffer (pH 8.0)
- Layer up to 1ml of the aqueous phase on a column of bio-gel A-150m or Sepharose CL-4B equilibrated in TE buffer (pH 8.0) and 0.1% sodium dodecyl sulphate (SDS).
- Wash the DNA into the column apply a reservoir or TE buffer (pH 8.0) containing 0.1% SDS and immediately begin to collect 0.5 ml fractions.
- When 15 fractions have been collected, clamp off the bottom of the column. Analyze 10 µl of each fraction by electrophoresis through a 0.7% agarose gel or by ethidium bromide fluorescence in order to locate the plasmid DNA.
- Pool the fractions that contain plasmid DNA. Recover the DNA by precipitating with 2 volumes of ethanol for 10 minutes at 4°C and centrifugation at higher than 10,000g for 15 minutes at 4°C.

Notes

Avoid any contamination while handling the live bacterial cells.

For successful lysis of the bacterial cells, the bacterial suspension should become highly viscous after treatment with detergent.

DNA precipitate, even if it is invisible in the centrifuge tubes, should be dissolved very gently to avoid shearing of DNA molecules.

PROTOCOL 9.3

LARGE-SCALE ISOLATION OF COSMID AND PLASMID DNA

The method used for the isolation of large scale double-stranded DNA is a modification of an alkaline lysis procedure followed by equilibrium ultracentrifugation in cesium chloride-ethidium bromide gradients. Briefly, cells containing the desired plasmid or cosmid are harvested by centrifugation, incubated in a lysozyme buffer, and treated with alkaline detergent. Detergent solubilized proteins and membranes are precipitated with sodium acetate, and the lysate is cleared first by filtration of precipitate through cheesecloth and then by centrifugation. The DNA-containing supernatant is transferred to a new tube, and the plasmid or cosmid DNA is precipitated by the addition of polyethylene glycol and collected by centrifugation. The DNA pellet is resuspended in a buffer containing cesium chloride and ethidium bromide, which is loaded into polyallomer tubes and subjected to ultracentrifugation overnight. The ethidium bromide stained plasmid or cosmid DNA bands, equilibrated within the cesium chloride density gradient after ultracentrifugation, are visualized under long wave UV light and the lower band is removed with a 5 ml syringe.

The intercalating ethidium bromide is separated from the DNA by loading the solution onto an equilibrated ion exchange column. The A260 containing fractions are pooled, diluted, and ethanol precipitated, and the final DNA pellet is resuspended in buffer and assayed by restriction digestion as detected on agarose gel electrophoresis.

Several modifications to the above protocol can be made. For example, initial cell growth times include three successive overnight incubations, beginning with the initial inoculation of 3 ml of antibiotic containing media with the plasmid or cosmid-containing bacterial colony, and then increasing the culture volume to 50 ml, and then to 4 litre. However, it was observed that recombinant cosmid DNA isolated from cell cultures grown under these conditions, in contrast to recombinant plasmid DNA, was contaminated with deleted cosmid DNA molecules. However, these deletions are avoided by performing each of the three successive incubations for 8 hours instead of overnight, although a slight yield loss accompanied the reduced growth time.

Recently, a diatomaceous earth-based method was used to isolate the plasmid or cosmid DNA from a cell lysate. The cell growth, lysis, and cleared lysate steps are performed as described above, but following DNA precipitation by polyethylene glycol, the DNA pellet is resuspended in RNase buffer and treated with RNase A and T1. Nuclease treatment is necessary to remove the RNA by digestion since RNA competes with the DNA for binding to the diatomaceous earth. After RNase treatment, the DNA containing supernatant is bound to diatomaceous earth in a chaotropic buffer of guanidine hydrochloride by incubation at room temperature. The DNA-associated diatomaceous earth then is collected by centrifugation, washed several times with ethanol buffer and acetone, dried, and then resuspended in buffer. The DNA is eluted during incubation at 65°C, and the DNA-containing supernatant is collected after centrifugation and separation of the diatomaceous earth particles. The DNA recovery is measured by taking absorbance readings at 260 nm. After concentration by ethanol precipitation, the DNA is assayed by restriction digestion.

Isolation

- Pick a colony of bacteria harbouring the plasmid or cosmid DNA of interest into a 12 x 75 mm Falcon tube containing 2 ml of LB media supplemented with the appropriate antibiotic (typically ampicillin at 100 μg/ml) and incubate at 37°C for 8-10 hours with shaking at 250 rpm.
- Transfer the culture to an Erlenmeyer flask containing 50 ml of similar media, and incubate further for 8-10 hours. Transfer 12.5 ml of the culture to each of 4 litre of similar media, and incubate for an additional 8-10 hours.

- Harvest the cells by centrifugation at 7000 rpm for 20 minutes in 500 ml bottles. Resuspend the cell pellets in old media and transfer to two bottles, centrifuge as before, and decant the media.
- The cell pellets can be frozen at –70°C at this point.
- Resuspend the cell pellets in a total of 70 ml of GET/Lysozyme solution (35 ml from each bottle) by gently teasing the pellet with a spatula and incubate for 10 minutes at room temperature. (Note: Do not vortex the lysate at any time because this may shear the chromosomal DNA).
- Add a total of 140 ml of alkaline lysis solution (70 ml for each bottle), gently mix, and incubate for 5 minutes in an ice-water bath.
- Add 105 ml of 3 M sodium acetate, pH 4.8 (52.5 ml for each bottle), cap tightly, gently mix by inverting the bottle a few times, and incubate in an ice-water bath for 30-60 minutes.
- Clear the lysate of precipitated sodium dodecyl sulphate (SDS), proteins, membranes, and chromosomal DNA by pouring through a double-layer of cheese-cloth. Transfer the lysate into 250 ml centrifuge bottle, centrifuge at 10,000 rpm for 30 minutes at 4°C.

Purification

For cesium chloride-gradient purification

- Pool the cleared supernatants into a clean beaker, add one-fourth volume of 50% PEG/0.5 M NaCl and swirl to mix, and incubate in an ice-water bath for 1-2 hours.
- Collect the PEG-precipitated DNA by centrifugation in 250 ml bottles at 7000 rpm for 20 minutes at 4°C.
- Dissolve the pellets in a combined total of 32 ml of 100:10 TE buffer, 5 ml of 5 mg/ml ethidium bromide, and 37 g cesium chloride (final concentration of cesium chloride should be 1 g/ml).
- Transfer the sample into 35 ml polyallomer centrifuge tubes, remove air bubbles, seal with rubber stoppers, and crimp properly.
- Centrifuge at 60,000 rpm to 16-20 hours at 15-20°C in an ultracentrifuge.
- Visualize the ethidium bromide stained DNA under long-wave UV light.
- Remove the lower DNA band using a 5 ml syringe with a 25 gauge needle. It may be helpful first to remove and discard the upper band. To remove the ethidium bromide, load the DNA sample onto an equilibrated 1.5 ml Dowex column, and collect 0.5 ml fractions.
- Equilibrate the Dowex AG resin by successive centrifugation, resuspension, and decanting with 1 M NaOH, water, and then 1 M Tris-HCl, pH 7.6 until the Dowex solution has a pH of 7.6.
- Pool those fractions which are having an A260 of 1 or greater, into 35 ml Corex glass tubes, add one volume of double distilled water and ethanol precipitate by adding 2.5 volumes of cold 95% ethanol.
- Incubate at least 2 hours at –20°C, centrifuge at 10,000 rpm for 45 minutes.
- Gently decant the supernatant. Add 80% ethanol, centrifuge as before.
- Decant, and dry the DNA pellet in a vacuum oven.
- Resuspend the DNA in 10:0.1 TE buffer.

For diatomaceous earth-based purification

- Pool the supernatants obtained after isolation into 500 ml bottles and add DNase-free RNase A and RNase T1 such that the final concentration of RNase A is 40 μg/ml and RNase T1 is 40 U/ml. Incubate in a 37°C water bath for 30 minutes.
- Add an equal volume of isopropanol and precipitate at room temperature for 5 minutes. Centrifuge at 9,000 rpm for 30 minutes. Decant the supernatant and drain the DNA pellet.
- Resuspend each DNA pellet in 20 ml 10:1 TE buffer, and add 40 ml of defined diatomaceous earth in guanidine-HCl (100 mg/ml) to each bottle. Allow the DNA to bind at room temperature for 5 minutes with occasional mixing. Centrifuge at 9,000 for 10 minutes.
- Decant the supernatant, resuspend each pellet in 40 ml of diatomaceous earth-wash buffer, and centrifuge as above.
- Decant the supernatant, resuspend each pellet in 40 ml of acetone, and centrifuge as above.
- Decant the supernatant and dry the pellet in a vacuum oven.
- Resuspend the pellet in 20 ml of 10:1 TE buffer, and elute the bound DNA by incubation at 65°C for 10 minutes with intermittent mixing.
- Remove the diatomaceous earth by centrifugation at 9,000 rpm for 10 minutes. Repeat if necessary.
- Combine the DNA-containing supernatants and precipitate the DNA in 35 ml Corex glass tubes adding 2.5 volumes of cold 95% ethanol/acetate.
- Resuspend the dried DNA pellet in 2 ml of 10:0.1 TE buffer and assay for concentration by absorbance readings at 260 nm or by agarose gel electrophoresis.

PROTOCOL 9.4

MINIPREP DOUBLE-STRANDED DNA ISOLATION

The standard method for the miniprep isolation of plasmid DNA includes the same general strategy as the large-scale isolation. However, smaller aliquots of antibiotic containing liquid media inoculated with plasmid-containing cell colonies, are incubated in a 37°C shaker for 12-16 hours. After collecting the plasmid containing cells by centrifugation, the cell pellet is resuspended in a hypotonic sucrose buffer. The cells are successively incubated with an RNase-lysis buffer, alkaline detergent, and sodium acetate. The lysate is cleared of precipitated proteins and membranes by centrifugation, and the plasmid DNA is recovered from the supernatant by isopropanol precipitation. The DNA is crudely checked for concentration and purity using agarose gel electrophoresis against known standards. A typical yield for this method of DNA isolation is 10-15 μg of plasmid DNA from a 6 ml starting culture.

Since highly supercoiled DNA is desired for double-stranded DNA sequencing, a modification of this method employing diatomaceous earth sometimes is used for isolation of double-stranded templates for DNA sequencing with fluorescent primers. After removal of the precipitated proteins and membranes, the plasmid containing supernatant is incubated with diatomaceous earth and guanidine hydrochloride and this mixture is added into one of the twenty-four wells in the BioRad Gene Prep Manifold. The supernatant is removed by vacuum filtration over a nitrocellulose filter. The DNA-associated diatomaceous earth is washed to remove the guanidine hydrochloride with an ethanol buffer, and then dried by filtration. Elution buffer is added to the wells, and the DNA-containing solution then is separated from the diatomaceous earth particles by filtration into a collection tube. The collected DNA is concentrated by ethanol precipitation and crudely assayed for concentration and purity by agarose gel electrophoresis against known standards. The approximate yield of double-stranded DNA is 3-5 µg of DNA from 6 ml of starting culture.

Isolation

- Pick a colony of bacteria harbouring the plasmid DNA of interest into a 17 X 100 mm Falcon tube containing 6 ml of TB media supplemented with the appropriate antibiotic (typically ampicillin at 100 µg/ml) and incubate at 37°C for 16-18 hours with shaking at 250 rpm.
- Harvest the cells by centrifugation at 3000 rpm for 5 minutes in a centrifuge and decant the supernatant. The cell pellets can be frozen at –70°C at this point.
- Resuspend the cell pellets in 0.2 ml of TE-RNase solution (50:10 TE buffer containing 40 µg/ml RNase A; some also add RNase T1 to a final concentration of 10 U/ µl) by gentle vortexing, add 0.2 ml of alkaline lysis solution, gently mix, and incubate for 15 minutes at room temperature.
- Add 0.2 ml of 3 M sodium acetate, pH 4.8, gently mix by swirling, transfer to 1.5 ml microcentrifuge tubes, and incubate in an ice-water bath for 15 minutes.
- Clear the lysate of precipitated SDS, proteins, membranes, and chromosomal DNA by centrifugation at 12,000 rpm for 15 minutes in a microcentrifuge at 4° C.
- Transfer the supernatant to a fresh 1.5 ml microcentrifuge tube, incubate in an ice-water bath for 15 minutes, centrifuge as above for an additional 15 minutes.
- Transfer the supernatant to a clean 1.5 ml tube.

Standard alkaline lysis purification:

- Precipitate the DNA by adding 1 ml of 95% ethanol, and resuspend the dried DNA pellet in 100-200 µl 10:0.1 TE buffer. Electrophorese an aliquot of the DNA sample on a 0.7% agarose gel to determine the concentration and purity.

Diatomaceous earth-base purification:

- Add 1 ml of defined diatomaceous earth in guanidine-HCl (20 mg/ml) and allow the DNA to bind at room temperature for 5 minutes with occasional mixing. Meanwhile soak the Prep-A-Gene nitrocellulose membrane in isopropanol for at least 3 minutes.
- Turn on the vacuum pump of Prep-A-Gene-manifold and adjust the vacuum level to 8-inch Hg, let the membrane dry for 1 minute, and then release the vacuum.
- Pour the well-mixed samples into the wells of the Prep-A-Gene manifold and filter at 8 inch Hg until all the liquid is filtered through.
- Wash the samples four times with 250 µl of diatomaceous earth-wash buffer, using a repeat pipette, allowing all of the liquid to filter through between washes.

- Reduce the vacuum to 5-inch Hg before turning the vacuum off. Without unscrewing the black clamps, release the white clamps and place the collection rack with clean 1.5 ml screw-capped tubes into the manifold. Clamp the manifold with the white clamps, and apply 300 µl of 10:1 TE buffer heated to 65°C and pull the eluted DNA through at 5 inch Hg. After the liquid has filtered through, raise the vacuum to 10-12 inch Hg, and let the membrane dry for 1 minute.
- Turn off the vacuum at the stopcock and remove the collection rack containing the tubes. Ethanol precipitates the DNA and resuspend the dried DNA pellet in 30 µl of 10:0.1 TE buffer.

PROTOCOL 9.5

MIDIPREP DOUBLE-STRANDED DNA ISOLATION

A midi-prep double-stranded DNA isolation has been developed to generate a sufficient amount of template DNA for several Sequenase^{TM} catalyzed fluorescent terminator reactions. Here, one bacterial colony, which harboured the plasmid of interest, is picked into 3 ml of liquid media containing ampicillin and incubated in a 37°C shaker for 8-10 hours. At this time, the culture is transferred into 50 ml of ampicillin-containing media and incubated further for 10-12 hours. After harvesting the cells by centrifugation, a diatomaceous earth-based alkaline-lysis purification method is performed, similar to that discussed above for large scale DNA isolation. The purified DNA is crudely assayed for concentration and purity by agarose gel electrophoresis against known standards. The approximate yield of double-stranded DNA using this method is 1 µg of DNA per ml of cell culture. For a 50 ml cell culture, about 50 µg of DNA are recovered, and 5 µg are used typically in a Sequenase^{TM} terminator reaction. This procedure is the method of choice for isolating double stranded plasmid-based templates for the Sequenase Dye-Labeled Terminator Sequencing Reactions.

Procedure

- Pick a colony of bacteria harbouring the plasmid DNA of interest into a 12 X 75 mm Falcon tube containing 3 ml of 2X TY media supplemented with the appropriate antibiotic (typically ampicillin at 100 µg/ml) and incubate at 37°C for 8-10 hours with shaking at 250 rpm. Transfer the culture to an Erlenmeyer flask containing 50 ml of similar media, and incubate further for 11-14 hours.
- Harvest the cells by centrifugation at 3000 rpm for 5 minutes using 50 ml conical tubes and decant the supernatant. The cell pellets can be frozen at –70°C at this point.
- Resuspend the cell pellets in 2 ml of GET/Lysozyme solution, add 4 ml of alkaline lysis solution, gently mix, and incubate for 5 minutes in an ice-water bath.
- Add 4 ml of 3 M sodium acetate, pH 4.8, gently mix by swirling, and incubate in an ice-water bath for 30-60 minutes.
- Clear the lysate of precipitated SDS, proteins, membranes, and chromosomal DNA by pouring through a double-layer of cheesecloth into a new 50 ml conical tube.

- Centrifuge at 3,000 rpm for 20 minutes at 4°C. Decant the supernatant to a 50 ml polypropylene centrifuge tube, add 20 µl of a 20 mg/ml DNase free RNase A and incubate in a 37°C water bath for 30 minutes.
- Add 7 ml (equal volume) of defined diatomaceous earth in guanidine-HCl (20 mg/ml) and allow the DNA to bind at room temperature for 5 minutes with occasional mixing. Centrifuge at 3,000 rpm for 5 minutes.
- Decant the supernatant, resuspend in 7 ml of diatomaceous earth-wash buffer, and centrifuge as above.
- Decant the supernatant, resuspend in 7 ml of acetone, and centrifuge as above. Decant the supernatant and dry in a vacuum oven. Resuspend the pellet in 0.6 ml of 10:1 TE buffer, and elute the bound DNA by incubation at 65°C for 10 minutes with intermittent mixing.
- Remove the diatomaceous earth by centrifugation at 3,000 rpm for 5 minutes in a centrifuge.
- Transfer the supernatant to a 1.5 ml microcentrifuge tube and centrifuge at 12,000 rpm for 5 minutes in a microcentrifuge at room temperature. Transfer the supernatant to a new 1.5 ml microcentrifuge tube and precipitate DNA by adding ethanol.
- Resuspend the dried DNA pellet in 40 µl of 10:0.1 TE buffer and assay for concentration by agarose gel electrophoresis.

PROTOCOL 9.6

PLASMID DNA ISOLATION (FROM LARGE CULTURE)

Materials

Stock solutions

TEG

50 mM Tris (pH 8.0), 25 mM EDTA, 1% Glucose.

5M Potassium acetate

Dissolve 295 g potassium acetate in 800 ml water, add 115 ml glacial acetic acid and fill up till 1 litre. Autoclave it.

Procedure

- Culture the bacteria overnight in 250 ml LC with antibiotics in 1 litre Erlenmeyer flask at 37°C.
- Spin down for 10 minutes at 6000 rpm and 4°C.
- Resuspend the pellets in 18 ml TEG buffer.
- Add 2 ml freshly prepared lysozyme solution in TEG (20 mg/ml) and incubate for 10 minutes at room temperature.
- Add 40 ml freshly prepared 0.2 M NaOH/1% SDS and mix carefully but thoroughly. Incubate for 5 minutes.

- Add 30 ml 5 M potassium acetate, mix very thoroughly and put on ice for 10-30 minutes.
- Spin down for 25 minutes at 10.000 rpm and 4ºC.
- Filter the supernatant over wet cheesecloth. Wash the buckets extensively with hot tap water.
- Pour the supernatant back into the bucket, add 60 ml of 2-propanol, and incubate for 10-30 minutes at room temperature and spin down for 30 minutes at 10,000 rpm.
- Completely remove the supernatant and resuspend the pellet in 3 ml water per bucket.
- Further purify the plasmid by CsCl/ethidium bromide centrifugation.

PROTOCOL 9.7

PLASMID MINIPREP I BY BIRNBOIM METHOD

Materials

Stock solutions

3 M Potassium acetate (pH 4.8)

Add 60 ml of 5 M potassium acetate and 11.5 ml glacial acetic acid. Make up to 100 ml.

Procedure

- Inoculate 3 ml LC with antibiotic with one colony using a toothpick. Grow overnight at 37ºC.
- Remove toothpick and spin down in a tabletop centrifuge for 10 minutes at maximum rpm. Suck off supernatent and resuspend the pellet in 200 µl TEG.
- Transfer to microvial. Add 400 µl freshly prepared 0.2 M NaOH, 1% sodium dodecyl sulphate (SDS) and mix well.
- Add 300 µl 3 M potassium acetate (pH4.8), mix well and spin for 5-10 minutes.
- Transfer 800 µl supernatant to a clean microvial and precipitate with 600 µl isopropanol.
- Spin for 10-20 minutes, remove supernatant carefully.
- Dissolve the pellets in 200 µl Tris-EDTA containing 20 µg/ml RNase.
- Incubate for 10 minutes at 37ºC.
- Extract once with phenol/sevag and once with sevag, add 10 µl of 7.5 M ammonium acetate and precipitate with 750 µl absolute ethanol.
- Spin for 20-30 minutes, carefully remove the supernatant.
- Dry the pellets briefly under vacuum.
- Resuspend the pellets in 50 µl water or Tris-EDTA. Store at –20ºC.
- Use 5-10 µl for restriction analysis.

PROTOCOL 9.8

PLASMID MINIPREP II BY BOILING METHOD

Materials

Stock solutions

STET buffer
10 mM Tris (pH 8.0)
50 mM EDTA
0.5% Triton X100
8% Sucrose

Procedure

- Inoculate 3 ml LC in which an antibiotic is present, with one colony using a toothpick. Grow overnight at 37ºC.
- Remove toothpick, spin down in tabletop centrifuge and resuspend cells in 700 µl STET buffer. Transfer to microvials.
- Add 125 µl freshly prepared lysozyme (10 mg/ml), place in boiling water for 40 seconds and spin down for 10 minutes.
- Remove the pellets from the microvials using a toothpick.
- Extract the aqueous layer with phenol/sevag and sevag.
- Add 350 µl, 7.5 M ammonium acetate and precipitate with 600 µl isopropanol during 10-30 minutes at room temperature.
- Spin for 20-30 minutes, wash the pellets with 70% ethanol, dry briefly under vacuum and resuspend in 50 µl Tris-EDTA containing 50 µg/ml RNase.
- Use 5-10 µl for gel analysis.

PROTOCOL 9.9

96 WELL DOUBLE-STRANDED TEMPLATE ISOLATION

A manual as well as an automated procedure is given below. The automated method is a modification of a previously reported procedure which allows simultaneous isolation of 96 double stranded DNAs per Biomek 1000 Automated Laboratory Workstation within two hours. Basically, colonies containing double-stranded plasmids are picked with sterile toothpicks into media and incubated at 37°C for 24 hours with shaking at 350 rpm. These cells are harvested by centrifugation and the pellets are either manually or robotically resuspended by the addition of TE-RNase solution. An alkaline lysis solution is used to lyse the cells and the lysate is precipitated with potassium acetate. The lysate is cleared by filtration and further concentrated by ethanol precipitation. An aliquot from each DNA sample is subjected to agarose gel eletrophoresis to crudely assay the concentration and purity. The yield of double stranded template is approximately 3 mg per sample.

Manual double stranded isolation method

The following is a manual for 96 well, double stranded sequencing template isolation procedure.

- Pick individual shotgun clones off from a plate with a sterile toothpick and deposit each separately into 96 well block containing 1.75 ml of TB media per well. Keep toothpick in media for about 5 minutes to allow the cells to defuse into the media, remove the toothpick, cover the 96 well block with the loose fitting lid, and allow the cells to grow for 24 hours in the 37°C shaker/incubator at 350 rpm.
- Remove block from the shaker/incubator and collect the cells by centrifugation at 2500 rpm for 7 minutes. The cells can be stored frozen at –20°C in the block at this stage. After thawing the cells, add 100 µl TE-RNase-A solution containing RNase T1, mix by pipetting up and down 4-5 times to resuspend the cell pellet and then incubate at 37°C incubator/shaker for 5 minutes at 350 rpm to mix more thoroughly.
- Remove the block from the incubator/shaker and then add 100 µl of alkaline lysis solution. Shake the block by hand to mix the reagents and then incubate at room temperature for 1 hour with intermittent swirling.
- Then add 100 µl of either 3M potassium or sodium acetate, pH 5, and place the block in the 37°C shaker/incubator for 5 minutes at 350 rpm to thoroughly mix and shear genomic DNA to reduce the viscosity of the solution. Place the block at –20°C for 30 minutes.
- Centrifuge the block in a centrifuge at 3000 rpm at 4°C for 30 minutes.
- Carefully remove 200 µl of the supernatant from each well in the 96 well block with the 12 channel pipetter and transfer them to a v-bottom microtitre plate, being careful not to transfer any cell debris.
- Transfer 10 µl of supernatant into the respective cycle sequencing reaction tubes, and precipitate with 150 µl of 95% ethanol (without added acetate). After storage at –20°C for 30 minutes, the pellet is collected by centrifugation, washed three times with 70% ethanol, and dried directly in the cycle sequencing reaction tubes.
- The dried templates should be stored at –20°C. An additional 75 µl of the supernatant is transferred to a Robbins PCR reaction tube (in 96 well tube format) and precipitated with 200 µl of 95% ethanol, washed three times with 70% ethanol, and stored dry at –20°C for future use.

Automated, 96 well, double stranded sequencing template isolation

- Pick colonies using a toothpick into 1.8 ml TB with TB salts containing appropriate antibiotic and shake for 22-24 hours at 350 rpm in a 96 well block with cover.
- Harvest cells by centrifugation at 1800 rpm for 7 minutes.
- Pour off supernatant and allow pellets to drain inverted. Cell pellets may be frozen at this point if necessary.
- Turn on Biomek, begin the program DSISOL2 and set up the Biomek as indicated in the configuration function on the screen. Specifically, put TE-RNase solution in the first module, alkaline lysis solution in the second reagent module and 3 M potassium acetate, pH 4.8 in the third module.

- Place the 96 well block containing cells onto the Biomek tablet at the position labeled "1.0 ml Minitubes". Place a Millipore filter plate in the position labeled 96 well flat bottomed microtitre plate.
- Start the program.
- First the Biomek will add 100 ml TE-RNase solution to the cell pellets and mix to partially resuspend.
- Next, the biomek will add 100 ml alkaline lysis solution to the wells of the filter plate.
- The Biomek then will mix the cell suspension again, transfer the entire volume to the filter plate containing alkaline lysis solution, and mix again. Set up the filtration apparatus with a clean 96 well block to collect the filtrate (wash and reuse the block used for growth).
- The Biomek will add 100 ml 3 M potassium acetate, pH 4.8 to the wells of the filter plate and mix at the sides of the wells. Some choose to place the filter plate at –20°C for 5 minutes at this point.
- Transfer the filter plate to the QiaVac Vacuum Manifold 96 and filter using water vacuum only (gentle filtration is needed as the plates are fragile and would loose their seal). This will typically take less than 20 minutes.
- The supernatant collected in the 96 well block is the crude DNA and must be ethanol precipitated before use by the addition of 1 ml 100% ethanol and incubation at –20°C for at least 30 minutes.
- Centrifuge for 25 minutes at 3000 rpm in a cooled centrifuge.
- Decant and wash with 500 ml 80% ethanol and centrifuge for an additional 5 minutes at 3000 rpm.
- Decant the supernatant, drain by inverting on a paper towel. Dry under vacuum.

PROTOCOL 9.10

CULTIVATION OF LAMBDA (λ) PHAGE

The mature virus particle consists of a linear double-helical DNA molecule surrounded by a protein coat. After it has infected a bacterium, two pathways are open to this virus: lytic or lysogenic. In the lytic pathway, the viral functions are fully expressed, leading to the lysis of the bacterium and the production of progeny virus particles. Alternatively, λ can enter the lysogenic pathway in which its DNA becomes covalently inserted into the host-cell DNA at a specific site. Lambda phage is used as a vector for cDNA. Bacteriophages are allowed to infect and multiply on bacterial cells. Then the bacterial cells are killed with chloroform and the phage particles are separated by centrifugation.

Materials

Any suitable strain e.g. *E. coli* LE 392.
Stock lambda phase (EMBL-3).
Sodium chloride
Chloroform

Polyethylene glycol (PEG 6000)
Pancreatic DNase and RNase
Cesium chloride

SM Buffer

Sodium chloride	5 g
Magnesium sulphate	1.2 g
1 M Tris (pH 8.0)	50 ml
Gelatin	0.1 g
Water q.s. to	1 litre

Sterilize it.

Luria Broth (LB)

Bacto-tryptone	10 g
Yeast-extract	5 g
Sodium chloride	5 g
D-glucose	1 g
Water q.s. to	1 litre

Sterilize it.

Procedure

- Inoculate 1 ml of overnight grown culture of LE 392 *E. coli* strain to 100 ml LB containing 10 mM $MgCl_2$ and 0.2% maltose (in triplicate). Grow for 2-3 hours till the OD600 reaches 0.4.
- Calculate the cell concentration taking OD600 equivalent to 8×10^8 cells/ml.
- Centrifuge the cell suspension at 4000 rpm for 10 minutes at room temperature and discard the supernatant.
- Suspend the bacterial cells again in 2 ml of SM buffer.
- Add bacteriophage from the stock to a concentration of 5×10^8 phage/ml and mix thoroughly. Incubate at 37°C for 20 minutes, shake intermittently.
- Add 1 ml of infected cells to 125 ml of LB containing 10 mM $MgSO_4$ and 0.2% maltose. Incubate at 37°C with vigorous shaking until the silkiness completely disappears (indication of complete lysis). It takes 7-9 hours for complete lysis.
- To check complete lysis, to 1 ml of the culture add few drops of chloroform. If it does not become clear (lysis is not complete), incubate it again till complete lysis is achieved.
- Add 2.5 ml chloroform to the flask and shake vigorously for 30 minutes at room temperature. Collect the supernatant and pool for virus particles.
- Add pancreatic DNase and RNase, both to a final concentration of 1 μg/ml to the culture, which was brought to room temperature. Incubate for 30 minutes at room temperature.
- Add NaCl to a final concentration of 1M (29.2 g in 500 ml of culture) and dissolve. Keep it for 1 hour on ice.
- Centrifuge at 11,000 rpm for 10 minutes at 4°C to remove white silky mass of bacterial cells. Collect the supernatant and repeat this step.
- Add solid polyethylene glycol (PEG 6000) in small quantities with shaking to the supernatant to a final concentration of 10% w/v. Cool in ice water and keep it overnight at 4°C.

- Centrifuge at 11,000 rpm at 4°C for 10 minutes and collect the precipitated phage particles.
- Suspend the bacteriophage pellet again in 7 ml SM buffer by gently shaking (i.e. 7 ml/500 ml of original supernatant). Add equal volume (7 ml) of chloroform to the suspension and mix. Centrifuge at 1600 rpm for 10 minutes and separate the aqueous phase, which contains bacteriophage.
- Measure the volume of this phage suspension and add 0.5 g/ml of solid cesium chloride and mix gently.
- Prepare cesium chloride solutions of 5 M and 3 M separately in distilled water. Transfer 10 ml of 5 M solution to the centrifuge tube (cellulose nitrate tube) and carefully transfer 10 ml of 3 M cesium chloride. Load the phage suspension over 3 M layer.
- Centrifuge at 25000 rpm for 3 hours at 4°C. Collect the bluish band of bacteriophage particles visible at the interface between 1.45 and 1.50 g/ml layers using siliconized Pasteur pipette and store at 4°C in tightly capped container.

Note

Cellulose nitrate tube should be filled full otherwise it will collapse during centrifugation

PROTOCOL 9.11

ISOLATION OF LAMBDA (λ)DNA

Material

Stock solutions

Lambda-dil

10 mM Tris (pH 7.5), 10 mM $MgSO_4$.

Procedure

- Grow LE 392 (or the appropriate host) in LC with 0.2% maltose and 10 mM $MgCl_2$.
- Prepare confluent lysis plates of lambda on LC with $MgCl_2$. Use LC-agarose with $MgCl_2$ and maltose as top.
- Cool the plates for a few hours at 4°C. Layer 5 ml PSB on the plate and incubate at 4°C overnight. Spin lysate for 15 minutes at 10000 rpm. Transfer the supernatant to a clean tube, add 1μl/ml DNase I (1mg/ml) and incubate for 1 hour at 37°C.
- Transfer to centrifuge tubes and sediment phages for 3 hours at 25000 rpm. Pour off the supernatant, dry the tubes with Kleenex and resuspend the pellet in 0.5-1 ml lambda-dil. Perform this step carefully.
- Transfer to microvial and spin for 15 seconds. Transfer supernatant to clean microvial and store at 4°C.
- Extract the phage DNA, after the addition of 1/10 volume 0.5 M EDTA and 1/50 volume 10% SDS, with phenol/ sevag and sevag.
- Precipitate the DNA with ethanol and resuspend in water or TE.

PROTOCOL 9.12

QUICK METHOD FOR ISOLATION OF LAMBDA (λ) DNA

Materials

Stock solutions

PSB buffer

10 mM Tris (pH 7.6), 10 mM $MgCl_2$, 100 mM NaCl, 0.05% Gelatin

Procedure

- Grow LE 392 (or the appropriate host) in LC with 0.2% maltose and 10 mM $MgCl_2$.
- Prepare confluent lysis plates of lambda on LC with $MgCl_2$. Use LC-agarose with $MgCl_2$ and maltose as top. Cool the plates for a few hours at 4ºC. Layer 5 ml PSB on the plate and incubate at 4ºC overnight.
- Transfer the lysate to a tube and add a drop of chloroform and store in refrigerator.
- Incubate 400 µl lysate with 10 µl DNase I (10 mg/ml) and 10 µl RNase (10 mg/ml) for 30 minutes at 37ºC.
- Add 1 µl DEPC (Diethylpyrocarbonate), shake for 1 minute and add 10 µl of 10% SDS. Mix carefully.
- Add 50 µl, 2 M Tris (pH 8.5), 0.2 M EDTA and heat for 5 minutes at 70ºC.
- Add 50 µl, 5 M Potassium acetate and incubate at least for 30 minutes on ice.
- Spin for 15 minutes and precipitate the supernatant with 1 ml ethanol at room temperature.
- Spin for 15 minutes, remove the supernatant, dry the pellet briefly and resuspend in 50 µl Tris-EDTA or water. Use 5 µl for gel analysis.

PROTOCOL 9.13

SINGLE-STRANDED M13 DNA ISOLATION USING PHENOL

This isolation procedure is the method of choice for preparation of M13-based templates to be used in Sequenase™ catalyzed dye-terminator reactions. A pre-incubated early log phase JM101 culture is prepared by transferring a thawed glycerol stock into 50 ml of liquid media and incubating for 1 hour at 37°C with no shaking. M13 plaques are picked with a sterile toothpick and placed into 1.5 ml aliquots of the early log phase JM101 culture, which are incubated in a 37°C shaker for 4-6 hours. After incubation, the bacterial cells are pelleted by centrifugation and the viral containing supernatant is transferred to a clean tube. The phage particles are precipitated with PEG, collected by centrifugation, and the pellet is resuspended in buffer. The phage protein coat is denatured and removed by one phenol and two ether extractions. After ethanol precipitation, the dried DNA pellet is resuspended in buffer, and the concentration and purity are assessed by agarose gel electrophoresis against known standards.

Procedure

- Prepare an early log phase culture of JM101, as above, and pick M13-based plaques with sterile toothpicks into 12 x 75 mm Falcon tubes containing 1.5 ml aliquots of the cells. Incubate for 4-6 hours at 37°C with shaking at 250 rpm.
- Transfer the culture to 1.5 ml microcentrifuge tubes and centrifuge for 15 minutes at 12000 rpm at 4°C.
- Pipette the top 1ml of supernatant to a fresh 1.5 ml microcentrifuge tube containing 0.2 ml 20% PEG/2.5 M NaCl to precipitate the phage particles. Mix by inverting several times and incubate for 15-30 minutes at room temperature.
- Centrifuge for 15 minutes at 12,000 rpm at 4°C to collect the precipitated phage. Decant the supernatant and remove residual PEG supernatant by suctioning twice.
- Resuspend the pellet in 100 µl of 10 mM Tris-HCl, pH 7.6 by vortexing, and add 50 µl of TE-saturated phenol.
- Extract the DNA with phenol and twice with ether, as discussed above and then by precipitating by adding ethanol.
- Resuspend the dried DNA in 6 µl of 10:0.1 TE for use in single-stranded Sequenase™ catalyzed dye-terminator sequencing reactions.

PROTOCOL 9.14

BIOMEK-AUTOMATED MODIFIED-EPERON ISOLATION PROCEDURE FOR SINGLE-STRANDED M13 DNA

This semi-automated method is a modification of a previously reported procedure and allowed the simultaneous isolation of 48 single-stranded DNAs per Biomek 1000 robotic workstation within 3 hours. Basically, M13 plaques are picked with sterile toothpicks into aliquots of early log phase JM101, prepared as discussed above. The phage infected cultures are incubated in a 37°C shaker for 4-6 hours, transferred into microcentrifuge tubes, centrifuged to separate bacterial cells from the viral supernatant, and then carefully placed on the Biomek table. For each sample, two 250 µl aliquots are robotically distributed into two wells of a 96-well microtitre plate, and this process is repeated for each of the 48 samples until the entire 96 wells are filled. A solution of polyethylene glycol (PEG) is then added robotically to each well and mixed. The microtitre plate is covered with an acetate plate sealer, incubated at room temperature to precipitate the phage particles, and then centrifuged. The supernatant then is removed by inverting the plate and gently draining on a paper towel, without dislodging the pellet. After placing the microtitre plate back on the Biomek, a more dilute PEG solution is robotically added to each well. The plate is then covered with another sealer and centrifuged again. This rinse step aided in the removal of contaminating proteins and RNA. After removing the supernatant, as before, and placing the microtitre plate back on the Biomek, a Triton X-100 detergent solution is robotically added to each well. The plate is agitated gently and the sample from each pair of wells is robotically transferred to microcentrifuge tubes, which then are capped and placed at 80°C water bath for 10 minutes to aid in the detergent solubilization of phage coat proteins. After a brief centrifugation to collect the condensate, the single-stranded DNA is precipitated dried, and resuspended. An aliquot from each DNA sample is subjected to agarose gel electrophoresis to assay the concentration and purity. The yield of single-stranded template is approximately 2-3 µg per sample.

Procedure

The entire procedure requires 9 rows of P250 tips (counting from the centre of the Biomek table towards the left) for the isolation of 48 templates (48ISOL). The reagent module should contain PEG-2000, Triton-X100, Tris-EDTA, and ethanol-acetate, respectively.

- Prepare an early log phase JM101 culture in 50 ml of 2X TY, as above.
- Using sterile toothpicks, transfer individual M13 plaques into 12 x 75 mm Falcon tubes containing 1 ml early log phase cell cultures.
- Incubate for 4-6 hours at 37°C with shaking at 250 rpm. (Growth for longer than 6 hours results in cell lysis and contamination of the phage DNA by cellular proteins and nucleic acids).
- Separate the bacterial cells from the viral-containing supernatant by centrifugation at 12000 rpm for 15 minutes at 4°C.
- Carefully open the tubes and place on the Biomek table.
- The Biomek will distribute two 250 µl aliquots of viral supernatant per sample into the wells of a 96-well flat-bottomed microtitre plate (Dynatech).
- The Biomek then will add 50 µl of 20% PEG/2.5 M NaCl solution to each well, and mix by pipetting up and down.
- Cover the plate with an acetate plate sealer and incubate at room temperature for 15 minutes.
- Pellet the precipitated phage by centrifuging the plate at 2400 rpm for 20 minutes. Remove the plate sealer and drain the PEG from the plate by gently draining upside down on a Kimwipe.
- Return the plate to the tablet, and the Biomek will robotically add 200 µl of PEG:TE rinse solution to each well.
- Cover the plate with a plate sealer, centrifuge, and drain, as above.
- Return the plate to the tablet, and the Biomek will add 70 µl of TTE solution to each well. Remove and gently agitate to resuspend.
- The Biomek then will robotically pool the contents from each pair of wells into 1.5 ml microcentrifuge tubes.
- Incubate the tubes at 80°C for 10 minutes to denature the viral protein coat and then centrifuge briefly to reclaim condensation.
- Ethanol precipitates the DNA by adding 500 µl ethanol/acetate to each tube, as described above.
- Resuspend the DNA templates in 20 µl of 10:0.1 TE buffer.

PROTOCOL 9.15

ISOLATION OF *ASPERGILLUS* DNA

Materials

Stock solutions

Triisopropyl naphthalene sulphonic acid (TNS) solution
20 mg/ml TNS in water, freshly prepared.
4-aminosalicylic acid (PAS) solution
120 mg/ml PAS in water, freshly prepared.
5X RNB
60.55g Tris, 36.52g NaCl, 47.55g Ethyleneglycol-bis-(β-aminoethylether)-N,N,N',N'-tetraacetic acid (EGTA) in 500 ml water (pH8.5)

Procedure

- Grind 0.5-1.0 g mycelium under liquid nitrogen using the membrane disrupter.
- Place polypropylene tubes with 1.5 ml water-saturated phenol, 1 ml TNS, 1 ml PAS and 0.5 ml 5X RNB in a water bath at 55°C, add the frozen mycelium to the tubes and vortex every 20 seconds for 2-4 minutes.
- Add 1 ml sevag and vortex with intervals for another 1-2 minutes.
- Centrifuge for 10 minutes at 4°C at maximum velocity.
- Extract the aqueous-phase once again with phenol-sevag and twice with sevag.
- Precipitate the DNA with 2 volume ethanol. Centrifuge for 10 minutes.
- Drain the tube, dry it with Kleenex and resuspend the pellet in 500 μl Tris-EDTA. Transfer to a microvial.
- Extract with phenol-sevag until interface stays clean. Then extract once with sevag.
- Precipitate with 2 volumes ice-cold ethanol, spin down and resuspend the pellet in 100-200 μl TE with 50 μg/ml RNase.

PROTOCOL 9.16

ISOLATION OF *ASPERGILLUS* DNA BY QUIAGEN METHOD

Materials

Stock solutions

Buffer B
750 mM NaCl, 50 mM MOPS, 15% ethanol (pH 7.0).
Buffer C
1000 mM NaCl, 50 mM MOPS, 15% ethanol (pH 7.0).

Buffer F

1500 mM NaCl, 50 mM MOPS, 15% ethanol (pH 7.5).

Buffer G

1500 mM NaCl, 50 mM MOPS, 30% ethanol (pH 7.0).

Procedure

- Grind 0.5-1.0 g mycelium under liquid nitrogen using the membrane disrupter. Place polypropylene tubes with 1.5 ml water-saturated phenol, 1 ml TNS, 1 ml PAS and 0.5 ml 5X RNB in a water bath at 55ºC, add the frozen mycelium to the tubes and vortex every 20 seconds for 2-4 minutes.
- Add 1 ml sevag and vortex with intervals for 2 minutes. Spin for 10 minutes in tabletop centrifuge at 4ºC with maximum velocity. Extract the water-phase once again with phenol-sevag and twice with sevag.
- Precipitate the DNA with 2 volumes ethanol. Spin directly for 10 minutes in the tabletop centrifuge. Drain the tube, dry with Kleenex, resuspend the pellet in 750 µl 50 mM MOPS (pH 7.0) and add 750 µl buffer G.
- Equilibrate a QUIAGEN-tip with 1 ml buffer B, add the sample and allow to flow through. Wash the resin 3-5 times with 1.5 ml buffer C.
- Elute the DNA with 500 µl buffer F and precipitate the DNA with 0.8 volume isopropanol, spin for 15 minutes, dry pellet briefly under vacuum.
- Resuspend the DNA gently in a small volume TE or water (preferably for overnight).

PROTOCOL 9.17

GENOMIC DNA ISOLATION FROM BLOOD

Genomic DNA isolation can be performed by given procedure. After the blood samples (stored at –70°C in EDTA vacutainer tubes) are thawed, standard citrate buffer is added, mixed, and the tubes are centrifuged. The top portion of the supernatant is discarded and additional buffer is added, mixed, and again the tube is centrifuged. After the supernatant is discarded, the pellet is resuspended in a solution of SDS detergent and proteinase K, and the mixture is incubated at 55°C for one hour. The sample then is extracted with phenol once with a phenol/chloroform/isoamyl alcohol solution, and after centrifugation the aqueous layer is removed to a fresh microcentrifuge tube. The DNA is ethanol precipitated, resuspended in buffer, and then ethanol precipitated a second time. Once the pellet is dried, buffer is added and the DNA is resuspended by incubation at 55°C overnight, the genomic DNA solution is assayed by the polymerase chain reaction.

Procedure

- Blood samples are obtained as 1 ml of whole blood stored in EDTA vacutainer tubes frozen at –70°C. Thaw the frozen samples, and to each 1 ml sample, add 0.8 ml 1X SSC buffer, and mix.

- Centrifuge for 1 minute at 12000 rpm in a microcentrifuge. Remove 1 ml of the supernatant and discard into disinfectant.
- Add 1 ml of 1X SSC buffer, vortex, and centrifuge as above for 1 minute and remove all of the supernatant.
- Add 375 µl of 0.2 M sodium acetate to each pellet and vortex briefly. Then add 25 µl of 10% SDS and 5 µl of proteinase K (20 mg/ml H_2O), vortex briefly and incubate for 1 hour at 55°C. Add 120 µl phenol/chloroform/isoamyl alcohol and vortex for 30 seconds.
- Centrifuge the sample for 2 minutes at 12,000 rpm in a microcentrifuge tube. Carefully remove the aqueous layer to a new 1.5 ml microcentrifuge tube, add 1 ml of cold 100% ethanol, mix, and incubate for 15 minutes at –20°C.
- Centrifuge for 2 minutes at 12000 rpm in a microcentrifuge. Decant the supernatant and drain. Add 180 µl 10:1 TE buffer, vortex, and incubate at 55°C for 10 minutes.
- Add 20 µl 2 M sodium acetate and mix. Add 500 µl of cold 100% ethanol, mix, and centrifuge for 1 minute at 12000 rpm in a microcentrifuge.
- Decant the supernatant and rinse the pellet with 1 ml of 80% ethanol. Centrifuge for 1 minute at 12000 rpm in a microcentrifuge. Decant the supernatant, and dry the pellet in a vacuum oven for 10 minutes (or until dry). Resuspend the pellet by adding 200 µl of 10:1 TE buffer. Incubate overnight at 55°C, vortexing periodically to dissolve the genomic DNA. Store the samples at –20°C.

PROTOCOL 9.18

RESTRICTION DIGESTION

Restriction enzyme digestions are performed by incubating double-stranded DNA molecules with an appropriate amount of restriction enzyme, in its respective buffer as recommended by the supplier, and at the optimal temperature for that specific enzyme. The optimal sodium chloride concentration in the reaction varies for different enzymes, and a set of three standard buffers containing three concentrations of sodium chloride are prepared and used when necessary. Typical digestions included a unit of enzyme per microgram of starting DNA, and one enzyme unit usually (depending on the supplier) is defined as the amount of enzyme needed to completely digest one microgram of double-stranded DNA in one hour at the appropriate temperature. These reactions usually are incubated for 1-3 hours, to insure complete digestion, at the optimal temperature for enzyme activity generally at 37°C.

Procedure

- Prepare the reaction for restriction digestion by adding the following reagents in the listed order to a micro-centrifuge tube:

Sterile double distilled water	q.s to 20 ml
10X assay buffer	one-tenth volume (2 ml)
DNA	1 µl
Restriction enzyme*	1-10 units per µg DNA

*If desired, more than one enzyme can be included in the digest if both enzymes are active in the same buffer and the same incubation temperature.

Note

The volume of the reaction depends on the amount and size of the DNA being digested. Larger DNAs should be digested in larger total volumes (between 50-100 µl).

Gently mix by pipetting and incubate the reaction mixture at the appropriate temperature (typically 37°C) for 1-3 hours.

Inactivate the enzyme(s) by heating at 70-100°C for 10 minutes or by phenol extraction (confirm the degree of heat inactivation for a given enzyme).

Prior to use in further protocols such as dephosphorylation or ligation, an aliquot of the digestion should be assayed by agarose gel electrophoresis versus non-digested DNA and a size marker, if necessary.

PROTOCOL 9.19

BACTERIAL CELL MAINTENANCE

Four strains of *E. coli* are used in these studies: JM101 for M13 infection and isolation, XL1BMRF' (Stratagene) for M13 or pUC-based DNA transformation, and ED8767 for cosmid DNA transformation. To maintain their respective F' episomes necessary for M13 viral infection, JM101 is streaked onto a M9 minimal media (modified from that given in reference plate and XL1BMRF' is streaked onto an Luria broth (LB) plate containing tetracycline. ED8767 is streaked onto an LB plate. These plates are incubated at 37°C overnight.

For each strain, 3 ml of appropriate liquid media are inoculated with a smear of several colonies and incubated at 37°C for 8 hours, and those cultures then are transferred into 50 ml of respective liquid media and further incubated for 12-16 hours. Glycerol is added to a final concentration of 20 %, and the glycerol stock cultures are distributed in 1.3 ml aliquots and frozen at –70°C until use.

Procedure

- Streak a culture of the bacterial cell strain onto an agar plate of the respective medium, listed below, and incubate at 37°C overnight.

E. coli strain	Agar media/liquid media
XL1BMRF' (Stratagene)	LB-Tet
JM101	M9
ED8767	LB

- Pick several colonies into a 12 x 75 mm Falcon tube containing a 2 ml aliquot of the respective liquid media, and incubate for 8-10 hours at 37°C with shaking at 250 rpm.

- Transfer the 2 ml culture into an Erlenmeyer flask containing 50 ml of the respective liquid media and further incubate overnight (12-16 hours) at 37°C with shaking at 250 rpm.
- Add 12.5 ml of sterile glycerol for a final concentration of 20%, and distribute the culture in 1.3 ml aliquots into 12 x 75 mm Falcon tubes.
- Store glycerol cell stocks frozen at –70°C until use.

Notes on Restriction/Modification Bacterial Strains

EcoK (alternate EcoB)-hsdRMS genes

Attack DNA not protected by adenine methylation (ED8767 is EcoK methylation).

mcrA (modified cytosine restriction), mcrBC, and mrr

Methylation requiring systems that attack DNA only when it is methylated. Ed8767 is mrr$^+$, so methylated adenines will be restricted. Clone can carry methylation activity. In general, it is best to use a strain lacking Mcr and Mrr systems when cloning genomic DNA from an organism with methylcytosine such as mammals, higher plants and many prokaryotes. The use of D (mrr-hsd-mcrB) hosts means general methylation tolerance and suitability for clones with N6 methyladenine as well as 5mC (as with bacterial DNAs).

Host mutation descriptions

ara	Inability to utilize arabinose.
deoR	Regulatory gene that allows for constitutive synthesis for genes involved in deoxyribose synthesis. Allows for the uptake of large plasmids.
endA	DNA specific endonuclease I. Mutation shown to improve yield and quality of DNA from plasmid minipreps.
F'	F' episome, male *E. coli* host. Necessary for M13 infection.
galK	Inability to utilize galactose.
galT	Inability to utilize galactose.
gyrA	Mutation in DNA gyrase. Confers resistance to nalidixic acid.
hfl	High frequency of lysogeny. Mutation increases lambda lysogeny by inactivating specific protease.
lacI	Repressor protein of lac operon. LacIq is a mutant lacI that overproduces the repressor protein.
lacY	Lactose utilization; galactosidase permease (M protein).
lacZ	β-D-galactosidase; lactose utilization. Cells with lacZ mutations produce white colonies in the presence of X-gal; wild type produces blue colonies.
lacZdM15	A specific N-terminal deletion which permits the α-complementation segment present on a phage mid or plasmid vector to make functional lacZ protein.
dlon	Deletion of the lon protease. Reduces degradation of β-galactosidase fusion proteins to enhance antibody screening of libraries.
malA	Inability to utilize maltose.
proAB	Mutants require proline for growth in minimal media.
recA	Gene central to general recombination and DNA repair. Mutation eliminates general recombination and renders bacteria sensitive to UV light.

recBCD	Exonuclease V. Mutation in recB or recC reduces general recombination to a hundredth of its normal level and affects DNA repair.
relA	Relaxed phenotype; permits RNA synthesis in the absence of protein synthesis.
rspL	30S ribosomal sub-unit protein S12. Mutation makes cells resistant to streptomycin. Also written strA.
recJ	Exonuclease involved in alternate recombination pathways of *E. coli*.
sbcBC	Exonuclease I. Permits general recombination in recBC mutants.
supE	Supressor of amber (UAG) mutations. Some phages require a mutation in this gene in order to grow.
supF	Supressor of amber (UAG) mutations. Some phage require a mutation in this gene in order to grow.
thi-1	Mutants require vitamin B_1(thiamine) for growth on minimal media.
traD36	mutation inactivates conjugal transfer of F' episome.
umuC	Component of SOS repair pathway.
uvrC	Component of UV excision pathway.
xylA	Inability to utilize xylose.
dam	DNA adenine methylase/mutation blocks methylation of adenine residues in the recognition sequence 5'-G*ATC-3' (*methylated)
dcm	DNA cytosine methylase/mutation blocks methylation of cytosine residues in the recognition sequences 5'-C*CAGG-3' or 5'-C*CTGG-3' (*methylated)
hsdM	*E. coli* methylase/mutation blocks sequence specific methylation AN6*ACNNNNNNGTGC or GCN6*ACNNNNNNGTT (*methylated). DNA isloated from a HsdM- strain will be restricted by a $HsdR^+$ host.
hsd R17	Restriction negative and modification positive. (rK^-, mK^+) Allows cloning of DNA without cleavage by endogenous restriction endonucleases. DNA prepared from hosts with this marker can efficiently transform rK^+ *E. coli* hosts.
hsdS20	Restriction negative and modification negative. (rB-,mB-) Allows cloning of DNA without cleavage by endogenous restriction endonucleases. DNA prepared from hosts with this marker is unmethylated by the hsdS20 modification system.
mcrA	*E. coli* restriction system/mutation prevents McrA restriction of methylated DNA of sequence 5'-C*CGG (*methylated).
mcrCB	*E. coli* restriction system/mutation prevents McrCB restriction of methylated DNA of sequence 5'-G5*C, 5'-G5h*C, or 5'-GN4*C (*methylated).
mrr	*E. coli* restriction system/mutation prevents Mrr restriction of methylated DNA of sequence 5'-G*AC or 5'-C*AG (*methylated). Mutation also prevents mcrF restriction of methylated cytosine sequences.

Other descriptions

cmr	Chloramphenicol resistance
kanr	Kanamycin resistance
tetr	Tetracycline resistance
strr	Streptomycin resistance
D	Indicates a deletion of genes following it

Tn10	A transposon that normally codes for tet^r
Tn5	A transposon that normally codes for kan^r
spi-	Refers to red-gam-mutant derivatives of lambda defined by their ability to form plaques on *E. coli* P2 lysogens.

PROTOCOL 9.20

DNA TRANSFECTION BY PROTOPLAST FUSION

Cloned DNA can be introduced into mammalian cells by protoplast fusion, prepared from bacteria carrying the plasmid DNA of interest, with cultured cells. The bacteria are grown in the presence of chloramphenicol to amplify the plasmid DNA and then treated with lysozyme to remove the cell wall. The resulting protoplasts are centrifuged onto a monolayer of mammalian cells and the resulting mixture is treated with polyethylene glycol (PEG) to promote fusion. During this process, bacterial and plasmid DNAs are transferred into the mammalian cell. PEG is then removed and the cells are incubated in fresh tissue culture medium containing kanamycin to inhibit the growth of any surviving bacteria.

Procedure

- Inoculate 100 ml of LB medium containing the appropriate antibiotic with a fresh overnight culture of bacteria containing the plasmid of interest. When the bacteria have grown to mid log phase (~ 2×10^8 bacteria/ml), chloramphenicol should be added from a stock solution (34 mg/ml in absolute ethanol and sterilized by passage through a 0.22 μ pore size filter) to a final concentration of 250 μg/ml. Incubate overnight.
- Recover the bacterial cells from 50 ml of the culture by centrifugation at 3000g for 10 minutes at 4°C and resuspend the pellet in 2.5 ml of an ice cold solution of 20% w/v sucrose in 50 mM Tris-HCl (pH 8.0).
- Add 0.5 ml of a fresh solution of lysozyme (5 mg/ml in 250 mM, Tris-HCl, pH 8.0). Incubate the suspension for 5 minutes at 4°C.
- Add 1 ml of ice cold 0.25 M EDTA (pH 8.0). Incubate on ice for 5 minutes.
- Slowly add 1 ml of ice cold 50 mM Tris-HCl (pH 8.0) and incubate the suspension for 15 minutes at 37°C. the bacterial cell wall is digested during this incubation. The resulting protoplasts are fragile and must be treated gently in all subsequent steps.
- Slowly add 20 ml of 10% w/v sucrose, 10 mM $MgCl_2$ made up in Dulbecco's modified Eagle's medium (DMEM) and equilibrated at 37°C. Gently swirl the tube to mix the solution. Incubate the suspension for 15 minutes at room, temperature. Check the protoplasts using the following criteria :
  a. The colour should be red orange.
  b. Upon swirling there should be turbidity but the viscosity should be low.
  c. Debris if present at all, should be minimal.

PROTOCOL 9.21

FRAGMENT PURIFICATION ON SEPHACRYL S-500 SPIN COLUMNS

DNA fragments larger than a few hundred base pairs can be separated from smaller fragments by chromatography on a size exclusion column such as Sephacryl S-500. To simplify this procedure, the following mini-spin column method has been developed.

Procedure

Thoroughly mix a fresh, new bottle of Sephacryl S-500, distribute in 10 ml portions, and store in screw cap bottles or centrifuge tubes in the cold room.

- Prior to use, briefly vortex the matrix and without allowing to settle, add 500 µl of this slurry to a mini-spin column (Millipore) which has been inserted into a 1.5 ml microcentrifuge tube.
- Following centrifugation at 2000 rpm in a tabletop centrifuge, carefully add 200 µl of 100 mM Tris-HCl (pH 8.0) to the top of the Sephacryl matrix.
- Centrifuge for 2 minutes at 2000 rpm. Repeat this step twice more.
- Place the Sephacryl matrix-containing spin column in a new microcentrifuge tube.
- Then, carefully add 40 µl of nebulized cosmid, plasmid or P1 DNA which has been end repaired to the Sephacryl matrix (saving 2 µl for later agarose gel analysis) and centrifuge at 2000 rpm for 5 minutes.
- Remove the column, save the solution containing the eluted, large DNA fragments (fraction 1).
- Apply 40 µl of 1X TM buffer and recentrifuge for 2 minutes at 2000 rpm to obtain fraction 2 and repeat this 1X TM rinse step twice more to obtain fractions 3 and 4.
- To check the DNA fragment sizes, load 3-5 µl of each elute fraction onto a 0.7% agarose gel that includes as controls, 1-2 µl of a φX174-HaeIII digest and 2 µl of unfractionated, nebulized DNA saved from above step.
- The fractions containing the nebulized DNA in the desired size ranges (typically fractions 1 and 2) are separately phenol extracted and concentrated by ethanol precipitation prior to the kinase reaction.

Agarose Gel Electrophoresis and Blotting

- Centrifuge samples for 10 seconds (14000 rpm, room temperature).
- Adjust control and marker DNAs to about the same LGT® agarose and BSA concentration as the samples (*Refer chapter 2, protocol 2.1*).
- Heat the samples to 65°C (1-2 minutes).
- Add 3.5 µl of loading solution (bromophenol blue, glycerol).
- Centrifuge for15 seconds (14,000 rpm, room temperature).
- Return to room temperature.
- Load the samples (0.7% agarose gel with ethidium bromide).
- Allow samples to set for at least 5 minutes before electrophoresis.

PROTOCOL 9.22

PCR AMPLIFICATION OF DNA

This assay has the potential to detect 1 molecule. It therefore becomes absolutely necessary that the DNA of each assay should not be contaminated.

Some suggestions for experimental procedure, to perform successfully:

- Do the controls last This will help cut down on the possibility of contamination. Use positive displacement pipetters such as a RmicroManS, as much as possible. If not 5% HCl-acid wash the pipettes for 10 minutes to avoid any DNA or oligonucleotides.
- After digestion with restriction enzymes (*i.e.*, EcoRI/BamHI) there will be about 35 μl of digestion mixture in agarose. Heat to 65°C for 5 minutes and spin in Eppendorf centrifuge at room temperature.
- Allow to solidify for 5 minutes on ice. Add 1 ml of sterile H_2O at 4°C to dialyze.
- Incubate the samples at 4°C with buffer changes after 1 hour, 18, and 24 hours (or at 1, 6, and 16 hours) as before for agarose dialysis. This is enough for 5-6 DNA samples.
- Remove the H_2O and then melt the sample at 65°C for 5 minutes.
- Mix with 150 μl H_2O also at 65°C. Vortex immediately.
- Take 30 μl of so prepared sample and use in the PCR reaction.

PROTOCOL 9.23

KINASE END-LABELING OF DNA

Typical 5'-kinase labeling reactions included the DNA to be labeled, [γ]-32-P-dATP, T4 polynucleotide kinase, and buffer. After incubation at 37°C, reactions are heat inactivated by incubation at 80°C. Portions of the reactions are mixed with gel loading dye and loaded into a well of a polyacrylamide gel and electrophoresed. The gel percentage and electrophoresis conditions varied depending on the sizes of the DNA molecules of interest (*see chapter 2*). After electrophoresis, the gel is dried and exposed to x-ray film, as discussed below for radiolabeled DNA sequencing.

Procedure

- Add the following reagents to a 0.5 ml microcentrifuge tube, in the order listed:

Sterile double distilled water	q.s
10X kinase buffer	1 μl
DNA	x μl (containing 1 μl)
[γ]-32-P-dATP	10 μCi
T4 polynucleotide kinase	1 μl (3 U/ μl)

- Incubate at 37°C for 30-60 minutes.
- Heat the reaction at 65°C for 10 minutes to inactivate the kinase.

PROTOCOL 9.24

ELUTION OF DNA FRAGMENTS FROM AGAROSE

DNA fragments are eluted from low-melting temperature agarose gels. Here, the band of interest is excised with a sterile razor blade, placed in a microcentrifuge tube, frozen at -70°C, and then melted. Then, TE-saturated phenol is added to the melted gel slice, and the mixture is again frozen and then thawed. After this second thawing, the tube is centrifuged and the aqueous layer removed to a new tube. Residual phenol is removed with two ether extractions, and the DNA is concentrated by ethanol precipitation (*for details refer chapter 2*).

Procedure

- Place excised DNA-containing agarose gel slice in a 1.5 ml microcentrifuge tube and freeze at –70°C for at least 15 minutes, or until frozen. It is possible to pause at this stage in the elution procedure and leave the gel slice frozen at –70°C.
- Melt the slice by incubating the tube at 65°C.
- Add one-volume of TE-saturated phenol, vortex for 30 seconds, and freeze the sample at –70°C for 15 minutes.
- Thaw the sample, and centrifuge in a microcentrifuge at 12000 rpm for 5 minutes at room temperature to separate the phases. The aqueous phase then is removed to a clean tube, extracted twice with equal volume of ether, ethanol precipitated, and the DNA pellet is rinsed and dried.

PROTOCOL 9.25

FUSION OF PROTOPLAST TO ADHERENT MAMMALIAN CELLS

Procedure

- Twenty four hours before transfection harvest exponentially growing cells by trypsinizaton and weed six well tissue culture plates with 7.5 x 10^5 cells/ well. Incubate the cultures overnight at 37°C in a humidified incubator in an atmosphere of 5-7% CO_2.
- Remove the medium by aspiration, rinse the wells once with DMEM and add 1.5 ml of the suspension of bacterial protoplasts . This corresponds to approximately 10000 protoplasts for every mammalian cell. Deposit the protoplasts onto the cells by centrifugation at 500g for 10 minutes at room temperature in a centrifuge.
- Immediately after centrifugation, remove the supernatant from the wells by aspiration without tilting the plate. Add 2 ml of 50% polyethylene glycol 1000 in DMEM minus fetal calf serum (equilibrated to 37°C) above the same spot used for aspiration. Incubate the plates for 1-2 minutes at room temperature.
- Add 5 ml of prewarmed (37°C) medium to each well at the same spot used for aspiration. Remove the medium from the plate by aspiration at the same spot. Do not agitate.

- Wash the monolayer of cells four times with prewarmed (37°C) DMEM without fetal calf serum.
- Add the appropriate amount of prewarmed (37°) tissue culture medium containing serum, penicillin (100 units/ml), streptomycin (100 µg/ml) and kanamycin (100 µg/ml).
- Incubate the dishes for 36-60 hours at 37°C in a humidified incubator in an atmosphere of 5-7% CO_2.
- Depending on the objective of experiment, continue with step* transient expression or * stable transformation.

* Transient expression: Harvest the cells 48-60 hours after transfection for analysis of RNA or DNA by hybridization. Newly synthesized protein may be analyzed by radioimmunoassay by Western blotting, by immunoprecipitation following *in vivo* metabolic labeling, or by assays of enzymatic activity in cell extracts. For assays that involve replicate samples or treatment of transfected cells under multiple conditions or over a time course it is desirable to avoid dish to dish variation in transfection efficiency. In these cases, it is best to transfect large monolayers of cells (90 mm dishes) and then to trypsinize the cells after 25 hours for incubation and distribute them among several smaller dishes.

** Stable transformation: Following 18-24 hours of incubation in non selective medium to allow expression of the transferred gene(s) to occur, the cells are trypsinized and replaced in the appropriate selective medium. This medium should be changed every 2-4 days for 2-3 weeks to remove the debris of dead cells and to allow colonies of resistant cells to grow. Individual colonies may be cloned and propagated for assay. A permanent record of the numbers of colonies may be obtained by fixing the remaining cells with ice cold methanol for 15 minutes and then stain them with 10% Giemsa for 15 minutes at room temperature before rinsing in tap water it is subsequently filtered through Whatman No.1 filter paper.

PROTOCOL 9.26

DELIVERY OF LIPOSOME-ENCAPSULATED RNA TO CELLS EXPRESSING INFLUENZA VIRUS HAEMAGGLUTININ

RNA Preparation

RNAs are synthesized in large quantities (several hundred micrograms) by *in vitro* transcription of linearized plasmid DNAs. The DNA templates contain the gene of interest under the transcriptional control of either an SP6 or T7 bacteriophage promoter. The transcription vector also contains 5' and 3' untranslated sequences derived from Xenopus β-globin mRNA. The genes encoding the enzymes chloramphenicol acetyltransferase (CAT) and luciferase are transcribed in the presence of 5' m7GpppG3', a cap analog.

Following transcription, template DNA is digested with RNase free DNase. After two phenol: chloroform (1:1) extractions, the RNA solution is brought to 0.3 M sodium acetate precipitated with pellet is either resuspended for immediate encapsulation into liposomes or stored in 70% ethanol at –70°C for later use.

Preparation of Liposomes

A lipid stock containing per ml, 0.75 μM each of cholesterol and phospholipids (egg phosphatidylcholine and plant phosphatidylethanolamine) is prepared in chloroform. One ml aliquots of this lipid stock are stored at –70°C under highest purity argon in acid cleaned glass screw capped tubes sealed with Teflon tape. For each preparation of liposomes 0.5 ml of methanol 3 μl of ^{14}C-cholesterol oleate and 20 μl of 10 mg/ml glycophorin are added to a tube of aliquoted lipid stock on ice. The tube is immersed in a bath sonicator at room temperature three to five times for 5 seconds each and then placed on evaporators at room temperature until the thin lipid film formed is completely dried for approximately 1-2 hours. Lipid films are used directly or after storing under high purity argon gas at –20°C for up to 2 weeks. The RNA to be encapsulated is resuspended to a final concentration of 0.8 to 10 μg/μl in 300-400 μl of calcium and magnesium free phosphate buffered saline (PBS-CMF) containing 10 mM dithiothreitol (DTT) and 1 unit RNase/μl and added to a lipid film. The solution is then flushed with argon, capped sealed with Teflon tape and rotated at 4°C overnight on a rotary apparatus. The apparatus is tilted at a slight angle so that the RNA solution in the tube just covers the entire lipid surface on rotation. The tube contents are then vortexed for 10 minutes until they become homogeneous and no patches of lipid remain adhering to the wall of the tube. The volume is recorded and a first aliquot is saved (about 3 μl). The rest of the solution is transferred to 11 x 34 mm polyallomer tube. A solution 5% w/v sucrose in PBS-CMF containing 10 mM DTT is underlaid with a 23-gauge syringe until the tube is nearly full. The liposomes are pelleted by centrifuging at 4°C for 90 minutes at 90000g. The supernatant is carefully removed and extracted with phenol: chloroform (1:1) to recover unencapsulated RNA. Typically only 1-2% of the total RNA gets encapsulated. The unencapsulated RNA can recovered and be used again. The liposomes pellet is washed twice, each time by resuspension with PBS- CMF and centrifugation at 4°C for 30 minutes as above. The final liposomes pellet is resuspended in about 300 μl PBS-CMF, the volume is recorded, and a second aliquot is removed. Both aliquots are analyzed in a scintillation counter. The % phospholipids recovered, and the phospholipid concentration of the final liposome solution, are calculated using a recorded volume and assuming that all 1.5 μM of phospholipid was present in the pregradient liposome preparation. Phospholipid recoveries range from 20-80%. The final liposomes are then stored at 4°C until used. RNA containing liposomes have been stored for over 2 months with good success.

Target Cells

Several stable cell lines expressing large numbers of HA molecules on their surfaces (> 3 x 10^6 HA trimers/cell) are available. These lines were derived from NIH3T3 (GP 4 f, HAb-2) and CHO (WTM) cells by transfection of HA structural gene and X:31 strains of influenza virus, respectively. For the studies described here GP4 cells are used. They are grown in complete medium [DME-H16, 1.0 g glucose per litre, 3.7 g $NaHCO_3$ per litre, 100 U penicillin/ml, 100 μg streptomycin/ml, 10% v/v fetal calf serum] in a 5% CO_2 incubator. Cells are typically plated at 100,000 cells/well in 6-well cluster dishes two days before use.

Fusion of Liposomes to Haemagglutinin Expressing Cells

Processing one plate at a time the cells are washed twice with DME-H16 containing no serum and incubated for 4 minutes at room temperature with 2 ml of a solution containing trypsin and neuraminidase (5 μg trypsin/ml, 1 mg neuraminidase/ml in DME-H16 without serum). Trypsin treatment cleaves the fusion inactive HA precursor, HA_0, to the fusion competent HA. Neuraminidase treatment of the target cells enhances binding of RBCs and glycophorin containing liposomes, presumably by decreasing electrostatic repulsion. Studies on fusion of RBCs to GP4 cells indicate that the amount of neuraminidase can be reduced to 0.2 mg / ml. After incubation with the trypsin/neuraminidase solution, the cells are washed twice with complete medium containing 20 μg soyabean trypsin inhibitor /ml. They are then returned to the incubator in complete medium for 45 to 90 minutes to allow the cells to reflatten. After washing twice with binding buffers [RPM1-1640, bovine serum albumin (BSA 0.2% w/v), 10 mM N-2-hydroxy ethyl piperazine-N-2-ethanesulphonic acid (HEPES) pH 7.4, 35 mM NaCl], 2 ml of liposomes solution (2.5-12.5 nM phospholipid /ml in binding buffer) is added per well. The plates are centrifuged twice for 5 minutes each time at 4°C and 500g with a 180°C rotation of the plates between spins. This centrifugation augments liposomes binding and fusion. Unattached liposomes are aspirated and the wells are washed once quickly but gently with fusion medium (binding buffer containing 10 mM succinate and brought to pH 4.75). 2 ml of fusion medium is then added and plate is held for 90 seconds in 37°C water bath. To ensure good temperature equilibration, care is taken to prevent the trapping of air bubbles between the plate and the water. After this brief incubation, the fusion medium is aspirated, 4 ml of complete medium is added and the plate is returned to the CO_2 incubator for the desired time.

Harvesting of the Cells and Analysis of RNA Expression

The cells are harvested by tripsinization, diluted in complete medium, pelleted, washed twice with PBS-CMF, and resuspended with 50 μl of sucrose lysis buffer [250 mM sucrose, 10 mM Tris (pH 7.4), 10 mM EDTA] in an Eppendorff centrifuge tube. After 3 freeze-thaw cycles each involving successive incubations in liquid nitrogen and 37°C water bath. The lysates are centrifuged at 9000g for 10 minutes at 4°C in a centrifuge. The supernatant are assayed for protein concentration and stored at –70°C until use. Chloramphenicol acetyl transferases activity is assayed by TLC or by phase extraction, using equal amounts of proteins from each samples.

PROTOCOL 9.27

RESISTANT BACTERIAL SYSTEM FOR DNA TRANSFORMATION

Genes control the traits that living organisms possess. Bacteria, such as *E. coli*, have genes on their chromosome and on a small circular piece of DNA called a plasmid. Genes can be transferred from one bacterium to another on the plasmid by a process known as transformation. In this experiment, a plasmid with a gene (DNA) for resistance to the antibiotic Ampicillin will be used to transfer the resistant gene into a susceptible strain of the bacteria. The same technique is used to transfer genes (DNA) for production of insulin, growth hormones, and other proteins into bacteria. The transformed bacteria are used in fermentation to produce commercial quantities of the protein for treating diabetes, dwarfism, or other uses.

Materials

2 Microcentrifuge tubes (1.5 ml) containing 2 drops of sterile $CaCl_2$ and labeled "$CaCl_2$"

1 Aluminum foil packet containing 4 sterile toothpicks.

4 Sterile plastic pipettes

1 Aluminum foil packet containing 4 sterile paper clips that are large and smooth. The clips should be opened into a 90° angle and the small end bent to close it.

1 Sharpie marking pen.

1 Glass test tube with a cap containing 2 ml of sterile nutrient broth and labeled "Broth".

2 Petri dishes containing only nutrient agar and labeled "No Ampicillin " on the bottom.

2 Petri dishes containing nutrient agar and the antibiotic Ampicillin. The dishes should be labeled "Ampicillin" on the bottom.

1 Petri dish containing colonies of *E. coli* (MM294)

1 Microcentrifuge tube (1.5 ml), labeled "P", containing 4 drops of plasmid DNA that is placed on ice to keep cold until used. The tube should be labeled "DNA".

1 Incubator for the Petri dishes set at 37°C or less.

It is difficult to maintain the temperature precisely unless a research incubator is used. Prolonged temperatures above 40°C will kill the bacteria, temperatures lower than 37°C will result in slower growth of the bacteria, but will not kill them.

Containers for placing tubes on ice after DNA has been added, such as a styrofoam cup.

Sterilization of Supplies

Sterilization of packets of microcentrifuge tubes, toothpicks, and paper clips can be accomplished by wrapping each item in aluminum foil, labeling the contents with a marking pen, and placing them in an autoclave for 15 minutes.

Calcium chloride

Dissolve 0.75 g of $CaCl_2$ into 50 ml of distilled water in a labeled 100 ml glass bottle with a cap. Keep the cap loose and place it in an autoclave for 15 minutes. Allow the bottle to cool until it is comfortable to hold, cap it tightly, and store in a refrigerator until used.

Ampicillin solution

For each 1,000 ml of Ampicillin agar to be prepared, dissolve 50 mg of Ampicillin (sodium salt) in 1 ml of cool sterile distilled water. The water can be sterilized by placing it in a glass bottle that is not more than half filled, putting the cap on loosely, and using the procedures described for the calcium chloride.

The sterile water should be stored in the refrigerator until it is used to make the Ampicillin solution. The Ampicillin solution should not be prepared and stored in advance for an extended period. The solution should be prepared and put in the refrigerator immediately before the nutrient broth solution and the agar plate solution are prepared.

Plasmid DNA solution

The plasmid DNA used in the laboratory has a gene for Ampicillin resistance. The plasma DNA is obtained from the supplier in a concentrated solution, which has to be diluted to

0.005 μg/μl for the DNA transformation experiment. The DNA should be kept in icebath. Any unused 0.005 μg/μl DNA can be stored in the freezer for future use. In a self-defrosting freezer, the DNA should be put on ice in an insulated container.

Nutrient broth solution

Calculate the amount of nutrient broth and add extra for spillage and other losses. Weigh 25 mg of LB premix /ml of distilled water into a bottle, make up the volume and label it. The bottle should not be more than half filled so that it does not boil over during sterilization. With the cap of the bottle loose, use one of the sterilization procedures described for the calcium chloride. After the LB has cooled and is comfortable to hold, cap it tight and store in a refrigerator.

Put 2 ml of the LB into glass test tubes, leave the caps loose, and place them in an appropriate rack in boiling water bath for 30 minutes to sterilize them. After the 30 minutes, remove the tube rack from the boiling water, let the tubes cool, then tighten the cap. Unused broth can be reboiled and stored in the refrigerator for future use.

Preparation of Ampicillin Agar Plates

Two types of agar plates should be prepared; with ampicillin and without ampicillin labeled “ampicillin” and “without ampicillin” respectively. Prepare separate solutions for the "No Ampicillin" and the "Ampicillin" plates. For each type of plate, 25 ml of agar solution will be required per plate. Label the plates on the underside, not the lid, before they are poured. Prepare three "No Ampicillin" plates: one for preparation of the starter culture and 2 for transformation. It is best to prepare about 5 extra plates for the entire class in case contamination occurs in one or more of them. Place the required volume of distilled water in one or more glass bottles with caps. The bottles should not be more than half full. Add 25 mg of LB premix and 15 mg of agar/ml of distilled water. With the caps loose, sterilize the solution by one of the methods described for the calcium chloride. After sterilization, the bottles should be swirled to mix the solution and cooled at room temperature to 55°C, which is when the bottles can be held without an insulated glove. The Petri dishes labeled "No Ampicillin" should be poured immediately. The bottom of the dish should be covered with the agar. Agar begins to solidify at about 45°C, therefore, it is important to pour the plates as rapidly as possible. If the "No Ampicillin" agar does solidify, it can be reboiled and used again. Rinse the bottle with a large amount of tap water immediately after use so that the agar does not solidify in it or in the sink. Prepare two "Ampicillin" plates. Follow the same procedure as for the "No Ampicillin" plates until the agar has cooled to 55°C. Add 1 ml of the Ampicillin solution per litre (1,000 ml) of solution, swirl to mix, and pour immediately the plates labeled "Ampicillin". If the agar solidifies, it cannot be reheated because the Ampicillin will be destroyed above 60°C. Allow the "No Ampicillin" and "Ampicillin" plates to solidify for about 30 minutes or until the agar has a milky or opaque appearance, then turn the dishes upside down (lid down, agar up). If they are to be kept for more than 2 days, store them upside down in a refrigerator. The plates can be kept refrigerated for a month.

Notes

Measures the temperature of the agar to determine when 55°C is reached, particularly for the solution to which Ampicillin is added. It is not possible to put a thermometer into the heated agar solution because it will become contaminated.

Preparation of *E. coli* Starter Plate

One Petri dish containing live *E. coli* is needed. A strain of *E. coli* should be used that does not have resistance to Ampicillin.

Use a sterilized transfer loop, a paper clip bent into a loop and sterilized, or a sterilized toothpick. Use the device to touch a colony of bacteria from a Petri dish or test tube. Spread the bacteria on the plate in a zig-zag pattern to obtain individual colonies as the concentration of bacteria on the transfer device becomes less. Incubate the plates at 37°C for 24-36 hours. Sterilize used toothpicks and 1.5 ml microcentrifuge tubes before placing them in the regular trash. Sterilize the pipettes before washing them. Sterilization can be achieved by placing them in an autoclave for 15 minutes. Wash glass bottles, pipettes, and paper clips for future use. Petri dishes can be burned, if convenient. If not, freeze the plates overnight or allow them to dry out in the refrigerator for 1 month, then wrap them securely in a plastic bag and place them in the regular trash.

Procedure

Day 1

- Use a separate sterile toothpick to transfer a colony of *E. coli* about the size of a small point into each of two tubes of calcium chloride. Use the toothpick to stir the cells vigorously and thoroughly into the solution. The solution should appear milky. Close the caps of both the tubes and discard the toothpicks into the container provided for that purpose. Label one of the tubes "B1" and other tube "B2".
- Place the tubes back in the ice and place the container of ice with tubes back in the refrigerator (Do not freeze as cold calcium chloride in the tube).

Day 2

- Finger flick the tube to resuspend the cells.
- Open the tube labeled "B1" and with a sterile pipette add one drop of solution from the "P" tube. Close the tube. Do not add anything to the tube labeled "B2". (The plasmid DNA, from the "P" tube, added to the tube has a gene for resistance to Ampicillin.)
- Place the tubes on ice for 15 minutes. (The cells are kept cold to prevent them from growing while the plasmids are being absorbed.)
- Remove the tubes from the ice and immediately hold them in a 42°C water bath for 90 seconds. (The marked temperature change causes the cells to readily absorb the plasmid DNA).
- Use a sterile pipette to add 5 drops of sterile nutrient broth. Close the tubes. Mix by tipping the tube and inverting it gently (The bacteria are provided nutrients to help them recover from the calcium chloride and heatshock treatments).

Note: For better results allow cell recovery at 37°C for any amount of extra time, 20 minutes preferred.

- On one "Ampicillin" plate, label "B1" and on the other "Ampicillin" plate label "B2". On one "No Ampicillin" plate label "B1" and on the other "No Ampicillin" plate label "B2".
- Use a fresh sterile pipette to place 3 drops of cell suspension from the tube labeled "B1" onto the centre of a Petri dish labeled "Ampicillin"/"B1" and 3 drops to the centre of a dish labeled "No Ampicillin"/"DNA". Use another fresh sterile pipette to place 3 drops of cell

suspension from the tube labeled "B2" onto the centre of the dish labeled "Ampicillin"/"B2" and 3 drops to the centre of the dish labeled "No Ampicillin"/"B2". Use a fresh sterile paper clip to spread the liquid evenly across the surface of each plate. Do not touch the part of the paper clip that comes in contact with the agar.

- Incubate the plates upside down for 24 hours at 37°C.
- Analyze the results of the transformation by placing the two plates labeled "Ampicillin" and the two plates labeled "No Ampicillin" together. The plate labeled "Ampicillin"/"B2" should not have bacterial growth because the bacteria are killed because they did not have resistance to the antibiotic Ampicillin. Bacterial growth on the "Ampicillin"/"B1" plate is from cells that took up plasmids and that became resistant to Ampicillin. There is extensive bacterial growth on both of the "No Ampicillin" plates because the antibiotic was not present and both resistant and nonresistant bacteria could grow.

PROTOCOL 9.28

DNA TRANSFORMATION OF BACTERIA RED COLONY

In this experiment, a plasmid with a gene (DNA) for resistance to the antibiotic Ampicillin and the lacZ gene will be transferred into a susceptible strain of the bacteria. The transformed bacteria are used in fermentation to produce commercial quantities of the protein for treating diabetes, dwarfism, or other uses. The cells that take up this plasmid will show resistance to the antibiotic protein produced by the lacZ gene.

Materials

Same as previous experiment except use *E. coli* (DH5 α strain) instead *E. coli* (MM294).

Sterilization of Supplies, Calcium chloride, Calcium chloride, Ampicillin solution, Plasmid DNA solution, Nutrient broth solution

Same as previous experiment (*protocol 9.27*).

MacConkey Agar Plates

Two types of agar plates should prepared, without ampicillin " No Ampicillin" and with Ampicillin "Ampicillin". Prepare separate solutions for the "No Ampicillin" and the "Ampicillin" plates. For each type of plate, 25 ml of agar solution is required per plate. Label the plates on the underside, not the lid, before they are poured. Prepare three "No Ampicillin" plates, one for preparation of the starter culture and 2 for transformation. It is best to prepare about 5 extra plates in case contamination occurs in one or more of them. Place the required volume of distilled water in one or more glass bottles with caps. The bottle should not be more than half full. Add 50 mg of lactose MacConkey medium per ml of distilled water. With the cap loose, sterilize the solution by one of the methods described for the calcium chloride.

Preparation of *E. Coli* Starter Plate

A strain of *E. coli* should be used that does not have resistance to Ampicillin. Use a sterilized transfer loop, a paper clip bent into a loop and a sterilized toothpick. Use the device to touch a colony of bacteria from a Petri dish or test tube. Spread the bacteria on the plate in a zig-zag pattern to obtain individual colonies as the concentration of bacteria on the transfer device becomes less. Incubate the plates at 37°C for 24-36 hours.

Preparation of Ampicillin Agar Plates

Prepare two "Ampicillin" plates. Follow the same procedure as for the "No Ampicillin" plates until the agar has cooled to 55°C. Add 1 ml of the Ampicillin solution per litre (1,000 ml) of solution, swirl to mix, and pour immediately the plates labeled "Ampicillin". If the agar solidifies, it cannot be reheated because the Ampicillin will be destroyed above 60°C. Allow the "No Ampicillin" and "Ampicillin" plates to solidify for about 30 minutes or until the agar has a milky or opaque appearance, then turn the dishes upside down (lid down, agar up). If they are to be kept for more than 2 days, store them upside down in a refrigerator. The plates can be kept refrigerated for a month.

Procedure

Day 1

- Use a separate sterile toothpick to transfer a colony of *E. coli* of about the size, of this into each of two tubes of calcium chloride. Use the toothpick to stir the cells vigorously and thoroughly into the solution. The solution should appear milky. Close the caps of both the tubes and discard the toothpicks into the container provided for that purpose. Label one of the tubes "B1"and the other tube "B2".
- Place the tubes back in the ice and place the container of ice with tubes back in the refrigerator. (Do not freeze the cold calcium chloride in the tubes.)

Day 2

- Finger flick the tube to resuspend the cells.
- Open the tube labeled "B1" and with a sterile pipette add one drop of solution form the "P" tube. Close the tube. Do not add anything to the tube labeled "B2". (The plasmid DNA, from the "P" tube, added to the tube has a gene for resistance to Ampicillin and lacZ.)
- Place the tubes on ice for 15 minutes. (The cells are kept cold to prevent them from growing while the plasmids are being absorbed.)
- Remove the tubes from the ice and immediately hold them in a 42°C water bath for 90 seconds. (The marked temperature change causes the cells to readily absorb the plasmid DNA).
- Use a sterile pipette to add 5 drops of sterile nutrient broth to each of the tubes. Close the tubes. Mix by tipping the tube and inverting it gently (The bacteria are provided nutrients to help them recover from the calcium chloride and heatshock treatments).

Note

For better results allow cell recovery at 37°C for any amount of extra time, 20 minutes preferred.

- Label the underside of the four Petri dishes. On one "Ampicillin" plate, label "B1" and on the other "Ampicillin" plate label "B2". On one "No Ampicillin" plate label "B1" and on the other "No Ampicillin" plate label "B2".
- Use a fresh sterile pipette to place 3 drops of cell suspension from the tube labeled "B1" onto the center of a Petri dish labeled "Ampicillin"/"B1" and 3 drops to the center of a dish

labeled "No Ampicillin"/"DNA". Use another fresh sterile pipette to place 3 drops of cell suspension from the tube labeled "B2" onto the center of the dish labeled "Ampicillin"/"B2" and 3 drops to the centre of the dish labeled "No Ampicillin"/"B2". Use a fresh sterile paper clip to spread the liquid evenly across the surface of each plate. Do not touch the part of the paper clip that comes in contact with the agar.

- Incubate the plates upside down for 24 hours at 37°C.
- Analyze the results of the transformation by placing the two plates labeled "Ampicillin" and the two plates labeled "No Ampicillin" together. (The plate labeled "Ampicillin"/"B2" should not have bacterial growth because the bacteria are killed because they did not have resistance to the antibiotic Ampicillin. Bacterial growth on the "Ampicillin"/"B1" plate is from cells that took up plasmids and that became resistant to Ampicillin and became dark red. There is extensive bacterial growth on both of the "No Ampicillin" plates because the antibiotic was not present and both resistant and nonresistant bacteria could grow. The resistant trait for the antibiotic Ampicillin is referred to as the "marker gene" or "selective marker".)

PROTOCOL 9.29

SOLUBILIZATION OF INCLUSION BODIES

A high level of expression of proteins in *E. Coli* often results in cytoplasmic granules that can be seen with a phase contrast microscope and that can be separated from crude cell lysates by centrifugation. Cells expressing high levels of foreign protein are concentrated by centrifugation and lysed by mechanical techniques, sonication or lysozyme plus detergents. The inclusion bodies are pelleted by centrifugation and washed with Triton-X 100 and EDTA or urea. To obtain soluble active protein the washed inclusion bodies must be solubilized and then refolded. Each protein may require a different procedure, which must be determined empirically. Various conditions (e.g., guanidine HCl 5-8 M, urea 6-8 M, SDS, alkaline pH, or acetonitrile/propanol) may be used to solubilize the inclusion bodies. The procedure given below has been used to solubilize prorennin inclusion bodies. After successful solubilization various refolding methods involving dilution or dialysis may be tried. The yield of active protein or of protein with the same disulphide bonds as the original protein depends on the concentration, purity and size of the polypeptide; the pH and ionic strength of the solvent and the rate of refolding. Other factors include the number of disulphide bonds and nature of the protein itself.

Procedure

Cell lysis

The following procedure utilizes lysozyme plus detergent for lysis

- Centrifuge one litre of cell culture at 500g for 15 minutes at 4°C.
- In the cold room remove the supernatant and weigh the *E. coli* pellet. For each gram (wet weight) of *E. coli*, add 3 ml lysis buffer. Resuspend the pellet.

- For each gram of *E. coli*, add 8 µl of 50 mM phenylmethylsulphonylfluoride (PMSF) and then 80 µl of lysozyme (10 mg/ml). Stir occasionally for 20 minutes.
- Add 4 mg of deoxycholic acid per gram of *E. coli* while stirring continuously.
- Place at 37°C and stir with a glass rod. When the lysate becomes viscous, add 20 µl of DNase I (1 mg/ml) per gram of *E. coli*.
- Place the lysate at room temperature until it is no longer viscous (about 30 minutes).

Purification and washing of inclusion bodies

- Centrifuge the cell lysate at 12000g for 15 minutes at 4°C in a microfuge.
- In a cold room decant the supernatant. Resuspend the pellet in 9 volumes of lysis buffer containing 0.5% Triton-X 100 and 10 mM EDTA (pH 8.0).
- Store at room temperature for 5 minutes.
- In a cold room, centrifuge at 12000g for 15 minutes at 4°C in a microfuge.
- Decant the supernatant and set aside for the next step. Resuspend the pellet in 100 µl of double distilled water.
- Remove 10 µl samples of the supernatant and the resuspended pellet. Mix each with 10 µl of 2X SDS gel loading buffer and analyze by SDS polyacrylamide gel electrophoresis to determine if most of the protein of interest is in the pellet.

Solubilization of inclusion bodies

- Suspend the washed pellet in 100 µl of lysis buffer containing 0.1 mM PMSF (added fresh), 8 M urea (deionized). Store for 1 hour at room temperature.
- Add this solution to 9 volumes of 50 mM KH_2PO_4 (pH 10.7), 1 mM EDTA (pH 8.0), 50 mM NaCl and store for 30 minutes at room temperature. Maintain the pH at 10.7 with KOH.
- Adjust the pH to 8.0 with HCl and store for at least 30 minutes at room temperature.
- Centrifuge at 12000 g for 15 minutes at room temperature in a microfuge.
- Decant the supernatant and set aside. Resuspend the pellet in 100 µl of 1X SDS gel loading buffer. Mix the pellet sample with 1X SDS gel loading buffer. Analyze both samples by SDS polyacrylamide gel elecrophoresis to determine the degree of solubilization.

PROTOCOL 9.30

SOLUBILIZATION OF RECOMBINANT PROTEINS FROM INCLUSION BODIES

Reagents

RIPA Buffer

0.1% SDS, 1% Triton X-100, 1% Sodium deoxycholate in PBS

10% SDS

Protease Inhibitors

PBS

Procedure

- Centrifuge protein suspension at 8000g for 10 minutes at 4°C to pellet the inclusion bodies.
- Wash the pellet twice by vortexing in fresh, ice cold RIPA containing 1mM PMSF, 1-5 µg/ml leupeptin, 1-5 µg/ml pepstatin, and 1-5 µg/ml aprotinin. Recentrifuge the inclusion bodies after each wash. At this stage the inclusion bodies should be quite pure.
- Estimate the volume of the inclusion bodies and add 2 volumes of 10% SDS. Transfer to Eppendorf tubes.
- Solubilize the pellet by gently pipetting up and down.
- Solubilization of the inclusion bodies can be facilitated by heating the sample to 95°C for a period of 1 hour.
- Once the inclusion bodies are in solution, dilute the sample with 9 volumes of PBS. The protein should stay in solution.
- Dialyze the protein solution overnight against a 100-fold volume of PBS containing 0.05% SDS and 1 mM PMSF. Perform this dialysis at room temperature as the SDS will come out of solution at 4°C.
- Change the dialysis buffer to PBS containing 0.01% SDS and 1 mM PMSF. Dialyze for several hours at room temperature. Some of the protein may precipitate during dialysis, but most will stay in solution
- Store the dialyzed solution at 4°C. Some fraction of SDS may separate come out of solution at this temperature, but it should go back in when the sample is warmed up to room temperature.
- Analyze a small aliquot of the preparation by SDS-PAGE along with protein standards to quantify the final protein concentration and yield (*Refer chapter 2*).

PROTOCOL 9.31

ASSAYS FOR GENE TRANSFER

There are several reliable methods to quantitate the presence of transferred DNA. These include Southern blot of genomic DNA, Polymerase chain reaction (PCR), Northern analysis of cellular RNA or by RNA driven PCR, assay of protein production using immunoprecipitation, assay (Western blot), assay of protein production by immunofluorescence analysis and bioassay of protein.

PCR is the method of choice for assay of DNA transfer as it has maximum sensitivity and speed. PCR can also be used for the quantitation of DNA, however Southern blot is less cumbersome to operate with. The major limitation of Southern Blot is that the samples to be tested must be in purified form while PCR analysis can be begun with crude cell homogenates. As far as result is concerned, Southern blot is more informative as it provides map information including information on junction fragments (regions of the host chromosomal DNA flanking the integrated DNA). Such analysis gives the information about overall arrangement of integrated DNA in the host chromosomes as well as about the number of copies of the integrated DNA present.

Southern Type Techniques

Composition of 20X SSC

Solution of 0.3 M trisodium citrate and 3 M sodium chloride

Final pH 7.0

Method I

- In a horizontal gel apparatus, prepare an agarose gel. The concentration of the agarose is dependent on the size of DNA fragments intended to be resolved (*see chapter 3, protocol 2.1*).
- Obtain 0.2-0.5 μg of restriction endonuclease digested recombinant plasmid DNA, which is more than sufficient to allow inserted DNA sequences to be easily detected by Southern hybridization. For restriction endonuclease digested mammalian genomic DNA, run 10-30 μg per lane in order to detect sequence that occurs as a single copy in a haploid genome.
- After electrophoresis stain the gel using 0.5 μg/ml ethidium bromide for 30 minutes and photograph the gel on ultraviolet light box with a fluorescent ruler alongside the gel. This will help orient the DNA bonding and migration pattern on the filter with respect to the gel.
- Transfer the gel in a glass baking dish to denature the DNA by soaking the gel in several volumes of 1.5 M NaCl/1.5 M NaOH for 1 hour at room temperature under constant motion.
- Pour off the denaturing solution and neutralize the gel by soaking it in several volumes of 1M Tris-HCl (pH 8.0)/1.5 M NaCl for 1 hour at room temperature, with constant motion.
- To set up the blot, use the acrylic gel tray to form the gel. Other supports can be used, such as a stack of glass plates. Place the gel support upside down in a glass Pyrex baking dish. Add 20X SSC to within ~1 cm of the top of the tray.
- Wet a piece of Whatman 3 MM paper approximately twice as long and of the same width as the gel. Wrap this over the support. This will function as a wick. Squeeze out any air bubbles that may have formed underneath the paper.
- Cut a piece of nitrocellulose filter approximately 2 mm wider and 2 mm longer than the gel. Place a pencil mark in the lower right hand corner of the filter to help orient the filter after hybridization. Prewet the nitrocellulose filter after hybridization. Prewet the nitrocellulose filter in H_2O, then add 2X SSC until the filter is completely wet.
- Invert the gel onto the Whatman wick so as to place the open wells in contact with the Whatman 2 MM paperwick. Gently squeeze out any air bubbles.
- Overlay the gel with the prewet nitrocellulose filter so as to position the pencil mark in the lower left-hand corner of the inverted gel. Make sure that the entire gel is covered with the filter. Remove any air bubbles that may have become trapped between the filter and the gel.
- Overlay the nitrocellulose filter with 2-3 pieces of Whatman 2 MM paper (prewet with 2X SSC) cut to the same size as the gel. Remove any air bubbles.
- Cut a stack of paper towels 6-8 cm high and 2-3 mm smaller in both the dimensions than the previous Whatman 3MM. Place on top of the Whatman 3 MM paper.

- Place a glass plate on top of the stack of paper towel, followed by a 500 g weight. The object is to set up a flow of liquid from the reservoir (in the glass baking dish) through the gel and the nitrocellulose filter, so that DNA fragments are eluted form the gel and deposited onto the nitrocellulose filter.
- Cover the blotting gel with plastic wrap to prevent evaporation of the 20X SSC transfer solution.
- The efficiency of DNA transfer is largely a function of the size of the DNA. As a matter of convenience, the transfer is allowed to proceed for ~16 hours (overnight).
- Remove the paper towels and Whatman 3 MM paper above the gel. Turn the dehydrated gel and filter over and lay them, gel side up, on a dry sheet of Whatman 3 MM paper. Mark the positions of the gel slots on the filter with soft pencil.
- Peel off the filter, rinse the filter with 2X SSC in squirt bottle and allow it to air dry.
- Bake the filter between two pieces of Whatman 3 MM paper for 1.5-2 hours at 80°C in a vacuum oven.

Method II

In this procedure a synthetic transfer membrane Gene Screen Plus™ is used instead of nitrocellulose. This membrane exhibits higher strength and higher capacity for nucleic acids without the need of backing.

- Electrophores the digested DNA into the gel. After electrophoresis, stain with 0.5 μg/ml ethidium bromide for 30 minutes.
- Photograph gel with a fluorescent ruler beside the gel to facilitate analysis of the DNA migration pattern.
- Incubate the gel in 0.4 N NaOH, 1.7 M NaCl for 30minutes, with constant rocking motion.
- Pour off previous solution and incubate gel in a solution containing 1.5 M NaCl, 0.5 M Tris-HCl, pH 7.5 for 30 minutes at room temperature, with constant rocking motion.
- Cut a Gene Screen Plus membrane 12 mm longer and 2 mm wider than the agarose gel. Label side B of the membrane it should be in contact with the gel. Use 10X SSC as the transfer solution.
- Assemble the gel support and set up the blot according to the same protocol used for nitrocellulose. Side B of the membrane should be in contact with the gel. Use 10X SSC as the transfer solution.
- Allow the transfer to occur for 16 hours or overnight.
- Remove the paper towels and Whatman membrane paper.
- Mark the wells with a soft pencil as needed to orient the membrane.
- Peel off the membrane and immerse in 0.4 N NaOH for 30-60 seconds.
- Remove the membrane and immerse in a solution containing 0.2 M Tris-HCl, pH 7.5, 2X SSC for 2-3 minutes.
- Place the membrane onto a piece of Whatman 3 MM paper, with the transferred DNA side up.
- Allow membrane to dry at room temperature.
- Proceed with prehybridization.

PROTOCOL 9.32

DNA TRANSFECTION IN RETROVIRUS STOCKS

Transfection Solutions

Prepare fresh solutions.

HBS solution

0.5 M HEPBS.	5.0 ml
2.0 M NaCl.	6.25 ml
0.15 M Na_2HPO_4.	0.5 ml

Add H_2O to ~45 ml.

Adjust pH to 7.05-7.10 with 1N NaOH.

Make up the volume to 50 ml. Filter and sterilize.

Procedure

- At day 1 plate retroviral packaging cells at 5x 10^5 cells/60 mm dish.
- At day 2 feed recipient cultures with 4 ml of fresh medium.
- Transfect with the calcium phosphate precipitation procedure:
  1. For each plasmid DNA sample, prepare a DNA/ $CaCl_2$ solution by mixing 25 µl of 2.0 M $CaCl_2$ and 10 µg of plasmid DNA. Bring to a total volume of 200 µl with distilled H_2O.
  2. For each sample, add 200 µl of DNA/ $CaCl_2$ solution drop by drop to the 2X HBS in to a clear plastic tube with constant agitation.
  3. After incubation at room temperature leave undisturbed for 30 minutes, add 400 µl of the fine precipitate to the recipient packaging line cells and swirl the medium to mix.
- At day 3 aspirate medium containing DNA. Feed cells with fresh medium.
- Plate corresponding packaging cells for infection on day 4 at 5 x 10^5 cells/60 mm dish.
- After not more than 16 hours of feeding on day 4, remove the viral supernatant from the transfected culture.
- Centrifuge for 5 minutes at 3000g at room temperature.
- Feed the recipient cells with 4 ml of fresh medium supplemented with polybrene to a final concentration of 4 µg/ml. Infect the recipient cells with samples of the virus containing medium.
- Infect multiple plates with increasing amounts (1 µl, 10 µl, 100 µl) of virus containing media.
- After virus addition, swirl the polybrene supplemented medium in the culture dishes to mix the virus.
- Incubate the infected cultures overnight at 37°C.
- At day 5 trypsinize the transfected cells 1:20 into selection medium.
- Change the selection medium every 3-4 days until colonies have formed.

PROTOCOL 9.33

TITRATION AND ANALYSIS OF RECOMBINANT RETROVIRUS STOCKS

Stock solutions

Polybrene stock (100 X)

400 μg/ml of polybrene in PBS. Sterilize by filtration and store at 4°C.

Procedure

- At day 1 plate viral producer cells at 2 x 10^5 cells/60 mm dish.
- At day 4 change media of producers. Plate recipient cells at 5 x 10^5 cells/60 mm dish.
- At day 5 after a 16 hours incubation, harvest the viral supernatant and centrifuge at 3000g for 5 minutes to remove cells and debris. Feed recipient cells with 4 ml of fresh medium supplemented with polybrene to a final concentration of 4 μg /ml. To titre a virus stock, assume a virus titer of 1 x 10^8 colony forming units CFU/ml. Prepare a dilution series (10^{-1} to 10^{-9}) of virus and infect with 100 μl of filtered virus. Incubate the infected cells overnight at 37°C.
- At day 6 trypsinize cells and seed 1:20 into appropriate selection medium. Feed cultures with selection medium every three days. When colonies appear, stain as described in the section on the propagation of cell lines. Virus titer is 20 x dilution x number of colonies.

PROTOCOL 9.34

ASSAY FOR GENE TRANSFER AND EXPRESSION BY PCR BASED TECHNIQUES

To detect the presence of nucleic acid sequence by PCR is a simple and reproducible method that is widely being used.

Method

- Prepare this PCR

Cell lysate	1 μl
10X PCR buffer	10 μl
10 mM dNTPs	10 μl
Upstream primer (30- 50 pmoles/μl)	1 μl
Downstream primer (30-50 pmoles/μl)	1 μl
Double distilled water	77 μl
Total	100 μl

Layer 100 μl of mineral oil.

Procedure

- Incubate the reaction mixture at 95°C for 5 minutes.
- Let the reaction cool to 80°C, then add one unit of Taq polymerase.

- Perform 25-35 cycles at:
  95°C, 30 seconds (denaturing step).
  50-72°C, 30 seconds (annealing step).
  72°C, 30-120 seconds (extension step).
- Extract the mineral oil by adding 300 µl of TE saturated chloroform.
- Extract any residual chloroform by ether extraction.
- Remove any residual ether by heating the tube, open at 68°C for 5 minutes.
- Add 2 µl of 6X LB to 10 µl of PCR reaction and load into a composite 3% NuSieve or 1% SeaKem agarose gel in TEA buffer.
- Electrophorese stain with 10 µg/ml ethidium bromide for 10 minutes.

PCR Based Techniques

Detection of the presence of nucleic acid sequence by PCR is a simple and reproducible method that is widely being used.

Reagents

Proteinase K

Dissolve proteinase K at a concentration of 20 mg/ ml in sterile water. Store the aliquots at –20°C.

Proteinase K

Digestion buffer: Prepare a solution containing 50mM Tris-HCl, pH 8.5, 1mM EDTA, 0.5% Tween 20.

Procedure

- Pellet approximately 10^4 mammalian cells by centrifugation, and wash twice in PBS. Add to the washed pellet 100 µl of proteinase K digestion buffer supplemented with proteinase K at a final concentration of 200 µg/ml.
- Incubate for at least 2 hours at 55°C or overnight at 37°C. Centrifuge the cell lysate to remove cell debris.
- Incubate the lysate supernatant at 95°C for 8-10 minutes to denature the proteolytic enzymes and nucleases.
- An aliquot of this supernatant may be used directly for PCR. The supernatant can be stored for future use at –20°C.

Analysis of protein by immunoprecipitation

In most cases the phenotype of a transferred gene is manifested by the protein encoded by that gene. To analyze protein two different methods are described below. Accomplished in four steps.

Preparation of protein A sepharose CL-4B beads

- Fill the bottle containing the beads with enough H_2O. Transfer 1 g of the beads quantitatively to a 15 ml test tube.
- Allow the beads to swell for 30 minutes on ice with occasional agitation to resuspend the beads.
- When the beads have settled, the beads and H_2O should be 50:50 v/v. Adjust the H_2O level if necessary. Freeze aliquots of the beads slurry at –20°C.

Labeling adherent cells

- Process immediately.

Labeling non adherent cells

- Wash the cells twice with PBS.
- Resuspend the cells in methionine minus or cysteine minus medium 5% dialyzed FCS. at a concentration range of 1.0 to 10.0 X10^6 cells/ml. Pipette cells into a 12 well plate, 1 ml of cell suspension per well.
- For 3 hours whirl the plate every 30 minutes.
- Transfer the cell suspension to a microfuge tube. Spin at 14 rpm for 1minute.
- Save the media supernatant for immunoprecipitation. Store at –70°C if not being processed immediately.
- Resuspend the cell pellet in 1 ml of lysis buffer. Incubate for 5 minutes at 4°C with occasional rocking.
- Spin the tube at 14 rpm for 5 minutes at 4°C. Transfer the supernatant to a new microfuge tube. Store at –70°C if not processing immediately.

Immunoprecipitation

- To each sample tube, add the appropriate amount of antibody (determined by antibody titration experiments).
- Incubate at 4°C for 60 minutes.
- Spin the sample tubes at 14 rpm for 15 minutes at 4°C.
- Transfer the supernatant to new microfuge tubes and add to each tube 30 µl of a protein A bead slurry (use disposable pipetteman tips whose tips have been cut off with a clean razor blade to create a larger orifice). The larger orifice ensures quantitative transfer and will keep the beads from being crushed during transfer.
- Incubate for 70 minutes at 4°C.
- Centrifuge for 15 seconds in a microfuge and discard the supernatant in a radioactive waste container.
- Rinse the beads three times with 1 ml of lysis buffer and twice with 1.0 ml of buffer B. The centrifugation should be for 15 seconds which should not be exeeded.
- Remove the supernatant from the final wash and leave the beads undisturbed in a volume of approximately 30 µl. Add 30 µl of 2X sample buffer. Boil for three minutes and load the samples on a polyacrylamide gel.
- Upon completion of immunoprecipitation the protein product is separated on a polyacrylamide gel.

SUGGESTED READINGS

Berger, S. L and Kimmel A. R, Methods in Enzymology, vol. 152, Academic Press, INC., San Diego, California, USA, 1987.

Jain, S. K, Text Book of Biotechnology, CBS Publishers and distributors, New Delhi, India, 2000,

Lehninger A. L., Nelson, D. L. and Cox, M., Principles of Biochemistry, 2nd Edition, CBS Publishers and Distributors, New Delhi, India, 1993.

Sadasivam, S. and Manickem, A., Biochemical Methods, 2nd Edition, New Age International Publishers, New Delhi, India, 1997.

Sambrook, J., Fritsch E. F. and Maniatis, T., Molecular Cloning: A Laboratory Manual, 2nd Edition, Cold Spring Harbor Press, NewYork, USA, 1989.

Vyas, S. P. and Dixit, V. K, Pharmaceutical Biotechnology, CBS Publishers, New Delhi, India, 1998.

CHAPTER 10

Hybridoma Cell Technology

- Introduction
- Polyclonal antibodies generation
- Production of murine monoclonal antibodies

INTRODUCTION

Antibodies are glycoproteins (globulins) present in the serum, which are also known as immunoglobulins (Igs) and are produced by a class of blood cells called B lymphocytes. These are secreted in response to antigens, which are either protein or polysaccharide molecule having the ability to provoke an immune response which may be foreign to the body. Antibodies production is triggered when body is invaded by foreign particle or organism and as a result, the B lymphocytes continue to produce antibodies until the stimulation persists. Using different types of stimulants one can produce different types of antibodies. Each antibody produced is specific to that particular antigen which has stimulated its production.

After injecting a particular antigen or when a particular antigen invades body, antibodies are produced. These antibodies are heterogeneous in nature. Most of antigens have many antigenic determinants or epitopes, each of which induces production of specific antibodies. The heterogeneity of antibodies increases immune protection *in vivo* and often reduces the efficacy of an antiserum for various *in vitro* uses. Conventional heterogenous antisera vary from animal to animal and contain undesirable non-specific antibodies. Removal of these non-specific antibodies with unwanted specification from a polyclonal antibody preparation is a time consuming task involving affinity chromatography and other repeated adsorption techniques. The elution of antibodies with desired specificity from such columns is, however, not easy. Moreover, large amount of the serum of immunized animal is required for the production of specific antibodies. These methods are seldom effective in reducing the heterogeneity of an antiserum and result in loss of much of the desired antibody. Scientists side stepped this difficulty by fusing normal B cells (plasma cells) with tumour cells (cancerous plasma cells) that grow easily and proliferate endlessly. The resulting hybrid cell is called a hybridoma that possessed the proliferating growth properties of cancerous plasma cells but secreted the antibody product of the B cells. Hybridoma cells produce large quantities of pure antibodies called monoclonal antibodies (MAbs) with a single antigenic specificity.

Principle of Generating Hybrid Cells

Formation and selection of hybrid cells is the most important aspect of hybridoma technology, which is based on the principle of synthesis of nucleotides by mammalian cells using two different pathways. One is the *de novo* pathway in which ribose 5-phosphate, some amino acids, carbon dioxide and ammonia serve as precursors of purine and pyrimidine nucleotides. Tetra-hydrofolate coenzymes are required in *de novo* pathway which are produced from di-hydrofolate using dihydrofolate reductase. The folic acid analogue aminopterin blocks *de novo* pathway by inhibiting dihydrofolate reductase. In the salvage pathway, free purine and pyrimidine bases and their corresponding nucleotides or deoxyribonuclesides are the precursors of nucleotides. The enzyme hypoxanthine guanine phosphoribosyl transferase (HGPRT) is essential for the salvage pathway. HGPRT deficient cells placed in aminopterin containing medium can not synthesize nucleotides and thereby can not survive. This redundant nature of nucleic acid biosynthesis has been exploited in the selection of hybrid cells.

Hybrid cells clones are generated by fusion of plasma cells with myeloma cells. Myeloma cells is HGPRT deficient, when cultured in a medium containing hypoxanthine, aminopterine and thymidine (HAT medium) would not survive since they could not overcome inhibition of nucleotide synthesis by aminopterin. Plasma cells are HGPRT positive but it is not able to multiply and its own life is limited. They also can not survive alone in HAT medium. Only hybrid formed by fusion of plasma cells with myeloma cells would proliferate in the HAT medium by virtue of genetic compensation by other partner. Thus HAT medium is used for the selection of desired plasma cells-myeloma cells A-B hybrid rather than A-A or B-B cells. The major steps involved in the production of antibodies are summarized in Figure 10.1.

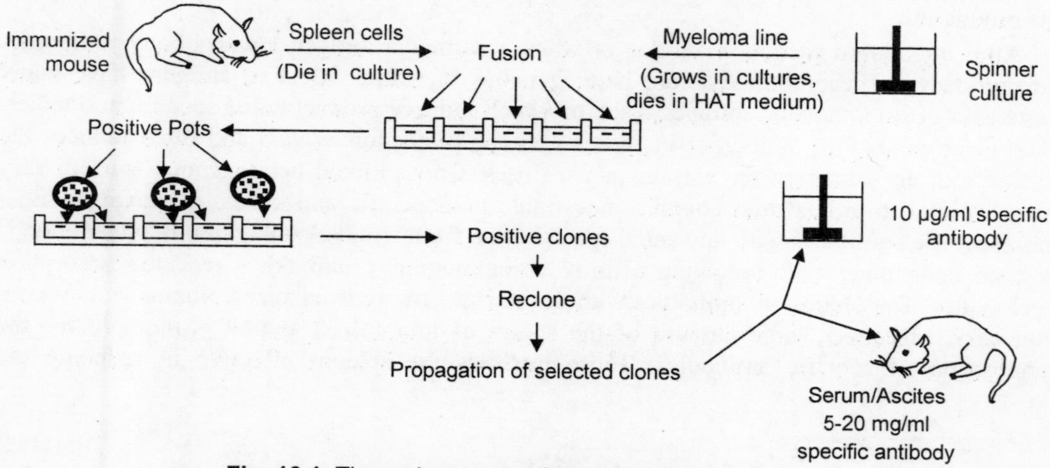

Fig. 10.1. The major stages of antibody production

PROTOCOL 10.1

POLYCLONAL ANTIBODIES GENERATION

Immunization of Animal

Mice

Injections should be made at intervals of at least two weeks. Either of the two following adjuvant can be used for successful immunization; Freund's adjuvant and MPL+TDM adjuvant. The MPL+TDM is less hazardous than the Freund's adjuvant.

- Preparation containing 15-50 μg antigen in 200 μl adjuvant is injected subcutaneously.
- 2 weeks later, booster injection containing 15-50 μg of antigen in adjuvant. (If time permits, boost again a month later).
- 7-10 days later bleed the mouse and test serum using the assay, which will be used for screening. If titre is not high enough, boost again two weeks after previous boost.

Rabbits

Rabbits are also immunized in the same manner as described above.

- First injection with Freund's adjuvant containing 100-200 μg/ml antigen, at two sites (over each shoulder).
- Second 1 month later in Freund's adjuvant.
- Bleed 2 weeks later. Boost 2 weeks later again
- If titre is not enough than repeat the booster in 2 weeks repetitive cycle.

Serum Preparation

- After collecting, blood should be allowed to clot for 60 minutes at 37°C or overnight at 4°C.
- Separate the clot from the sides of the tube (ringing) using a Pasteur pipette.
- Place clot at 4°C overnight.
- Centrifuge at 10000g for 10 minutes at 4°C to separate the serum. Serum can be stored at –20°C after adding glycerol to 50%.

Note

Sterile incomplete Freund's adjuvent (without mycobacteria) are to be used for this protocol.

PROTOCOL 10.2

PRODUCTION OF MURINE MONOCLONAL ANTIBODIES

If monoclonal antibodies are to be prepared, the primary requisite is to generate polyclonal antibodies and then a reliable screening method could be adopted for the selection of monoclonal antibodies.

If titre is positive against some antigen follow one of the following 2 weeks later

- Boost tail vein with 20-50 μg of antigen in PBS and proceed with fusion on 4th day or
- Boost subcutaneously with 50-100 μg of antigen in PBS and proceed with fusion 4 days later or
- Boost 3 days in a row with 15 μg antigen in PBS and proceed with fusion on 4th day.

Cell Lines

Some myeloma cell lines that are used for the production of monoclonal antibodies are as follows:

Myeloma P3X63-Ag8.653
Myeloma fox-NY
Macrophage-derived J774A1

Macrophage Feeder Cells

- Seed macrophages at a density of 1.5 x 10^5 cells/ml in the medium. Add 2.5 μg/ml lipopolysaccharides (LPS), which induces differentiation. Collect supernatant after 2-3 days, or when medium is getting too yellow.
- Induce 2 more times, each time with 1 μg/ml LPS and collect supernatant after 2 days each. Pool the supernatant, filter and use. (could be aliquoted and stored at -20°C.)

Stock Solutions

IMDM
Fetal Calf Serum (FCS)
Transferrin Iron saturated. 1000X stock is equivalent to 1 mg/ml
HT supplement 50X stock (Store at –20°C)
2-Mercaptoethanol 1000X stock equivalent to 0.05 M (Store at 4°C)
AT 50X stock (Store at –20°C.)
Kanamycin Sulphate 100X (Store at –20° C)
Macrophage Conditioned Medium (MCM)

Preparation of Media

For P3X63-Ag8.653 and J774A.1

IMDM complete medium

425 ml of IMDM
0.5 ml 1000X Transferrin
0.5 ml 1000X 2-Mercaptoethanol
10 ml 50X HT
5 ml 100X Kanamycin Sulphate
75 ml FCS (final 15%)

For fox-NY

IMDM or RPMI supplemented with

10 % FCS
1X AT supplement
Transferrin
Kanamycin

Maintenance of Cells

Growth conditions

All cell lines mentioned above are to be grown at 37°C supplying 7% CO_2.

The myelomas optimal density is 3.5 x 10^5/ml

The macrophages optimal density is 1.5 x 10^5/ml. When expanding them, scrape them from the Petri dishes at this stage.

Freezing Hybridoma /Myeloma /Macrophages

Freezing solution
90 % FCS
10 % Dimethyl sulphoxide (DMSO) ice cold.

Procedure

- Centrifuge 10^7 cells (10^6 minimum) at 1200 rpm for 5 minutes.
- Aspirate the medium and resuspend in 1 ml of ice cold freezing solution.
- Transfer the vial to an insulated freezing box and place at –70°C for at least 1 hour however, this could be kept for a couple of days.
- Transfer the vial from the freezing box to the liquid nitrogen tank.

Thawing Cells

- Take the vial out of liquid nitrogen tank and thaw it immediately in a 37°C bath for about 1 minute.
- When there is still a small piece of ice left, dilute the cells by transferring them into a conical tube containing 10 ml of the growth medium at 37°C.
- Centrifuge at 1200 rpm for 5 minutes.
- Aspirate the medium and resuspend cells in 5 ml of medium, in a 25 ml flask.

Cell Fusion and Selection

Solutions

IMDM-m
  IMDM complete
  15% Macrophage condition medium (MCM)
Phosphate buffered saline (PBS)
50% (w/v) Polyethylene glycol 4000 (PEG 4000)

Procedure

- Prepare a T-150 flask with 170 ml of IMDM complete with MCM, and keep it in the incubator for fused cells.

Isolation of spleen cells

- Sacrifice mouse by cervical dislocation. Immerse mouse in 70% ethanol.
- Remove spleen (on the left side) and transfer into a small Petri dish, which contains IMDM at room temperature.
- Clean fat from the spleen and transfer the spleen into an empty dish. Using sharp tipped forceps, one end is punctured. A curved forceps is used to hold down the intact end, and

the spleen is gently rubbed towards the opened end with another set of forceps. The cells from inside the spleen will ooze out with very little damage.

- Stop the process when nearly empty, transparent skin is left.
- Collect the cells by rinsing with IMDM. Transfer cell suspension to a 15 ml conical tube and let the cell debris settle out (approximately 5 minutes).
- Remove the cell suspension (without disturbing the settled cell debris) and transfer to a 50 ml conical tube.
- Add an additional 30 ml of IMDM and pellet the cells at 1200 rpm for 5-10 minutes.
- Aspirate the medium, resuspend pellet and wash again with 30 ml of IMDM. One immunized spleen has approximately 10^8 cells. After this wash the cells are ready for the fusion.

Myeloma cell preparation

- It is essential that the myeloma be free of debris, rounded and refractive under phase contrast, and that they are harvested in log or late log phase growth (between 3.5-9 x 10^5 cells/ml).
- Thaw cells 7 days before scheduled fusion. Myeloma do not grow well after being in culture for more than a few weeks.
- Refreeze cells for future use.
- The ratio of 2 spleen cells:1 myeloma cell has been used. However, a ratio from 1 to 10 spleen cells per myeloma has been used successfully. For used spleen harvested 5 x 10^7 cells are harvested. Centrifuge at the same time while the second wash of the spleen cells is done.

The fusion

- The washed myeloma and spleen cells are pooled in 30 ml of PBS (room temp.) and spun gently at 1000 rpm for 10 minutes.
- Aspirate the PBS and resuspend pellet gently by tapping the tube. Volume should be approx. 0.8 ml.
- Set a timer.
- Add an equal volume of PEG solution, slowly, dropwise, with gentle tapping for over 1.5 minutes at room temperature. Then gently wiggle the tube for 1.5 minutes at 37°C. Some cell clumping will be evident.
- The suspensions spun at 1000 rpm for 3-4 minutes (at this point see the different layers of cells with PEG on top).
- Slowly add 37°C IMDM to 10 ml, without disturbing pellet.
- After adding, swirl the tubes gently to mix and dilute the PEG. Do not disturb the cells.
- Spin at 1000 rpm for 5 minutes.
- Aspirate medium, resuspend cells by tapping. Slowly add 5 ml of 37°C IMDM-m.
- Bring to 20 ml and add to the flask in the incubator. (If using feeder cells, add them at this point; 10^6 cells/ml).
- Add aminopterin (2 ml to 200 ml of medium). (alternatively, leave the cells at this point for 24 hours before adding aminopterin)
- Seed the cells in 96 well microtitre dishes, 250 µl per well, 8 plates per fusion.

- First clones may be seen in 7-10 days. First screen will usually start after 2 weeks, with a second and third, if necessary, a few days later.

Expanding hybridoma clones

- Transfer the strongest positive clones to a 24 well plate by scraping the adhering cells with a truncated yellow tip.
- Make up the volume to 1 ml using the IMDM-m medium. When cells gets confluenced, freeze them (about 10^6 cells per full well). Scrape them using a blue tip.
- Add 1 ml of IMDM-m to cells left in the well, let them grow and repeat the freezing.
- While the cells are growing, save their supernatant at each freezing. Use the supernatant to do the other tests required such as western, immunofluorescence and others. (If supernatant is not used under sterile conditions, add 0.02% azide and keep at 4°C for months)
- Transfer the cells to a 25 ml flask in 4 ml of IMDM-m and continue to expand as desired. The cells at this point are "addicted" to the macrophage supplement and then it is possible to wean them by gradually reducing the amount of MCM. It should be done only if very large volumes are needed.
- After selecting best clones, recloning should be done so as to ascertain their homogeneity by isotying.

Cloning of hybridoma

- Make an accurate cell count of cells in log phase ($3x10^5$-$1x10^6$ cells/ml).
- Determine the volume needed to give 100 cells.
- Add the 100 cells to 25 ml of IMDM-m and plate 250 ml of the suspension in each well. Therefore, 1 cell should be delivered into it each well.
- Clones should be visible and ready to screen in 10 to 14 days.

Ascites production

- 7 days before injection of cells, inject 0.5 ml of Pristine (Tetramethyl pentadecane), intraperitoneally.
- Prepare cells in log phase.
- On day of injection, spin 1-2 x 10^6 cells per mouse.
- Resuspend in IMDM or PBS at 1-2 x 10^6 cells/0.5ml (do not leave the cells without serum for more than 1 to 2 hours). Transfer cells to syringe using a 16 gauge needle.
- Inject 0.5 ml per mouse, using a 20G needle, intraperitonealy.
- Collect ascites when animals are ready (swollen abdomen), 10 days to 15 days after injection.
- Centrifuge the fluid at 3000g for 10 minutes to remove the cells. If there is oil layer, remove it and discard. Carefully remove the supernatant from the cells.
- For storage, add sodium azide to 0.02%. Store at –20°C.
- The screening of antibodies is done by ELISA.

SUGGESTED READINGS

Campwell, P., Monoclonal Antibodies, 2000.

Goding J.W., Monoclonal Antibodies: Principle and Practice, 2001.

Harlow, E. and Lane, D., Antibodies: A Laboratory Manual, Cold Spring Harbor Laboratory Press, New York, 1992.

Kemmemy, D. M. and Challacombe, S. J, ELISA and other Solid Phase Immunoassay: Theoretical and Practical Aspects, John Wiley and Sons, New York, 1989.

Perlmann, H. and Perlmann, A Laboratory Handbook, 1992.

Talwar, G. P. and Gupta, S. K., A Handbook of Practical and Clinical Immunology, 2nd Edition, CBS Publishers and Distributors, New Delhi, 1992.

Trehan, K., Biotechnology, Wiley Eastern Limited, New Delhi, India, 1991.

Vyas, S. P. and Dixit, V. K, Pharmaceutical Biotechnology, CBS Publishers, New Delhi, India, 1998.

CHAPTER 11

Immunological methods

INTRODUCTION

Immunology is concerned with the specific mechanisms by which body reacts to foreign biological material (including invading microorganisms) so that resistance or immunity develops whereas, serology deals with the laboratory study of the activities of the components of blood serum that contribute to immunity. The basis of immunology and serology, especially its specific aspects, is essentially chemical.

Natural and Acquired Immunity

Immunity in most general sense may be defined as natural or acquired resistance to disease and may be classified as natural immunity and acquired immunity. Natural immunity is further subdivided into three classes: Species immunity, Racial immunity, and Individual immunity. Acquired immunity is attributed to antibodies produced or the altered responsiveness of body cells to the infectious agent and classified as passive acquired and active acquired immunity (Fig. 11.1).

An antigen is a substance that provokes an immune response by producing antibodies (immunoglobulins) or sensitizing lymphoid cells, in an immunologically competent individual.

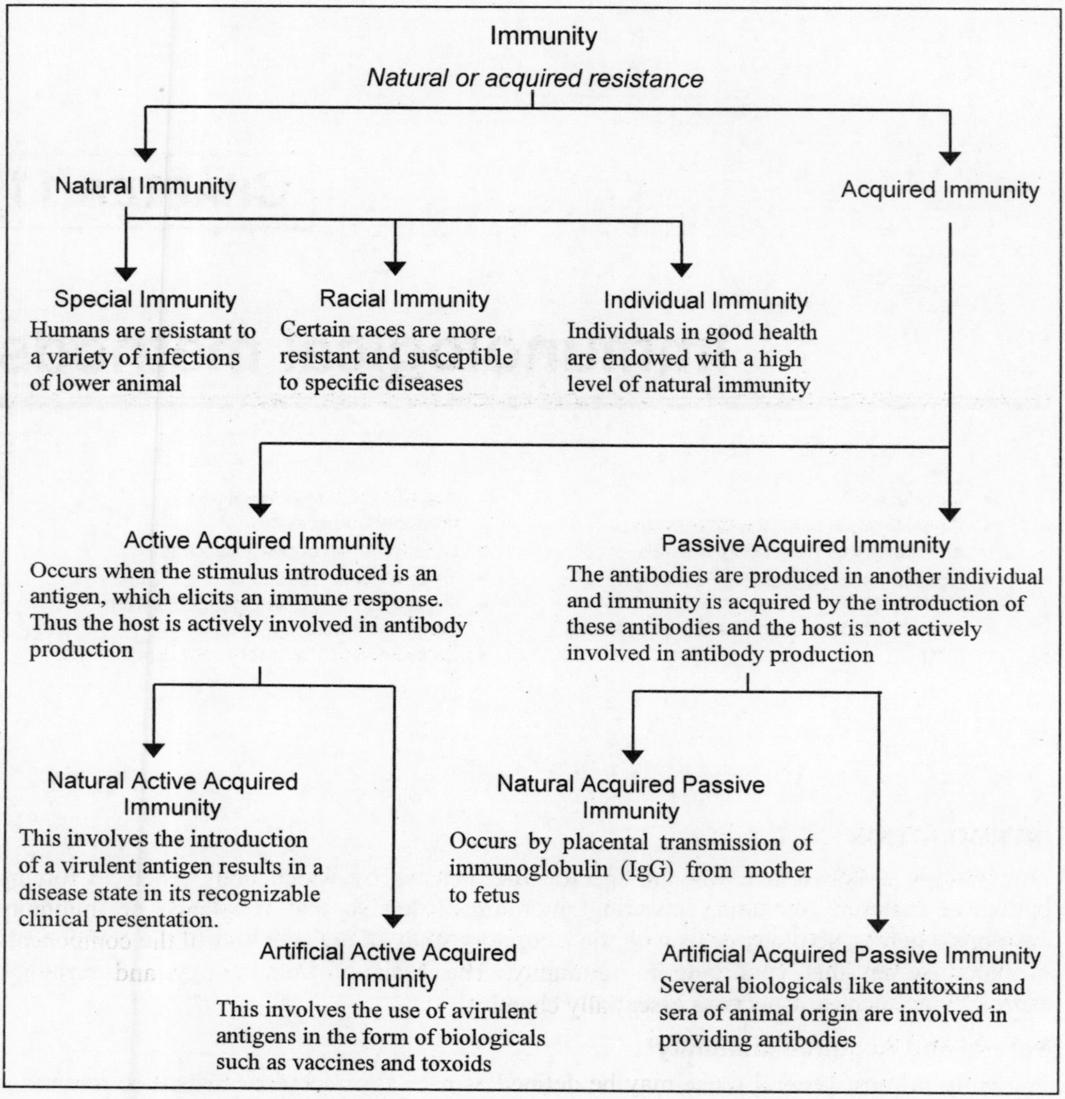

Fig. 11.1. Schematic showing various kinds of natural and acquired immunity

Chemically, vast majority of antigens are proteins, nucleoproteins, glycoproteins, and certain large polysaccharides. In general, they have molecular weight of 10,000 or greater. The entire microbes, such as bacterium or virus, or component of microbes, and nonmicrobial material such as pollen grains, egg white, incompatible blood cells, transplanted tissues or organ may act as antigen. Antibodies do not form against the whole antigen. There are various specific regions or chemical groups on the surface of the antigen, which are called antigenic determinants sites. They specifically combine with the antibody. It is possible to separate these determinant sites with intact ability to react with an antibody in response to the original antigen (reactivity), but does not have the ability to stimulate the production of antibodies (immunogenicity) when injected into an animal. A determinant site that has reactivity but not immunogenicity is called a partial antigen or hapten.

Antibodies are protein molecules of the globulin fraction of blood serum, also known as immunoglobulins, produced by the body in response to an antigen and are capable of combining specifically with an antigen. The formation of antibody is a function of cells associated with lymphoid tissue and found especially in lymph nodes, spleen, liver and bone marrow. Most antibodies contain four polypeptide chains in which two of the chains are identical to each other and are called heavy (H) chains, each chain consists of 450 amino acids. Other two chains are also identical to each other and are called light (L) chains, each chain consists of 220 amino acids. Antibodies are classified under five major classes which are IgG, IgA, IgM, IgD & IgE .

Cellular and Humoral Immunity

Body defends itself against invading agents by two closely allied components, cellular immunity and humoral immunity. Cellular (cell mediated) immunity is concerned with the formation of especially sensitized lymphocytes that have the capacity to attach to the foreign material and destroy it. Cellular immunity is particularly effective against fungi, parasites intracellular viral infections, cancer cells, and foreign tissue transplant. T cells are responsible for cellular immunity, whereas B cells for humoral immunity and both are derived from lymphocytic stem cells in bone marrow (Fig. 11.2).

T cells are classified mainly in four categories: killer T cells destroy antigen directly; helper T cells cooperate with B cells to help amplify antibody production; Supressor T cells help to regulate the immune response; and memory T cells initiate response to subsequent invasions by the antigen. Humoral immunity is the production of antibodies that are capable of attacking an invading agent and is particularly effective against bacterial and viral infections. B cells develop into antibody-producing plasma cells with the help of thymic hormones and memory B cells, which recognize the original, invading antigen (Fig. 11.3).

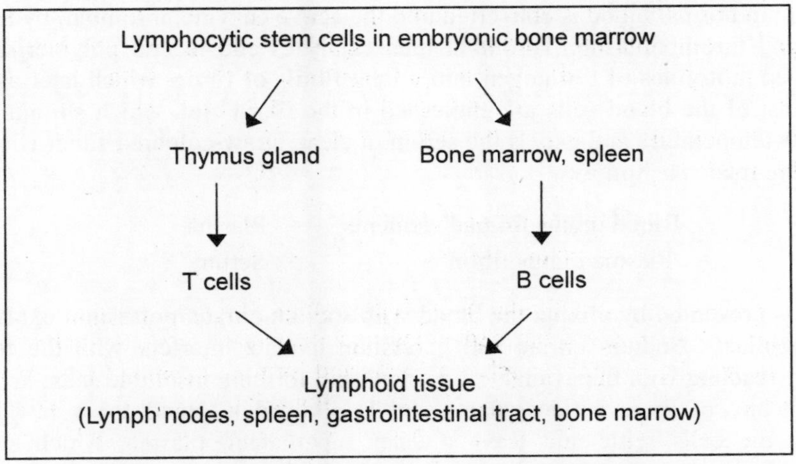

Fig. 11.2. Origin and differentiation of T cells and B cells

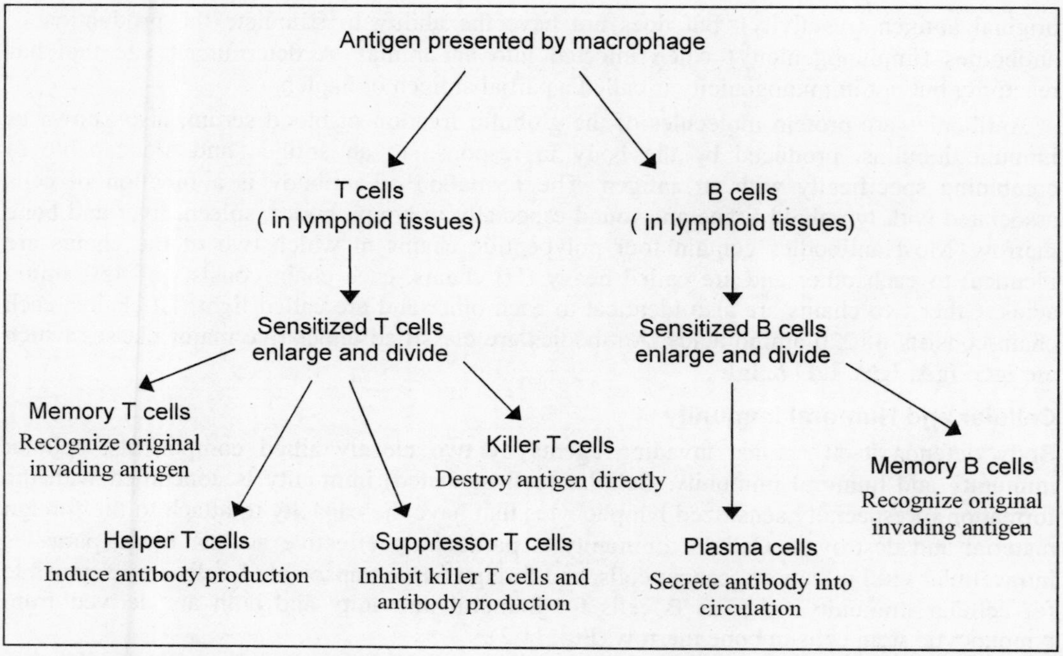

Fig. 11.3. Schematic showing role of T cells in cellular immunity and B cell in humoral immunity

The Composition of Blood

Blood, plasma, and serum: blood is composed of formed elements (cells and cell-like structures) and plasma (liquid containing dissolved substances).

Freshly drawn blood clots within a few minutes. Formation of the clot is a complex process in which a protein, fibrinogen, is converted into insoluble fibrin. Enzyme precursor, prothrombin, in normal blood is converted into the active enzyme, thrombin, by reaction with Ca^{++} ions and thromboplastin. Thrombin then catalyzes end to end polymerization of the needle shaped molecules of fibrinogen into a long fibrils of fibrin, which later associate into bundles. Most of the blood cells are enmeshed in the fibrin clot, which shrinks after a few hours at low temperature and expels the serum, a clear, straw-coloured fluid. Blood, plasma, and serum are related as follows:

Blood minus formed elements	=	Plasma
Plasma minus fibrin	=	Serum

Clotting is prevented by mixing the blood with sodium citrate, potassium oxalate, heparin, or other chemicals. Sodium citrate and potassium oxalate interfere with the formation of thrombin by reacting with the available Ca^{++} ions and forming insoluble salts. When blood is treated with any of these anticoagulants and is allowed to stand for a few hours or is centrifuged, the cells settle and leave a clear supernatant, plasma, which still contains fibrinogen. The serum proteins contain about 7% of the weight of serum. Normal serum contains several proteins distinguishable by their "salting out" properties with sodium or ammonium sulphate, their precipitability with alcohol under various conditions of pH and electrolyte concentration, their electric charges, and their molecular weight.

Normal human blood contains between 4.8 to 5.5 million red erythrocytes, per cubic millimeter. These cells are about 7.5 μ in diameter and 2 μ in thickness. They are formed in the bone marrow and have average life span in the circulation, of 100 to 120 days. The white blood cells are an important defense tool of immune system. Their number varies between 5000 to 9000 per cubic millimeter. The several kinds of leukocytes are classified according to their size (7 μ to 22 μ), presence and type of granules, shape of nucleus, and character of cytoplasm, and are usually present in fairly constant percentage (Fig. 11.4).

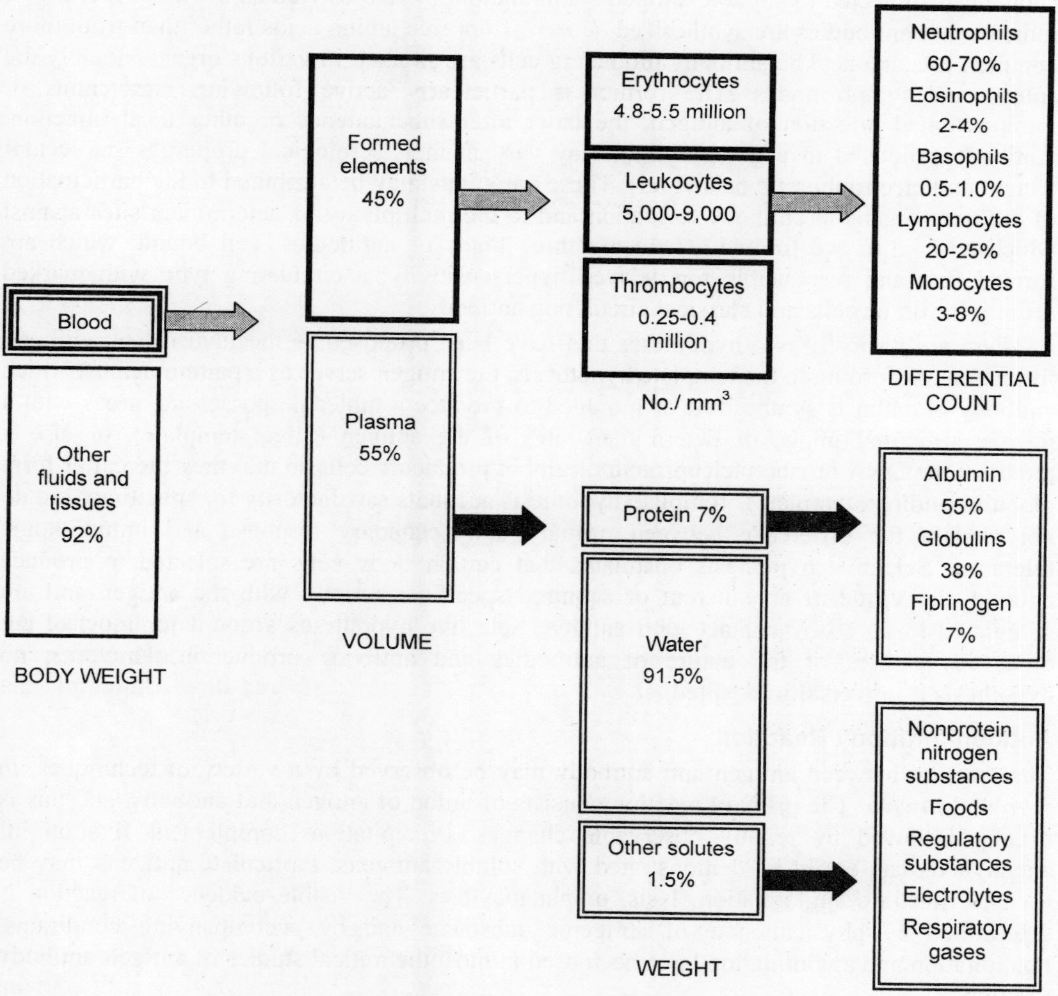

Fig. 11.4. Composition of blood in a normal adult

Production of Antibodies

Primary antigenic stimulation of an immunologically mature animal is followed, after an induction period of several days, by slight to moderate liberation of antibody into the circulating blood; the antibody titre then decreases rapidly. Secondary antigenic stimulation after a suitable interval promptly incites a steep (logarithmic) rise in antibody titre to a higher level, which is maintained for longer duration than that of a primary response. A series of injections of antigen induce stepwise increase of antibodies in circulating blood, but eventually a maximum is reached beyond that further injection produces no increase in antibody titre.

Antibodies are formed in cells of the lymphoid series, which appear to develop into plasma cells when subjected to suitable antigenic stimulation. *In vivo* as well as *in vitro* experiments indicate that antibodies are synthesized *de novo* from free amino acids rather than from more complex precursors. The antibody producing cells are situated in various organs, notably the spleen and lymph nodes. The former is particularly active following intravenous or intraperitoneal injection of antigen, the latter after subcutaneous or other local injection. Antibody produced in a given animal may vary in their serological properties (molecular weight and electrophoretic behaviour). These variations may be attributed to the participation of different organs in antibody formation and to the multiplicity of determinant sites against which antibodies are formed. There are three kinds of antibodies: cell bound, which are formed first and responsible for delayed hypersensitivity; a circulating type with marked affinity for tissue cells and classical circulating antibody.

There are basically two hypotheses that have been proposed as mechanisms of antibody formation. According to the template hypothesis, the antigen serves as a pattern against which antibody globulin is synthesized or moulded to produce a molecule possessing areas with a reverse structural image of determinant sites of the antigen (direct template), or else it modifies the DNA or ribonucleoprotein of globin producing cells so that they thereafter form globulin (indirect template). Template hypothesis accounts satisfactorily for specificity but do not explain the difference between primary and secondary response and immunologic tolerance. Selective hypothesis postulates that certain body cells are selected to produce antibody by virtue of an inherent or acquired specific reactivity with the antigen and are stimulated to do so by contact with antigen. Selective hypotheses account for most of the observed features of the nature of antibodies and antibody production. However, no hypothesis is universally accepted.

Antigen-antibody Reaction

The reaction between antigen and antibody may be observed by a variety of techniques, *in vitro* and *in vivo*. The primary reaction consists of union of antigen and antibody, and this is usually followed by readily observable changes. Precipitation, complement fixation, or anaphylaxis can easily be demonstrated with soluble antigens. Particulate antigens may be used to illustrate agglutination, lysis, or phagocytosis. The visible evidence of reaction is determined by physical state of antigenic substance and by accompanying conditions. Precipitation and agglutination have been used in most theoretical studies of antigen-antibody reactions.

There are various hypotheses for the demonstration of antigen-antibody reaction like the lattice hypothesis, Ehrlich's side chain hypothesis, Arrhenius' and Madensen's mass action hypothesis, and Bordey's absorption hypothesis. The lattice hypothesis is the most widely favoured. It is described by Marrack in 1938, and modification were proposed by Heidelberger, Pauling, and various other workers. The basic concept is that an antigen-antibody aggregate consists of a lattice or framework of alternating antibody molecules and antigen or particles. Marrack regarded that the solubility of antibody globulin is attributable to its polar radicals, and that these are brought into close apposition and attract each other instead of water molecules when antibody combine with antigen. This complex precipitates if the surface potential is below a critical level. Assuming that both antigen and antibody are multivalent, large complexes may be build up through specific links provided by further antigen molecules and thus form a network or lattice. Pauling supported the lattice hypothesis, but saw no need for multivalent antibody except in certain situations involving polyhaptenic antigens. He postulated that antibody is bivalent and antigen may be multivalent. The reactive sites of an antigen and its antibody correspond closely in physical configuration, and the molecules join alternately to form large aggregates.

The agglutination of cells was represented diagrammatically in Figure 11.5, the cells being held together at the region of "contact" by antibody molecules. The relative sizes of antigen and antibody obviously limit the effective valence of antibody to two. Precipitation under optimal conditions was represented as in Figure 11.6.A. A network formed with a greater than optimal proportion of antibodies is depicted in Figure 11.6.B, and network and complexes with less than optimal antibodies in Figure 11.6.C.

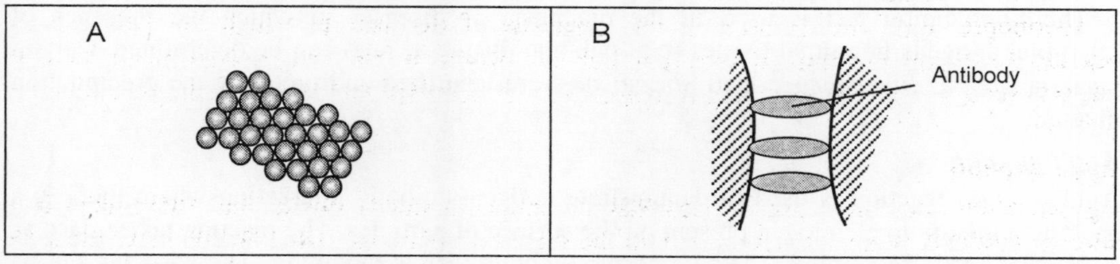

Fig. 11. 5. Schematic diagram showing (A) agglutination of cells and (B) the region of contact of two cells and mode of action of agglutinin molecules

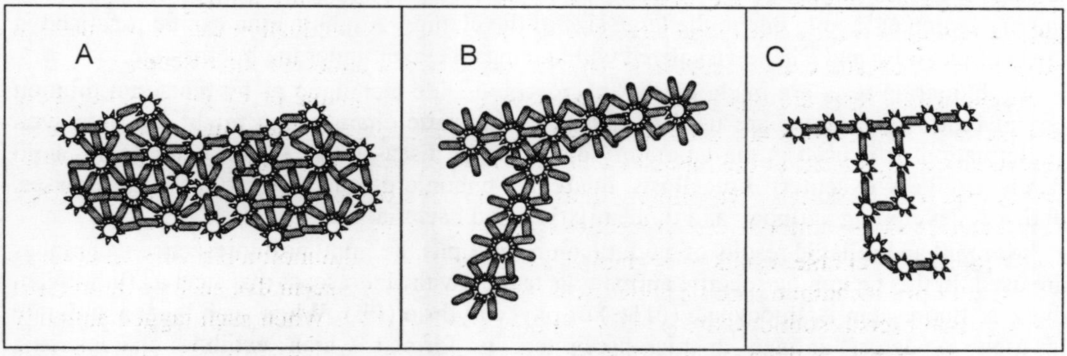

Fig. 11. 6. Complexes formed with soluble antigen and antibody. A, an ideal framwork. B, a network formed with antibody excess. C, a network formed with antigen excess.

Precipitation

Precipitation is considered the basic serological reaction. It has been used in much of the theoretic study of antigen-antibody interaction. Qualitative or semiquantitative precipitin tests can very easily be made by mixing undiluted or slightly diluted (e.g., 1:3 to 1:5) antiserum with antigen. Sufficient dilutions of antigen are employed to ensure a positive result that might otherwise be missed because of inhibition by too concentrated antigen.

Quantitative precipitin tests initially developed by Heidelberger and Kendall, gives an accurate measure of antibody concentration in serum. It is based on the observations that, addition of increasing amounts of soluble antigen to a series of tubes containing a constant volume of antisera, the amount of precipitate formed increases to reach an optimum after which consistently less precipitate is formed. There are numerous procedures, each useful for some particular purpose:

- Simple mixtures of antigen and antibody, observed by the naked eye, provide rough information regarding the presence and amount of antibody in an antiserum; with the aid of photoelectric measuring devices, considerable information can be obtained about the composition of an antigen-antibody system.
- The interfacial ring test is a sensitive method of detecting specific antigens.
- Gel diffusion tests (e.g., double immunodiffusion technique popularly known as Ouchterlony technique) are used for the determination of antigenic complexity of natural materials such as sera, polysaccharides and tissue extracts.

Thermoprecipitin test is used in the diagnosis of diseases in which the presence of microbial antigens in animal tissues (e.g. bubonic plague in rats) can be determined. Certain bacteria such as *Pneumococci* and S*treptococci* are identified and typed by the precipitation methods.

Agglutination

Agglutination reaction is used to demonstrate antigen-antibody interaction where there is a specific antibody to an antigen present on the surface of particles. The reaction takes place as a result of particles coming together and producing a visible clumping. The particles can be bacteria, cells of higher plants or animals, microfungi, or rickettsiae. Agglutination starts with the linking of different particles or cells by antibody molecules and form large lattices through the cross-linking by the antibody molecules. Large lattices are formed through cross-linking sediment readily due to the large size of the clumps. Agglutination can be practiced in tubes or on slides and can be visualized with the naked eye or under the microscope.

Agglutination tests are made by the macroscopic slide technique or by the serial dilution test method. Electrolytes are used to reduce electrostatic charges that might interfere with agglutination. It is used in the laboratory diagnosis of diseases like typhoid and paratyphoid fevers, bacillary dysentery, brucellosis, tularemis, bubonic plague and various viral diseases, to detect developing antibody and to identify isolated bacteria.

For rapid and reliable results of agglutination reactions the immunofluorescence techniques are used. In this technique specific antibody is tagged with fluorescent dye such as fluorescent dye e.g. fluorescein isothiocynate (FITC) or phycoerythrin (PE). When such tagged antibody is used to detect antigen a microprecipitate is formed which exhibits characteristic fluorescence when view under the fluorescence microscope.

Phagocytosis

Phagocytosis is the ingesion and destrucion of microbes or any particulate matter by certain cells called phagocytes. It is one of the principal body defenses against infection. Phagocytic cells include the circulating blood leukocytes and the fixed and wandering macrophages of the reticuloendothelial system.

Phagocytosis mainly involves two phases: adherence and ingestion. Adherence or attachment is the formation of firm contact between the cell membrane of phagocyte and the microbe. In some cases adherence occurs easily but in other cases, adherence is more difficult and particles or microbes can be phagocytozed if the phagocyte traps the particles to be ingested against a rough surface, like a blood vessel or connective fibre tissue, where it can not slide away. This is called nonimmune or surface phagocytosis. Microbes can also be phagocytosed if they are first coated with complement or antibody to promote the attachment of the microbe to the phagocyte. This is referred to as opsonization or immune adherence. A final factor that help in adherence, is chemotaxis. Ingestion occurs after adherence in which projections of the cell membrane of the phagocyte, called pseudopodia, engulf the microbe. Once the microbe is surrounded, the membrane folds inward, forming a sac around the microbe called a phagocytic vacuole. The vacuole pinches off the membrane and enters the cytoplasm. The cytoplasm vacuole interacts together with lysosomes that contain digestive enzyme. After interaction it fuses together to form a larger structure called phagolysosome. Within the phagolysosome most microbes are killed within 10 to 30 minutes by the lactic acid which lowers the pH in phagolysosome, lysozyme that degrades carbohydrates, proteins, lipids and nucleic acids (Fig. 11.7).

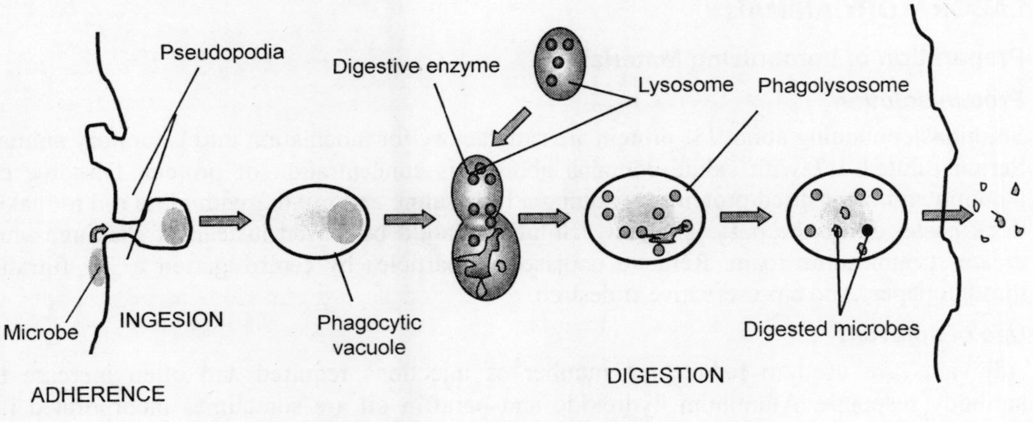

Fig.11. 7. Phases of phagocytosis

Toxins and Antitoxins

The components of bacteria that are toxic to higher forms of life include exotoxin, endotoxins, and certain hydrolytic and other enzymes. Exotoxins are proteins, typically released during the life of the bacterial cell. Endotoxins are polysaccharide-phospholipid-protein complexes, also called somatic antigens, and are normally part of the cell wall of gram negative bacteria, from which they are set free or liberated by autolysis of the dead cells. Exotoxins have marked affinity for particular tissues and produce specific damage. Endotoxins from all sources produce the same effects like marked changes in body temperature, increasing in circulating white blood cell counts and possibly diarrhea, weakness, irreversible shock and even death. Exotoxins and their nontoxic denatured products, toxoids, are highly antigenic and induce formation of antitoxin, which neutralize the homologous toxins completely according to the law of multiple proportions. Antibodies against endotoxins neutralize their toxins only partially, but usually agglutinate the corresponding intact cells strongly. Toxicity is titrated by laboratory animal inoculation, and the potency of antitoxin is also assayed in animals by comparison with "standard" antitoxin of the known protective power. Antitoxin can combine with toxin in varying proportions, according to the ratio in which they are mixed, to yield complexes that produce no effects when injected. Flocculation may also occur if the reagents are mixed in optimal proportions, as in the case of the precipitin reaction.

Toxins and toxoids are used for active immunization of animals and man and in small doses for testing susceptibility to certain diseases (diphtheria, scarlet fever). Small amounts of antitoxins are injected into individuals exposed to the corresponding pathogenic agents for prophylactic purposes, and larger doses are administered therapeutically.

PROTOCOL 11.1

GENERAL PROTOCOL FOR THE PRODUCTION OF ANTIBODIES FROM LABORATORY ANIMAL

Preparation of Immunizing Materials

Protein solution

Solutions containing about 1% protein are satisfactory for inoculation into laboratory animals. Serum diluted 1:7 with saline contains about this concentration of protein. Dissolve egg albumin and other dried proteins by adding a little saline and mixing with glass rod to make a thick paste, dilute the paste gradually. Solution should be stirred instead of shaking, which creates troublesome foam. Remove undissolved particles by centrifugation or by filtration through paper. Add a preservative if desired.

Use of adjuvant

Adjuvants are used to reduce the number of injections required and often increase the antibody response. Aluminum hydroxide and paraffin oil are sometimes incorporated into materials for animal inoculation for this purpose.

Alum precipitation

Prepare 50 ml of bacterin or other immunizing agent and its preservative (if any) in double strength. Add 2.33 ml of 10% $AlCl_3$ and sufficient 20% NaOH to bring the reaction to pH 7.0. Dilute to 100 ml with saline.

Oil in water (Freund's adjuvant)

Prepare the immunizing material and preservative in double strength. Sterilize good quality light paraffin oil and Arlacel A by autoclaving. Mix 8.5 volumes of the paraffin oil with 1.5

volumes of Arlacel A, using a warring blender or by aspirating it repeatedly in to syringe without needle. Add 10 volumes of antigen and mix as before. Test the emulsion by allowing a drop to fall from an applicator stick onto the surface of water. If the drop remains perfectly formed and does not spread over the surface, the emulsion is ready for use.

An additional adjuvant effect is sometimes provided by incorporation of killed acid fast bacteria. Dried *Mycobacterium tuberculosis* or *M. bytyricum* that have been killed by heat (70°C for 30 minutes) are added to the paraffin oil at concentration 10 mg/100 ml and thoroughly mixed by grinding in a mortar. Aracle A and antigen are then added as described previously.

Inoculation and Bleeding of Animals

Rabbit

For antisera production usually young adult rabbit of 2-4 kg body weight, are used. Inoculations may be done by using intravenous, intraperitoneal or subcutaneous route. The intravenous route is commonly used for this purpose. For the production of antibacterial sera in rabbits, the schedule of inoculation of killed suspensions of gram negative rod bacteria consists of following intravenous injections (Table 11.1).

Table 11.1. Intravenous injections for the production of antibacterial sera in rabbits.

Day	Inoculum size in ml
1	0.1
4	0.3
8	0.5
11	1.0
15	2.0

Serum of high titre value is usually secured 3 to 5 days after the last injection. For living bacteria closely spaced intravenous injections are satisfactory. Stock saline suspension having any visible are tested employing antigen-agglutination test. Fresh stock suspensions are prepared as indicated in Table 11.2 and refrigerated when not in use. Anti-erythrocyte effect is produced by a series of twice weekly intravenous injections of 1 ml of 50% suspension of red blood cells. Animal serum is then titrated 3 or 4 days after the fourth injection and if the titre is not satisfactory additional incubations are conducted.

Another injection routine consists of four daily intravenous injections of 1 ml of 10% red blood cells per kg body weight followed by six injections every second day. Peak titre is usually found about 2 weeks after the first injection and is often maintained for several days.

Protein solutions, 1% are injected intravenously once or twice a week. The number of injections is determined by the results of trial titrations of the animal's serum. After the first 2 weeks, injections are given following a rest period of a week or more by intraperitoneal route to reduce the likelihood of anaphylactic shock. One or two 0.5 ml subcutaneous injections of antigens emulsified in paraffin oil are usually followed which produce antisera of high titre. A trial titration is performed 3 or 4 weeks after the first injection, and if the antibody titre is not sufficiently high, a second injection is given.

Table 11.2. Preparation of stock solutions

Day	Inoculum size	Dilution
1	0.1	Fresh stock suspension 1:1000
2	0.2	Suspension 1:100
3	0.3	Suspension 1:100
4	0.1	Fresh stock solution undiluted
5	0.2	Suspension undiluted
6	0.3	Suspension undiluted
11	0.5	Fresh stock solution undiluted
16	0.5	Trial titration, if titration is satisfactory, bleed from the heart otherwise, inject 0.5 ml fresh undiluted stock suspension and titrate after an additional 5 days

Intravenous injection

The marginal ear vein of the rabbit located at the outer edge of the dorsal side of the ear is readily accessible. One ear is reserved for injection and the other for bleeding. The first injection of a series is always made as near the tip of the ear as possible, succeeding injections being made closer towards the animal's head, so that scar tissue will not prevent injected material from entering the circulation.

- Hold the animal on the lap facing the operator and shave the skin over the vein. Rub vigorously with 70% alcohol. Hold the ear with left hand so that the middle finger supports the area to be injected. Insert the inoculating needle, bevel up, in the direction of blood flow through the skin and into the vein at a very acute angle to the vein so that it does not pass completely through.
- Inject the inoculum slowly. When the injection is made correctly the inoculum can be seen passing towards the heart as it partially replaces the blood. If the needle is not within the vein, the antigen will produce a blanched, raised area in the neighboring tissue. Gentle massage is used to force the material out of the needle puncture, and injection should be made at another site.
- Firmly apply cotton moistened with alcohol after the inoculation is completed and withdraw the needle.

Intraperitoneal injection

- Clip the hair in the median abdominal line and disinfect with alcohol. Pinch up a fold of skin and peritoneum between the thumb and forefinger and insert the needle into the ridge of the skin, and through the fold of peritoneum, release the peritoneum and skin to make an successful inoculum.
- Wash the area with alcohol.

Subcutaneous injection

- Clip the hair and shave the hair on the side of the back and disinfect with alcohol. Pinch up a fold of skin between the thumb and forefinger and insert the needle into the ridge of the skin, release the skin and make the injection.
- Wash the area with alcohol.

Bleeding from the ear vein

Marginal vein of the ear is used to collect small amount of blood. The first bleeding of the series is made near the base of the ear and succeeding punctures are made towards the distal end from the head.

- Hold the animal on the lap facing away from the operator and rub the ear vigorously to increase the blood circulation. A drop of xylol can also be placed on the tip of the ear to produce mild inflammation. Xylol must be removed by washing three times with alcohol before animal is returned to cage.
- Shave the area and place an artery clamp over the vein proximal to the site to be punctured.
- Hold the ear so that middle finger of the left hand supports the site of puncture and make a short cut with a sharp razor blade. Collect the desired amount of the blood in a centrifuge tube and move the artery clamp distal to the puncture and hold dry cotton firmly over the puncture until bleeding stops.
- Remove the clot by centrifugation and collect the serum carefully with pipette.

Bleeding from the heart

Large quantity of the blood can be collected from the heart or jugular vein. Cardiac bleeding is usually simpler and can be repeatedly performed on the same animal if proper technique is used.

- Clip the area over the sternum and disinfect with alcohol and tincture of iodine.
- Insert the needle between two ribs in the area of maximum pulsation, usually about midway of the sternum and slightly to the left and advancing the needle in a straight line towards the right shoulder. Blood will appear in the needle as soon as needle punctures the heart. 50 ml may safely be collected from an average rabbit.
- If finding the heart is difficult, withdraw the needle and reinsert in another direction. Twisting the needle with the pericardial cavity can tear the heart and cause immediate death.
- Collect the blood in a centrifuge tube and remove the clot by centrifugation and collect the serum with pipette.
- Serum is stored in glass bottles in the refrigerator and can be preserved with methiolate (1:10,000) or phenol (0.5%).

Mice

- Intraperitoneal injections are usually employed with mice. Hold the mouse by its tail with the right hand and grasp it firmly between the ears with the thumb and forefinger of the left hand and turn it over.
- Hold the tail with the help of little finger of the left hand. Hold the animal's head down so that the intestine falls forward.
- Make the injection in the posterior region of the abdomen.

PROTOCOL 11.2

DOUBLE IMMUNODIFFUSION (OUCHTERLONY TECHNIQUE)

Ouchterlony technique is used to analyze complex mixtures of antigens and to make serological comparisons with related antigens. The formation of precipitin band between the antigen and the antibody depends upon the concentrations of the reactants. If the system is "balanced" a precipitate is formed between two wells containing the antigen and the antiserum.

Materials

Agar

Borate buffer

Boric acid	6.184 g
$Na_2B_4O_7.10\ H_2O$	9.536 g
NaCl	4.384 g
Distilled water up to	1000 ml

Saline

1% Methiolate

Procedure

- Heat 0.85 g agar of refined grade in 99 ml of borate saline prepared by adding 5 ml of borate buffer, pH 8.4-8.5 to 94 ml of saline.
- Pour agar containing buffered saline and a preservative, 1 ml of 1% methiolate in a Petri dish or glass plate and allow it to harden.
- Make the holes using a cork borer 7 mm in diameter and fill antiserum and antigen solutions in holes. Then keep the plates in humid boxes for several days to weeks.
- Under favourable conditions bands of precipitates appear within few hours between wells containing homologous reagents.

The number of lines of precipitates indicate the minimum number of distinct antigenic substances present in the antigenic solution. When antigen and antibody are in reservoirs of identical size and shape, the curvature of the precipitate band depends upon the relative molecular weights of antigen and antibody. Line is usually straight in the case of same molecular weight of antigen and antibody, otherwise the line tends to be concave toward the reagent of higher molecular weight.

Ouchterlony distinguished three principal types of reactions that may be observed when related antigens in adjacent wells react with antibodies against the various determinants diffusing from central reservoir. If two antigens, a and b are loaded in wells arranged equidistant from the central well containing antiserum, AB, two bands are obtained corresponding to the reactions of a and b with the respective antibodies. If a and b are serologically identical, both bands fuse completely and it is called reaction of complete identity. If a and b are not identical bands crosses each other and it is called reaction of non-identity. If a and b are partially related, a spur is formed with one of the arcs. Double spur is formed when each of the cross-reacting antigens is somewhat different from the antigen used to produce antiserum (Fig. 11.8).

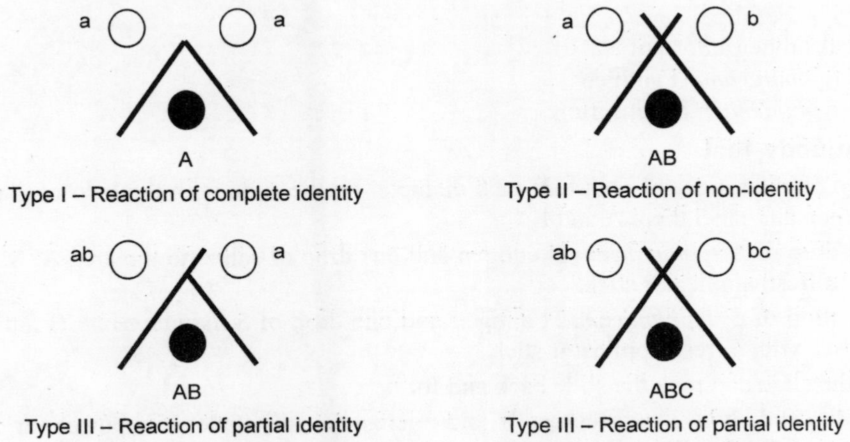

Fig. 11.8. Types of reaction in Ouchterlony gel diffusion precipitation tests.

PROTOCOL 11.3

AGGLUTINATION REACTION (THE FEBRILE ANTIBODY TEST)

Febrile antigens, such as endotoxins, enzymes and other toxic end products are elaborated upon some of the microorganisms such as salmonellae, brucellae and reckettsiae. These antigens produce febrile (fever) symptoms and febrile antibody test is used in the diagnosis of diseases that give such symptoms. These antigens are used specifically to detect or exclude the homologous antibodies that develop in response to these antigens during infection. In febrile antibody test the antigen is mixed on a slide with the serum being observed. Cellular clumping indicates the presence of homologous antibodies in the serum while the absence of antigen is indicated when no clumping of cells takes place. Febrile antibody test can also be used to detect and identify the unknown microorganism through serotyping. For this a specific antiserum is mixed with variety of unknown bacterial antigen preparations on slides. The bacterial antigen that is giving agglutination reaction is identified as a causative organism for the infection. For quantitative assay antibody titre test can be performed.

Equipment

Bunsen burner, Inoculation loop, Glass slides, Test tubes, Sterile 1ml pipettes, Mechanical pipetting device, Applicator sticks, Glassware marking pencil, Microscope.

Materials

Cultures

Suspension of *Escherichia coli*, *Proteus vulgaris*, *Shigella dysenteriae* and *Salmonellae typhimurium*.

Reagents

Physiological saline (0.85% of NaCl)
Salmonella typhimurium H antigen
Salmonella typhimurium H antiserum.

Febrile Antibody Test

- Mark two circular areas of bout half-inch diameter on the slide with the help of glassware marking pen and label them A and B.
- Add one drop of *S. typhimurium* H antigen and one drop of saline to the area A. Mix with the help of fresh applicator stick.
- Add one drop of *S. typhimurium* H antigen and one drop of *S. typhimurium* H antiserum. Mix the two with a fresh applicator stick.
- Pick up the slide and rock the slide back and forth.
- Observe the slide both macroscopically and microscopically under low power for cellular clumping or agglutination.
- Record the observations.

Serological Identification of an Unknown Organism

- Prepare two microscope slides as in the previous procedure and label four areas on the slides with the name or number code of the four unknown cultures. Into each area on both slides place one drop of *S. typhimurium* H antiserum.
- With a sterile inoculating loop, suspend a loopful of each number coded unknown culture in the drop of antiserum in its appropriately labeled area on the slides.
- Pick up the slides and slowly rock them back and forth.
- Observe both slides macroscopically and microscopically under low power for agglutination.
- Record the observation.

Determination of Antibody Titre

- Take a series of 10 test tubes in a rack and number the tube 1 to 10. Pipette 1.8 ml of 0.85% saline into the first tube and 1 ml into each of remaining nine tubes.
- Pipette 0.2 ml *Salmonella typhimurium* H antiserum in the tube 1. Mix thoroughly by pulling the fluid up and down in the pipette. The antiserum has now been diluted 10 times. Using a clean pipette, transfer 1 ml from tube 2 to tube 3.
- Continue this procedure through tube 9 and discard 1 ml from tube 9. Tube 10 will serve as the antigen control and therefore will not contain antiserum. The antiserum has been diluted during this twofold dilution to give final dilutions of 1:10, 1:20, 1: 40, 1:80, 1: 160, 1:320, 1: 640, 1:1280 and 1:2560.
- Add 1 ml of the *Salmonella typhimurium* H antigen suspension adjusted to an optical density of 0.5 at 600 nm to all tubes.
- Mix the contents of the test tubs by shaking the rack vigorously.
- Incubate the test tubs in 55°C water bath for 2 to 3 hours.

PROTOCOL 11.4

AGGLUTINATION DETERMINATION USING IMMUNOFLUORESCENCE

Material

Equipment

Micorscope slides, Petri dishes, U-shaped glass rods to fit into Petri dishes, Filter paper, Coplin jar, Glassware marking pen and fluorescence microscope.

Cultures

24 hours brain-heart infusion broth cultures of group A *Streptococcus pyogens* and group D *Enterococcus faecalis*, numbered, unknown mixed broth cultures of group A *S. pyogens*/ *E.coli* and group D *E. faecalis*/*E.coli*.

Reagents

Fluorescent antibody *Streptococcus* group A
Fluorescent antibody *Enterococcus* group D
Phosphate buffered saline (PBS)
Buffered glycerol.

Procedure

- Label two slides , *S. pyogenes* and *E. faecalis*, respectively with a glass marker pen.
- Label the third slide as unknown and mark an equal division with glass marker pen.
- Prepare a heat fixed smear of each known test organism on its appropriately labeled slide.
- On the labeled slide mix unknown and make a smear on each half of the slide using the unknown mixed culture.
- On slides labeled *S. pyogenes* and *E. faecalis*, add one drop of each respective fluorescent antibody.
- Spread gently over the surface of the smear, on the slide of the mixed unknown smears.
- Allow to spread evenly over the smears.
- Place moistened filter paper in the Petri dishes, insert the U-shaped glass rod (slide support).
- Place the prepared slides on the slide supports.
- Cover the Petri dishes and incubate for 35 minutes at 25°C.
- Remove the slides from the Petri dishes and wash away excess antibody with 1% phosphate buffered saline for 10 minutes at 25°C.
- Blot the slides dry with bibulous paper.
- To each slide add one drop of buffered glycerol, cover with a coverslip and examine under a fluorescence microscope.
- Record the observations.

PROTOCOL 11.5

DETERMINATION OF PHAGOCYTIC INDEX

Phagocytosis of Artificially Opsonized Staphylococci

- Prepare the antigen on well-grown tryptose agar slants of *Staphylococcus aureus*. Wash the organisms from each slant with about 2 ml of saline. Pool and add equal volume of 1% chrome alum in saline. Suspend them in saline and incubate at 37°C for 2 hours.
- Centrifuge at high speed and discard the supernatant liquid, then wash the cells two times by centrifugation with saline and resuspend the organisms in saline to a concentration of about 1 billion cells per ml.
- Mix 0.2 ml heparinized human blood with 0.2 ml *staphylococcus* antigen in an agglutination tube and incubate in water bath at 37°C for 30 minutes. Make smears from each tube by the usual blood smear technique, stain by the Wright's method* and examine with the oil immersion objective.

  (*Wright's method for staining: Flood with Wright's stain and after 1 minute add an equal amount of distilled water. When a greenish metallic scum or sheen appears on the surface wash with running water until the smear appears pink.)
- Count the bacteria ingested by each of the first 25 polymorphonuclear leukocytes encountered. The average number of bacteria ingested is the phagocytic index.

Opsonizing Antibodies in Serum

Opsonins for *Brucella* or *S. aureus* can be demonstrated in suitable human or animal sera. The pooled sera of about five normal individuals are used as a control.

- Cultivate the organisms on an appropriate agar medium and suspend them in saline then wash the cells three times by centrifugation with saline. Resuspend them to a concentration of about 1 billion bacteria per ml in saline or Krebs-gelatin solution, composition of which is given in Table 11.2.

Table 11.2. The composition of Krebs-gelatin solution

Material	Quantity
Gelatin (6% in 0.9% NaCl)	50 parts
0.9% NaCl	50 parts
1.15% KCl	4 parts
1.22% $CaCl_2$	3 parts
2.11% KH_2PO_4	1 part
3.82% $MgSO_4.7H_2O$	1 part
5% $NaHCO_3$	4.6 parts

- Mix 0.1 ml heparinized human blood, 0.1 ml of patient serum and 0.1 ml of bacterial suspension in an agglutination tube. Prepare a control using pooled normal serum.
- Make smears from each tube by the usual blood smear technique, stain by the Wright's method and examine with the oil immersion objective. Calculate the opsonic index of the patient's serum by dividing its phagocytic index by that of the normal serum.

PROTOCOL 11.6

TOXIN-ANTITOXIN REACTIONS

Tetanus toxin, toxoid, and antitoxin can be used to demonstrate the determination of the minimum lethal dose (M.L.D.) of toxin, neutralization of toxin by antitoxin and immunizing action of toxoid. Mice or guinea pigs can be utilized for tetanus toxin.

M.L.D. of Tetanus Toxin

- Prepare decimal dilutions of toxin from 1:100 to 1:1,000,000 using a diluent consisting of NaCl containing 1% peptone to increase the stability of toxin.
- Inject pairs of mice (approximately 20 g weight) intramuscularly in the right hind leg with 0.5 ml of toxin dilutions.
- Observe the mice at frequent intervals and note the time of paralysis and death.
- Determine the approximate M.L.D. of the toxin from the average death time of the pair of mice that received the smallest fatal dose by reference to Table 11.3. For example, if both mice injected with 0.5 ml of 1:100,000 toxin survived, and the 1:10,000 toxin contained about 4.5 M.L.D. One M.L.D. is therefore equivalent 0.5 ml of 1: 45,000 toxin
- Prepare three dilutions, one consisting of the estimated M.L.D. dilution and other differing by about 10% above and below. In the above example, dilutions of 1:40,000, 1;45,000 and 1:50,000 are employed.
- Repeat the inoculations and observations using 10 mice for each dose.

Table 11.3. Death time of mice and dosage of tetanus toxin

Death Time (hours)	No. of M.L.D.	Death Time (hours)	No. of M.L.D.	Death Time (hours)	No. of M.L.D.
12	282	60	2.3	108	1.10
18	45	66	2.0	114	1.05
24	18	72	1.74	120	1.00
30	9.8	78	1.55	126	0.96
36	6.3	84	1.41	132	0.93
42	4.5	90	1.30	138	0.90
48	3.4	96	1.21	144	0.87
54	2.8	102	1.15	150	0.85

Neutralization of Toxin by Antitoxin

- Prepare a dilution of the tetanus toxin previously titrated in saline-peptone so that each ml contains 10,000 M.L.D and dilute the tetanus antitoxin to contain 0.4 antitoxin unit per ml.
- Pipette 1.0 ml of the antitoxin dilution into each of the 6 test tubes.
- Add saline peptone as indicated in Table 11.4, then add toxin and mix the contents of each tube immediately. Allow the mixture to stand 1 hour at room temperature.
- Inject the mixture intramuscularly into two or more mice and record reaction during the next 5 days.

- Calculate the indicated free toxin (in M.L.D. units) from the observed death times and subtract from the corresponding doses of toxin injected to determine the quantity neutralized by 0.1 unit of antitoxin.

Immunizing Action of Toxoid

- Inject a dose of toxoid containing 20 flocculating units (Lf) to each of four mice subcutaneously in the back and inject an equal number of mice with 2 Lf of toxoid.
- Challenge all mice by intramuscular injection of 10 M.L.D. of tetanus toxin after 14 days and at the same time inject the same dose of toxin as a control to third group of immunized mice.
- Record reaction during the next 5 days and compare the survival times of mice immunized with the two dosage of toxoid.

Table 11.4. Neutralization of tetanus toxin by antitoxin

Antitoxin (1:) (1 ml = 0.4 unit)	Saline Peptone	Toxin (1:) (1 ml = 10,000 M.L.D.)	Dose per mouse (0.5 ml) Antitoxin	Toxin
1.0 ml	0.92 ml	0.08 ml	0.1 unit	200 M.L.D.
1.0 ml	0.87 ml	0.13 ml	0.1 unit	325 M.L.D.
1.0 ml	0.80 ml	0.20 ml	0.1 unit	500 M.L.D.
1.0 ml	0.68 ml	0.32 ml	0.1 unit	800 M.L.D.
1.0 ml	0.50 ml	0.50 ml	0.1 unit	1250 M.L.D.
1.0 ml	0.00 ml	1.00 ml	0.1 unit	2500 M.L.D.

Flocculation of Toxin or Toxoid by Antitoxin

Flocculation can be demonstrated by mixing varying amount of antitoxin with a constant amount of toxin or toxoid. The mixture is then incubated and observed constantly. The first mixture that shows visible flocculation is called indication mixture and is neutral when tested by animal inoculation. The relationship between toxin and antitoxin in the indication mixture is expressed as follows:

$$\text{ml antitoxin} \times \text{antibiotic units/ml} = \text{ml toxin} \times \text{Lf units/ml}$$

If the approximate Lf value of the toxin or toxoid is not known, preliminary titration over wide range is performed to establish the zone in which the end point is expected. Antitoxin of the known potency is used in the experiment.

- Measure antitoxin into agglutination or Wassermann tubes, the amounts varying from tube to tube by increments of 25 to 30% (e.g., 0.010 ml, 0.013 ml, 0.016 ml etc.) and add 1 to 4 ml toxin in constant amounts.
- Shake the tubes and incubate in constant temperature water bath at about 42°C. Cloudiness and fine granular precipitate appears within few minutes in some tubes and then flocculation occurs in one or more test tubes. Flocculation time may vary from few minutes to several hours. Some toxins and toxoids with low Lf value flocculate slowly and requires higher temperature.

- Calculate the approximate Lf value of the toxin or toxoids from the above equation.
- If toxin is employed, rather than toxoid, centrifuge the indication mixtures on either side and inject liquids into experimental animals to test residual toxicity.

PROTOCOL 11.7

SEPARATION OF MONONUCLEAR CELLS FROM PERIPHERAL BLOOD

Method for the separation of lymphocytes by sedimentation through a high-density medium (1.077 g/ml for human cells) is most commonly used. Mononuclear cells are obtained by centrifuging whole blood on a Ficoll-Hypaque (2.4:1) gradient (Fig. 11.9). For this premixed commercial preparations of Ficoll are also available.

Materials

Sterile balanced salt solution (BSS)
RPMI-1640 containing 2 g/l sodium bicarbonate and 20 mM HEPES heat inactivated Fetal calf serum (FCS)/pooled human AB serum
Preservative free heparin
Ficoll-Hypaque density 1.077 g/ml
Trypan blue (1.2% in BSS) for cell counting
Centrifuge
Laminar flow hood/bench
Microscope
Haemocytometer
Sterile pipettes and tips

Procedure

- Collect heparinized (10-50 U/ml) peripheral blood by vein puncture.
- Dilute the blood 2 times with balanced salt solution (BSS). Layer not more than three times the volume of diluted blood or leukocyte rich plasma (obtained by letting the blood stand for not more than an hour to allow the erythrocytes to settle down) on to a given volume of Ficoll-Hypaque. With the tube held at an angle gently layer diluted blood with a pipette on top of the Ficoll-Hypaque. Take care that the ficoll and blood do not mix while layering.
- Centrifuge at room temperature at 400g for 30 minutes using a centrifuge with brakes off so that it does not decelerate too rapidly.
- Mononuclear lymphocytes and monocytes are recovered at the ficoll plasma interface where they form a white band. The erythrocytes and polymorphonuclear cells sediment through Ficoll-Hypaque and form a pellet. Aspirate the cells at the interface without taking out too much of the ficoll as it may lead to granulocytes contamination.
- Wash the cells with large volume (3 times the volume of the suspension to be washed) of saline at 600-700g (2000-2500 rpm) for 10 minutes. (The first wash should be at a higher speed if high concentration of ficoll is used, since the increased fluid density requires either longer time or higher 'g' forces to pellet the cells.

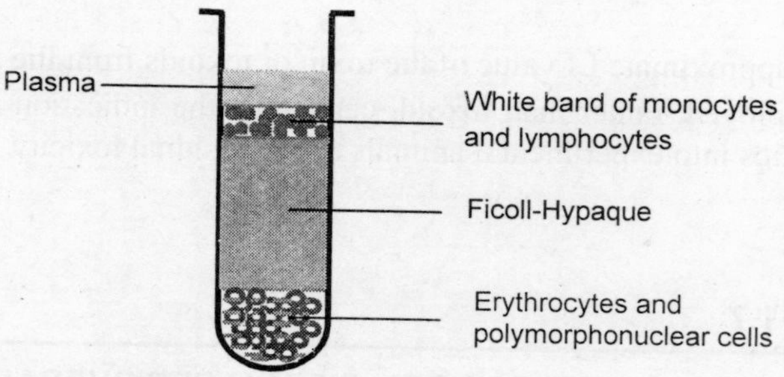

Fig. 11.9. Separation of mononuclear cells from peripheral blood by gradient centrifugation

- Remove the supernatant and mix the pellet. Add RPMI and wash twice at 100g (800-1000 rpm) for l0 minutes.
- Discard the supernatant and suspend the pellet in an appropriate medium.

This procedure yields 90-95% pure mononuclear cells with more than 98% viability.

Counting of the Lymphocytes

The haemocytometer can be used to count the lymphocytes. For details see chapter 1, Cell Culture Techniques, page no.9.

Determination of Viability

Viability of the cells can be assessed by Trypan blue exclusion. Viable cells exclude the dye thereby enabling a visual distinction between unstained viable cells and blue stained nonviable cells. Cells are stained with Trypan blue (final concentration 0.1%), and must be counted within 3 minutes as after that time viable cells may also begin to take up the dye. Since Trypan blue has a great affinity to proteins, elimination of serum from the cell diluent allows a more accurate determination of cell viability.

PROTOCOL 11.8

SEPARATION OF T AND B LYMPHOCYTES

A variety of cell separation procedures are available which can separate the various lymphocyte populations. These procedures make it possible to remove one or more cell populations from a heterogeneous population. The most commonly used procedures for separation are

- E-rosette method: for enrichment/depletion of T cells based on the affinity of sheep red blood cells (SRBC) to the CD2 antigen
- The nylon wool separation procedure: which utilizes the property of B cells and other accessory cells adherence to the nylon wool.

E-rosette Assay

This widely used technique takes advantage of the natural affinity of a component of sheep erythrocytes (SRBC) for the CD2 antigen expressed on human T cells from other species including sheep themselves also form these rosettes. Best results are obtained when incubation is carried out at 4°C, as the E-rosettes formed by normal peripheral blood lymphocytes are labile at 37°C (Fig. 11.10).

This procedure can be used to prepare either purified T or T depleted cells. These cells can be used for assays where the marker to be studied is present on both B cells and certain T cells (e. g. class II molecules).

Materials

SRBC

Alsever's solution

2-Aminoethylisothiouranium bromide

Centrifuge tubes

Tris-Ammonium Chloride lysis buffer

NH_4Cl 0.16 M (8.3 g/l)

0.17 M Tris, pH 7.65

Dissolve 20.6 g Tris base in 900 ml water; adjust pH to 7.65 with HCl. Make upto 1000 ml.

Working solution

Mix 90 ml of NH_4Cl solution and 10 ml of Tris buffer and adjust to pH 7.2 with HCl.

Preparation of SRBC

Collect sheep blood in Alsever's solution. Wash the blood to obtain erythrocytes. Carefully remove buffy-coat cells pellet to avoid spontaneous rosette formation by the sheep leukocytes themselves. Either suspend erythrocytes (final concentration 20%) in 2-aminoethyl isothio uranium bromide (0.14 M, pH 9.0) for 15 minutes at 37°C and wash 4 times or treat a 5% suspension of erythrocytes with neuraminidase (0.005 to 0.12 units per ml) for 20-60 minutes at 37°C and wash.

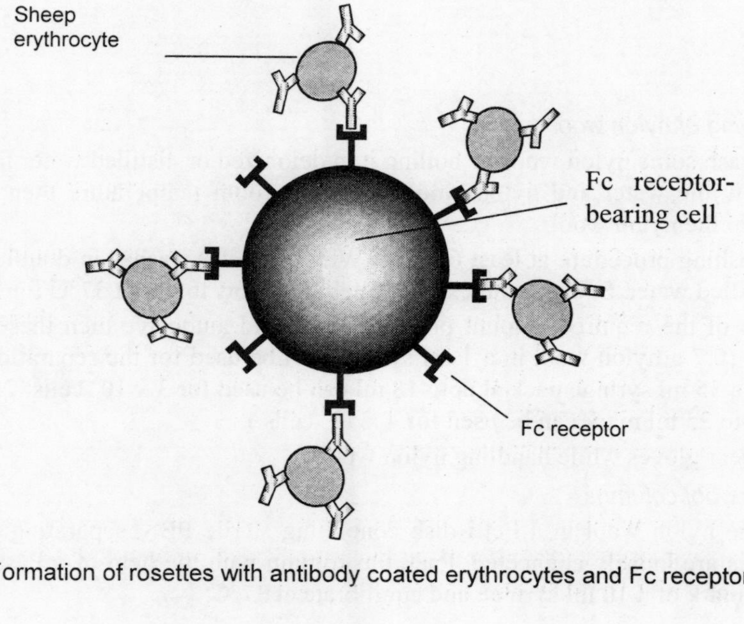

Fig.11.10. Formation of rosettes with antibody coated erythrocytes and Fc receptor bearing cells

Procedure

Lymphocytes and erythrocytes are washed immediately before use and mix erythrocytes in a ratio of 50:1 or 100:1 (optimum concentration of lymphocytes is 5-10 x 10^6 cells per ml; 1% v/v sheep erythrocyte is about 2 x 10^8 per ml). After rosette formation (60 minutes at 4°C) the cells in a centrifuge tube are gently pelleted. The supernatant will be T depleted. To obtain purified T cells the pellet is lysed with Tris buffered ammonium chloride (lysis buffer). 1ml of lysis buffer is then added to 0.1 ml packed cells. Now hold at room temperature for 2-5 minutes. dilute the sample with medium and spin down. The pellet contains RBC free T cells.

Nylon Wool Separation

The passage of cells through a nylon wool column is a simple and an effective method of obtaining a population enriched with T cells. B cells, plasma cells and some null cells pass through the column. Dead cells adhere to the column. The passed fraction therefore contains of relatively uncontaminated T cells (purity about 95-98% of input T cells). In general higher the intrinsic viability better the yield and purity. The T cells present in the effluent are representative of all T cells subpopulations. Variation in retention of cells, if observed, could be due to variation in nylon wool batches, the degree to which the column is packed, and/or the preparative washing procedures used.

Material

Nylon wool
Aluminum foil
Disposable syringe
Disposable gloves
Forceps
Sterile PBS (50 mM phosphate, 0.15 M NaCl, pH 7.4)
RPMI-1640 supplemented with 5% FCS
Pasteur pipettes
Centrifuge tubes

Procedure

Washing and drying of nylon wool

- Thoroughly wash some nylon wool by boiling it in deionized or distilled water for about 10 minutes. Allow the water and nylon wool to cool at room temperature then decant the water and drain the nylon wool.
- Repeat the washing procedure at least 6 times. With the last 2 washes in double deionized or double distilled water. Squeeze out excess water and allow to dry at 37°C for 2-3 days.
- Prepare packs of the required amount of nylon wool and autoclave then these packs are ready for use. (0.7 g nylon wool in a 1 ml syringe can be used for the separation of 4x10^7 cells; 1.8 g in a 35 ml syringe packed upto 18 ml can be used for 3 x 10^8 cells; 2.4 g in a 35 ml; packed upto 25 ml mark can be used for 4 x 10^8 cells.)

  Precaution: Wear gloves while handling nylon wool.

Packing of nylon wool columns

- Tease apart the nylon wool in a Petri dish containing sterile PBS, separating the strands until the pieces are loosely connected. Pack the column with the help of a Pasteur pipette upto the 6 ml mark of a 10 ml syringe and equilibrate at 37°C.

- Rinse the column with 5-10 ml of prewarmed (37°C) RPMI-FCS. Allow the medium run through, then load approximately 5x 10^7-10^8 cells suspended in 1 ml of prewarmed RPMI-FCS, close the stopcock after the cells have penetrated. Add an additional 0.5 ml of medium-FCS, and incubate for 30-45 minutes at 37°C.
- Collect non-adherent cells in a centrifuge tube by washing with about 20 ml of prewarmed RPMI-FCS and forcibly push fluid out with the plunger.

  (Nylon wool can be recycled by rinsing in saline followed by soaking it overnight in 0.1M HCl. Repeat the washing steps as outlined above.)

  Note : For sterile work pack syringes in autoclaved aluminium foil for all the incubations.

SUGGESTED READINGS

Cappuchino, J. G. and Sherman, N., Microbiology: A Laboratory Manual, 4th Edition, Addison-Wesley Longman, Inc. Harlow, England, 1993.

Carpenter, P. L., Immunology and Serology, Toppan Company Ltd., Tokyo, Japan, 1965.

Kemmemy, D. M. and Challacombe, S. T. (Eds.), ELISA and other Solid Phase Immunoassay: Theoretical and Practical Aspects, John Wiley and Sons, NewYork, USA, 1989.

Talwar, G. P. and Gupta, S. K. (Eds.), A Handbook of Practical and Clinical Immunology, 2nd Edition, CBS Publishers and Distributors, New Delhi, 1992.

Trehan, K., Biotechnology, Wiley Eastern Limited, New Delhi, India, 1991.

Vyas, S. P. and Dixit, V. K, Pharmaceutical Biotechnology, CBS Publishers, New Delhi, India, 1998.

Glossary

Adjuvant: Insoluble substance that increases the formation and persistence of antibodies when injected with an antigen.

Aerobic: Needing oxygen for growth.

Affinity chromatography: Used to isolate pure antibodies. A column is prepared from antigen covalently coupled to an inert solid phase such as cross-linked dextran beads. The antibody-containing solution is run into the column in neutral buffer. Specific antibody binds to the antigen, while unbound antibody and other proteins are washed through. The specific antibody is eluted using a buffer that dissociates the antigen/antibody bond. By using antibody bound to the solid phase, the technique can be used to isolate antigens. Affinity chromatography is used in bioprocess engineering for separation and purification of almost any biomolecule on the basis of its biological function or chemical structure. The molecule to be purified is specifically and reversibly absorbed by a complementary binding substance (ligand) and immobilized on a matrix. The substance of interest is first bound to the immobilized ligand and then dissociated to recover by changing experimental conditions.

Affinity labeling: Used to identify specific amino acid residue at the site where an antibody molecule binds to an antigen (paratope) by means of special haptens. These haptens have a highly reactive bond, which is activated by illumination with UV light. When bound to the antibody these bonds attach to the amino acids forming the paratope; the antibody is then denatured and the location of the covalently coupled hapten determined. See also *paratope*.

Agarose: A galactan polymer purified from agar, which forms a rigid gel with high free water content. Primarily used as electrophoretic support.

Agglutination: See *agglutinin.*

Agglutinin: An antibody that, when stimulated by the presence of the appropriate antigen, causes the clumping (agglutination) of bacteria and other cells.

Allogenic: Of the same species but with different genotype.

Amino acids: Building blocks of proteins.

Amplification: The process of increasing the number of copies of a particular gene or chromosomal sequence.

Anaerobic: Growing in absence of oxygen.

Anchorage-dependent cells or cultures: Cells, or cultures derived from the source, which will grow, survive, or maintain function only when attached to an inert surface such as glass or plastic.

Aneuploid: The nucleus of a cell when does not contain an exact of the haploid number of chromosomes, one or more chromosomes being represented more or less times than the rest is referred to as aneuploid. The chromosomes may or may not show rearrangements.

Anther culture: Refers to culture of single pollen grains or of the anther, containing the male gametophytes or microspores, with the objective of producing monoploid plants.

Antibiotic: One of many natural organic substances secreted by plants or microorganism that are toxic to other species, retard or prevent their growth and presumably function as defense mechanisms.

Antibody: Protein produced by humans and higher animals in response to the presence of a specific antigen.

Anticodon: Triplet of nucleotide bases (codon) in tRNA that pairs with its complementary triplet in mRNA. See also *Base*; *Base pair*; *Complementary*.

Antigen: A substance that, when introduced into the body, induces an immune response by a specific antibody.

Antigen-antibody binding: The binding of antibody and analyte is reversible process characterized by an association rate constant k_1 and dissociation rate constant k_2. The rate of formation of the antibody-analyte complex (Ab-Ag) is dependent on the concentration of the bound and free species.

Antigenic determinant: See *Hapten*.

Antioxidants: A substance, which is sometimes added to the sterilizing solution or to isolation medium to inhibit or prevent oxidative browning of the culture media.

Antiserum: Blood serum containing specific antibodies against an antigen. Antiserum is used to confer passive immunity to many diseases.

Antibiotic: Chemical substance formed as a metabolic byproduct in bacteria or fungi and used to treat bacterial infections. Antibiotics can be produced naturally, using microorganisms, or synthetically.

Aseptic: Free of pathogens, contaminants, algae, bacteria, fungi, viruses etc. Absence of all organisms.

Aspirate: To draw something in or out, up or through using suction or a vacuum.

Assay: To test or evaluate.

Attenuated: Weakened form of pathogenic organisms that have been treated so as to render them avirulent.

Autoclave: A closed chamber in which substances to be sterilized, are heated under pressure to above their boiling points.

Autoimmune disease: A disease in which the body produces antibodies against its own tissues.

Autoimmunity: A condition in which the body mounts an immune response against one of its own organ or tissues.

Autoradiography: Detects radioactive labeled molecules by the effect in creating an image on photographic film.

Autosome: Any chromosome other than sex chromosome.

Avirulent: Unable to cause disease.

Axillary bud proliferation: Propagation in culture by protocol and media, which promotes axillary lateral shoot growth.

Axis: The main plant stem.

B lymphocytes (B cells): A class of lymphocytes released from the bone marrow that produce antibodies.

Bacillus subtilis: A bacterium commonly used as a host in recombinant DNA experiments. Important because of its ability to secrete proteins.

Bacteriophage: Virus that lives in and kills bacteria. Also called phage.

Base: One of the four chemical units on the DNA molecule, that, according to their order and pairing, represent the different amino acids. The four bases are adenine (A), cytosine (C), guanine (G), and thymine (T). In RNA, uracil (U) substitutes for thymine.

Base pair: Two nucleotide bases on different strands of the nucleic acid molecule that bond together. The bases can pair in only one way: adenine with thymine (in DNA) or uracil (in RNA), and guanine with cytosine.

Batch culture: A cell suspension grown in liquid medium of a set volume. Inocula of successive subcultures are of similar size and cultures contain about the same cell mass at the end of each passage.

Batch processing: Growth in a closed system with a specific amount of nutrient medium. In bioprocessing, defined amounts of nutrient material and living matter are placed in a bioreactor and removed when the process is completed. See also *continuous processing*.

Bioassay: A biological assay or assessment procedure, performed on living cells or on a living organism, sometimes used to detect minute amounts of substances which influence or are essential for growth.

Biocatalyst: In bioprocessing an enzyme that activates or speeds up a biochemical reaction.

Bioconversions: Chemical restructuring of raw materials by using a biocatalyst.

Biologic response modulators: A substance that alters the growth of functioning of a cell. It includes hormones and compounds (e.g., cytokines and lymphokines) that affect the nervous and immune systems.

Biomass: The total biological matter in a given area. As commonly used in biotechnology, it refers to the total cell mass in a fermentor or bioreactor.

Bioprocess: A process in which living cells, or components thereof, are used to produce a desired end product.

Biosysthesis: Production of a chemical by a living organism.

Biotechnology: Development of products by using biological process. Production may be carried out by using intact organisms, such as yeasts' and bacteria, or by using natural substances (e.g., enzymes) from organisms.

Buffer: A substance in solution, or system that resist pH change.

Callus: Disorganized tumour like masses of plant cells that form in culture.

Capping: Occurs when antibodies bind and cross-link the surface antigens on a living cell. The antigens aggregate at one pole of the cell, appearing as a fluorescent cap. The cap is then internalized (capped off).

Captured immunoassays: Use antigen or antibody bound to the solid phase to capture molecules from the test solution that are then detected with the labeled reagents. For example, solid phase anti-IgM captures IgM from the test solution, and the antigen specific IgM is detected with a labeled antigen.

Catalyst: An agent (such as an enzyme or a metallic complex) that facilitates a reaction but is not itself changed during the reaction.

Cell count: The number of cells per unit suspension volume or callus weight. The number of cells is counted by using haemocytometer.

Cell culture: Growth of cells under laboratory conditions.

Cell fusion: See *fusion*.

Cell generation time: The interval between consecutive divisions of a cell.

Cell hybridization: The fusion of two or more dissimilar cells leading to the formation of a synkaryon.

Cell line: A cell line arises from a primary culture at the time of the first subculture. The term cell line implies that cultures from it consist of numerous lineage of cells originally present in the primary culture. The terms finite and continuous are used as prefixes if the status of the culture is known. If not, the term line will suffice. The term 'continuous line' replaces the term 'established line'.

Cell mediated immunity: Acquired immunity in which T lymphocytes play a predominant role. Development of the thymus in early life is critical to the proper development and functioning of cell mediated immunity.

Cell number: The absolute number or approximation of the number of cells per unit area of a culture or medium volume.

Cell selection: Selection of genetically different cells within a group of genetically different cells.

Cell strain: A cell strain is derived either from a primary culture or from a cell line by the selection or cloning of cells having specific properties or markers. The properties or markers must persist during subsequent cultivation. In describing a cell strain, its specific features must be defined.

Chemically defined medium: A nutritive solution for culturing cells, which contains each component of a known chemical structure is referred to as chemically defined medium. Although it is recognized that even the purest chemical compounds may have some contaminants, high quality chemicals should be used provided with analytic data, if possible, on contaminants.

Chromosomes: Threadlike components in the cell that contain DNA and proteins. Genes are carried on chromosomes.

Cistron: A length of chromosomal DNA representing the smallest functional unit of heredity, essentially identical to a gene.

Clone: A group of genes, cells, or organisms derived from a common ancestor. Because there is no combining of genetic material (as in sexual production), the members of the clone are genetically identical to the parent.

Co-capping: Used to determine whether two different cell surface antigens are independent, in which case they form separate caps with specific antibodies, or associated, when they form a single cap (co-cap).

Codon: A sequence of three nucleotide bases that specifies an amino acid or represents a signal to stop or start a function.

Coenzyme: An organic compound that is necessary for the functioning of an enzyme. Coenzyme is smaller than the enzymes themselves and sometimes separable from them.

Cofactor: A nonprotein substance required for certain enzymes to function. Cofactors can be coenzyme or metallic ions.

Colony-stimulating factors (CSFs): A group of lymphokines that induce the maturation and proliferation of white blood cells from the primitive cell types present in bone marrow.

Complement fixation test: Detects antibody (or antigen). Test antibody is mixed with the antigen and a small amount of active complement. If antibody is present, complexes form and fix the complement; if none are present, active complement remains. Active complement is detected (if complexes did not form) by adding antibody-sensitized red cells (EA), that lyse if complement is present. (To detect antigen specific antibody is mixed with the test solution and complement.)

Complementary: The relationship of the nucleotide bases on two different strands of DNA or RNA. When the bases are paired properly (adenine with thymine in DNA or uracil in RNA; guanine with cytosine), the strands are said to be complementary.

Complementary DNA (cDNA): DNA synthesized from a messenger RNA rather than from a DNA template. This type of DNA is used for cloning or as a DNA probe for locating specific genes in DNA hybridization studies.

Continuous processing: A method of bioprocesing in which new materials are added and products removed continuously at a rate that maintains the volume at a specific level. See also *Batch processing.*

Coomb's test (direct and indirect): The original haemagglutination tests to detect antibodies to red cell antigens. The direct Coomb's test identifies antibodies that are themselves capable of cross-linking the red cells. The indirect Coomb's test detect antibodies that can not crosslink the cells alone (e.g., because there are too few antigens). This is achieved by the addition of a second layer anti-antibody.

Crossed electrophoresis (Laurell): First separate antigens according to their charge in an electric field in the first dimension. Then the antigens are electrophoresed into an antibody containing gel at right angles to the first separation. In this case the area under the precipitin arcs is proportional to the antigen concentration. This technique is useful for quantitating the different forms of an antigen, or example C3 and C3c that share epitopes but have different charges.

Culture: Cultivation of living organisms in prepared medium.

Culture medium: Any nutrient system for the artificial cultivation of bacteria or other cells; usually a complex mixture of organic and inorganic materials.

Cyto: Referring to cell of cell plasma.

Cytochrome: Haem containing proteins, which transport electron by way of iron atom valency changes.

Cytogenetics: Study of the cell and its heredity-related components, especially chromosomes.

Cytoplasm: Cellular material that is within the cell membrane and surrounds the nucleus.

Cytotoxic: Able to cause cell death.

De novo: Arising sometimes spontaneous from very unknown or very simple procedure.

Deoxyribonucleic acid (DNA): The molecule that carries the genetic information for the most living systems. The DNA molecules consist of four bases (adenine, cytosine, guanine and thymine) and a sugar phosphate backbone, arranged in two connected strands to form a double helix. See also *Comlementary DNA (cDNA); Double Helix; Recombinant DNA (rDNA)*.

Diagnostic: A product used for the diagnosis of disease or medical condition. Both monoclonal antibodies and DNA probes are useful diagnostic products.

Diploid: The state of the cell in which all chromosomes, except sex chromosomes, are two in number and are structurally identical with those of the species from which the culture was derived. See also *haploid*.

Direct immunoflurescence: The antibody is covalently coupled to a fluorescent molecule, such as fluorescein or rhodamine, that is then incubated with the cells or a frozen tissue section. The antibody binds to the antigen and this is then visualized by observing the material under a microscope with incident UV light.

DNA: See *Deoxyribonucleic acid.*

DNA probe: A molecule (usually a nucleic acid) that has been labeled with a radioactive isotope dye, or enzyme and used to locate a particular nucleotide sequence or gene on a DNA molecule.

DNA sequencing: Determine the order of nucleotide bases in a DNA molecule.

Double helix: A term often used to describe the configuration of a DNA molecule. The helix consists of two spiraling strands of nucleotides (a sugar, phosphate and base) joined crosswise by specific pairing of the bases. See also *Deoxyribonucleic acid; Base pair*.

Double immunodiffusion (Ouchterlony): Used to distinguish antigens in the mixtures. The reactants are placed in holes punched in the gel and diffuse together. The precipitin arcs may show one of three patterns. When two arcs are fused this indicated identity between the antigens. If the arcs form independently the antigens are not identical. If the arcs are fused but with a spur, then the antigens are partially identical, but one antigen contains epitopes that the other lacks.

Downstream processing: The stages of processing that take place after the fermentation of bioconversion stage, which includes separation, purification and packaging of the product.

Electrophoresis: A technique used for separating different types of molecules based on their patterns of movement in an electric field.

Endonuclease: An enzyme that breaks nucleic acids at specific interior bonding sites; thus producing nucleic acid fragments of various lengths. See also *Exonuclease*.

Enzyme: A protein catalyst that facilitates specific chemical or metabolic reactions necessary for cell growth and reproduction.

Enzyme linked immunosorbant assay (ELISA): Used for detecting antibody. Antigen is adsorbed to a solid phase and test antibody is added as in radioimmunoassay; the ELISA ligand used to detect the antibody is an enzyme linked to a molecule specific for the bound antibody. Enzymes such as peroxidase and phosphatase are often used. In the final stage a chromogenic substrate is added, generating a coloured endproduct in the presence of the enzyme portion of the ligand. The optical density of this solution is measured after a defined period. This is proportional to the amount of enzyme, which in turn is related to the amount of the test antibody. By comparison with RIA, this test has the advantage of stable reagents, but is usually less sensitive.

Enzyme-mediated immunologic technique (EMIT™): In EMIT™ tests the enzyme activity corresponds to the concentration of the drug to the sample and is measured by a change in absorbance resulting from the enzyme's catalytic action on the substrate. A common coenzyme is used in NAD^+ (the oxidized form of nicotinamide adenine dinucleotide). Acting as a coenzyme, NAD^+ is converted to NADH (the reduced form of nicotinamide adenine dinucleotide), and absorbs light in the range of 450-570 nm. EMIT is a trademark of the Syva Corporation.

Equilibrium dialysis: The reference method for determining antibody affinity in which an antigen or hapten that can be separated by dialysis and the test antibody are placed in chambers on opposite side of the dialysis membrane. The system is left until the concentration of the free antigen is the same on the either side of the membrane (equilibrium), and then the solution is sampled. The average affinity (k_0) is defined as the reciprocal of the free antigen concentration when half of the antibody's combining sites are occupied, so for IgG with two sites:

$$k_0 = 1/[Ag_{free}]$$

Erythropoietin: A protein that boosts production of red blood cells. It is clinically useful in treating certain types of anaemia.

***Escherichia coli* (*E. coli*):** A bacterium that inhibits the intestinal tract of most vertebrates. Much of the work using recombinant DNA technique has been carried out with this organism because it has been well characterized genetically.

Eukaryote: A cell or organism containing a true nucleus, with a well-defined membrane surrounding the nucleus. All organisms except bacteria, virus, and blue-green algae are eukaryotic. See also *Prokaryote*.

***Ex vivo*:** Organisms removed from cultures and transplanted generally on soil or potting mixture.

Exon: The part of the gene in eukaryotic cells that is transcribed into messenger RNA and encodes a protein. See also *Intron; Splicing*.

Exonuclease: An enzyme that breaks down nucleic acids only at the ends of polynucleotide chains, thus releasing one nucleotide at a time in sequential order. See also *Endonuclease*.

Explant: Tissue taken from its original sites and transferred to an artificial medium for growth.

Explant culture: The maintenance or growth of an explant in a culture.

Expression: In genetics, manifestation of characteristics that is specified by a gene. With hereditary diseases, for example, a person can carry the genes for the disease but not actually has the disease. In this case, the gene is present but not expressed. In industrial biotechnology, the term is often used to mean the production of a protein by a gene that has been inserted into a new host organism.

Factor VII: A large, complex protein that aids in blood clotting and is used to treat haemophilia.

Fermentation: An anaerobic process of growing microorganisms for the production of various chemicals or pharmaceutical compounds. Microbes are normally incubated under specific conditions in the presence of nutrients in large tanks called fermenters.

Fluorescence enhancement: The increased fluorescence produced by haptens when bound to antibody. The energy is absorbed from the antibody and emitted with the wavelength characteristic of the hapten.

Fluorescence immunoassays (FIAs): Immunoassays analogous to RIAs, but substitute fluoresceinated reagents for the radiolabeled material. The method has the advantage that fluorescent reagents may be detected instantaneously; problems can arise with the intrinsic fluorescence of the test material and also with the availability of suitable reagents. Some fluorescent reagents respond differently when they are bound to antibody then when free. In this case it is not necessary to separate bound and free fractions of the fluorescence enhancement, fluorescence polarization, and fluorescence quenching. See also *fluorescence enhancement, fluorescence polarization, and fluorescence quenching.*

Fluorescence polarization: If polarized light is directed at a fluorescent molecule it is absorbed and emitted shortly afterwards, during which time the molecules move at random so that the fluorescent emission shows reduced polarization. If, however, the fluorescent molecule is bound to an antibody, it has less rotational freedom and the polarization of the emission will be retained to greater degree. These properties of fluorescent reagents are used in the determination of antibody affinity and avidity. The determination of the antibody affinity requires that the antigen and antibody react and reach a state of equilibrium. Since it is possible to determine the concentration of bound and free fluorescent reagents without separating them, this is a great advantage because physical separation of the free and bound antigen may disturb the equilibrium conditions. Unfortunately suitable fluorescent reagents are available for a new antigens and antibodies.

Fluorescence quenching: The reduction of fluorescence emitted by an antibody (or antigen) when it forms a complex. For example, this occurs when a hapten, that absorbs radiation at 350 nm, binds to an antibody. Normally, antibody illuminated at 280 nm fluoresces at 350 nm; but if the hapten is bound at the binding site, some of the fluorescence is absorbed (quenched).

Frameshift: Insertion of deletion of one or more nucleotide bases such that incorrect triplets of bases are read as codons.

Fusion: Joining of the membrane of two cells, thus creating a daughter cell that contains the nuclear material from parent cells. Used in making hybridoma.

Fusogen: A fusion-inducing agent used for protoplast agglutination in somatic hybridization studies e.g. PEG or Sendai viruses.

Gene: A segment of the chromosomes. Some genes direct the syntheses of proteins, while others have regulatory functions. See also *Operator gene; Regular gene; Structural gene; Suppressor gene.*

Gene machine: A computerized device for the synthesizing genes by combining nucleotides (bases) in the proper order; also used by Pharmacia/LKB Biotechnology as the trade name for their automated synthesizer unit.

Gene mapping: Determination of the relative position of genes in DNA or RNA.

Gene sequencing: Determination of the sequence of the nucleotide bases in a strand of DNA; also called DNA sequencing.

Gene therapy: The replacement of a defective gene in an organism suffering from a genetic disease. Recombinant DNA techniques are used to isolate the functioning gene and insert it into cells. Over 300 single-gene genetic disorders have been identified in humans. A significant percentage of these may be amenable to gene therapy.

Genetic code: The mechanism by which genetic information is stored in living organisms. The code uses sets of three nucleotide bases (codons) to make the amino acids that, in turn, constitute proteins.

Genetic engineering: A technology used to alter the genetic material of living cells in order to make them capable of producing new substances or performing new functions.

Genome: The total hereditary material of a cell, comprising the entire chromosomal set found in each nucleus of a given species.

Genotype: Genetic make-up of an individual or group. See also *Phenotype*.

Growth hormone: Proteins produced from the pituitary gland and involved in cell growth. Growth hormones are sometimes added to mammalian cell cultures, *in vitro,* to increase cell and/or endproduct yield in a given time. Also called somatotropins.

Haploid: A cell with half the number of chromosomes, or only one chromosome set. Sex cells are haploid. See also *Diploid.*

Hapten: The portion of an antigen that determines its immunological specificity (antigenic determinant). When coupled to a large protein, a hapten stimulates the formation of antibodies to the two molecule complex. Also called antigenic determinant.

Haemagglutination: Clumping (agglutination) of red blood cells.

Haemagglutination test: This term covers a number of techniques for detecting antibodies, based on the agglutination of red blood cells. The antigen may either be a red cell antigen, or the antigen (sensitizing antigen) required can be chemically linked to the cell surface. For the test, the antibody is titrated in wells and red cells added. If antibody to the red cell is present the cells are agglutinated and sink as a mat to the bottom of the well, but if it is absent they roll down the sloping sides of the well to form a pellet.

Heterokaryon: Genetically different nuclei, irrespective of their number, in a common cytoplasm, usually derived as a result of cell to cell fusion.

Heteroploid: The term is referred to a cell culture where the cells constituting the culture possess nuclei containing chromosome numbers other than the diploid number. This is a term used only to describe individual cells. Thus, a heteroploid culture should be one, which contains aneuploid cells.

Histocompatibility: Immunological similarity of tissues such that grafting can be done without tissue rejection.

Histocompatibility antigen: An antigen that causes the rejection of grafted material from an animal different in genotype from the host animal.

Homokaryon: Genetically identical nuclei, irrespective of their number, in a common cytoplasm, usually derived as a result of cell fusion.

Homologous: Corresponding or alike in structure, position, or origin.

Hormone: A chemical that acts a messenger or stimulator signal, relaying instructions to stop or start certain physiological activities. Hormones are synthesized in one type of cell and then released to direct the function of other cell types.

Host: A cell or organisms used for growth of a virus, plasmid, or other form of foreign DNA, or for the production of cloned substances.

Host-vector system: Combination of DNA receiving cells (host) and DNA reporting substances (vector) used for introducing foreign DNA into a cell.

Humoral immunity: Immunity resulting from circulating antibodies in plasma protein.

Hybridization: Production of offspring, or hybrids, from genetically dissimilar parents. The process can be used to produce hybrid plants (by crossbreeding two different varieties) or hybridomas (hybrid cells formed by fusing two unlike cells, used in producing monoclonal antibodies). The term is also used to refer to the binding of complementary strands of DNA or RNA.

Hybridomas: The cell produced by fusing two cells of different origin. In monoclonal antibody technology, hybridomas are formed by fusing an immortal cell (one that divides continuously) and an antibody-producing cell. See also *Monoclonal antibody*; *Myeloma.*

Immune system: The aggregation of cells, biological substances (such as antibodies), and cellular activities that work together to provide resistance to disease.

Immunity: Non-susceptibility to a disease or to the toxic effect of antigenic material. See also *Active immunity; Natural passive immunity; Passive immunity.*

Immunoabsorbents: Solid phase antigens or antibodies including cells, chemically cross-linked antigen precipitates, and proteins coupled to solid supports.

Immunoabsorption: Used to specifically remove particular antibodies from a solution, by the addition of a solid phase antigen immunoabsorbants.

Immunoassays: Techniques for identifying substances based on the use of antibodies.

Immunodiagnostics: The use of specific antibodies to measure a substance. This tool is useful in diagnosing infectious disease and the presence of foreign substances in a variety of human and animal fluid (blood, urine, etc.). It is currently being investigated as a way of locating tumour cells in the body.

Immunoelectrophoresis (EIP): A technique in which mixture of antigens are first separated in an electric field according to their charge, and are then precipitated with antiserum from a trough lying parallel to the separated antigens.

Immunofluorescence: Technique for identifying antigenic material that uses antibody labeled with fluorescent material. Specific binding of the antibody and antigen can be seen under a microscope by applying UV light rays and noting the visible light that is procured.

Immunogen: Any substances that can elicit an immune response.

Immunoglobulin: General name for proteins that function as antibodies. These proteins differ somewhat in structure and are grouped into five categories on the basis of these differences: (1) Immunoglobulin G (IgG), (2) Immunoglobulin M (IgM), (3) Immunoglobulin A (IgA), (4) Immunoglobulin D (IgD), and (5) Immunoglobulin E (IgE).

Immunology: Study of all phenomena related to the body's response to antigenic challenge (i.e., immunity, sensitivity, and allergy).

Immunomodulators: A diverse class of proteins that boost the immune system. Many are cell growth factors (e.g., cytokines, lymphokines) that accelerate the production of specific cells that are important in mounting an immune response in the body.

Immunoradiometric assay (IRMA): A test for antigen in which excess specific labeled antibody is added to the test antigen. The test antigen binds and neutralizes some of the antibody. The remaining free antibody is removed by adding solid phase antigen. The labeled antibody still in solution is the proportion bound to the test antigen; the radioactivity of the solution is proportional to the amount of test antigen.

Immunotoxins: Specific monoclonal antibodies that have a protein toxin molecule attached. The monoclonal antibody is targeted against a tumour cell and the toxin is designed to kill that cell when the antibody binds to it. Immunotoxins have also been termed magic bullets.

In situ: In the natural, original place or position.

***In vitro*:** Literally, in glass. Performed in test tube or other laboratory apparatus.

***In vivo*:** In the living organisms.

Incubate: To maintain under conditions favourable for development often in an incubator. The process is called as incubation.

Incubation: See *incubate*.

Inducer: A molecule or substance that increases the rate of enzyme synthesis, usually by blocking the action of the corresponding repressor. See also *Repressor*.

Inoculate: To introduce something into.

Interferon: A class of lymphokine proteins important in the immune response. There are three major types of interferon: alpha (leukocyte), beta (fibroblast) and gamma (immune). Interferons inhibit viral infections and may have anticancer properties.

Interleukin: A type of lymphokine whose role in the immune system is being extensively studied. Two types of interleukins have been identified. Interleukin 1 (IL-1), derived from macrophages, is produced during inflammation and amplifies the production of other lymphokines, notably interleukin 2 (IL-2). IL-2 regulates the maturation and replication of T lymphocytes.

Intron: A sequence of DNA in eukaryotic cells that is contained in the gene but does not encode for protein. The presence of intron "splits" the coding region of the gene into segments called exons. See also *Exon*; *Splicing*.

Isoenzymes: One of the several forms that a given enzyme can take. The forms may differ in certain physical properties, but function similarly as biocatalysts.

Isogenic: Of the same genotype.

Kidney plasminogen: A pecursor to the enzyme urokinase that has blood-clotting properties.

laurell electrophoresis: See *Crossed electrophoresis; Rocket electrophoresis*.

Lecithin: A naturally occurring choline containing phospholipid present in animal and plant tissue.

Leukocyte: A colourless cell in the blood, lymph, and tissues that is an important component of the body's immune system; also called white blood cell.

Library: A set of clone DNA fragment.

Ligand conjugates: Two molecules covalently coupled together (e.g., RIA ligands are usually antibody molecules or protein-A, covalenly bound to ^{125}I or another tracer).

Ligase: An enzyme used to join DNA or RNA segments together; called DNA ligase and RNA ligase respectively.

Linkage: The tendency for certain genes to be inherited together due to their physical proximity of the chromosome.

Linker: A fragment of DNA with a restriction site that can be used to join DNA strands.

Lipoproteins: A class of serum proteins that transport lipids and cholesterol in the bloodstream. Abnormalities in the lipoprotein metabolism have been implicated in certain heart diseases.

Liposomes: Thermodynamically stable vesicular structures consisting of one or more concentric spheres of lipid bilayers separated by water or aqueous compartments.

Lymphokine: A class of soluble proteins produced by white blood cells that play a role, as yet not fully understood, in the immune response. See also *Interferon*; *Interleukin.*

Lymphoma: Form of cancer that affects the lymph tissue.

Lysis: Breaking apart of cells.

Lysozyme: An enzyme present in, for example, tears, saliva, egg whites, and some plant tissues, that destroys the cells of certain bacteria.

Macrophage: A type of white blood cell produced in blood vessels and loose connective tissues that can ingest dead tissue and cells and is involved in producing interleukin-1 (IL-1). When exposed to the lymphokine " macrophage-activating factor," macrophage also kills tumour cells. See also *Phagocyte*.

Macrophage-activating factor (MAF): An agent that stimulates macrophages to attack and ingest cancer cells.

Messenger RNA (mRNA): Nucleic acid that carries instructions to a ribosome for synthesis of a particular protein.

Monoclonal: Highly specific, purified antibody that is derived from only one clone of cells and recognizes only one antigen. See also *Hybridoma*; *Myeloma.*

Monoclonal antibody: An antibody produced from a clone of cells making only that particular antibody.

Monolayer: A single layer of cells growing on a surface.

Multigenic: Of hereditary characteristics, one that is specified by several genes.

Mutagen: A substance that induces mutations.

Mutaion: A change in genetic material of a cell.

Mutant: A cell that manifests new characteristics due to change in DNA.

Muton: The smallest element of chromosomes whose alteration can result in a mutation or a mutant organism.

Myeloma: A type of tumour cell that is used in monoclonal antibody technology to form hybridoma.

Natural active immunity: Immunity that is established after the occurrence of a disease.

Natural killer (NK) cell: A type of leukocytes that attacks cancerous or virus-infected cells without previous exposure to the antigen. NK cell activity is stimulated by interferon.

Natural passive immunity: Immunity conferred by the mother on the foetus or newborn.

Nuclease: An enzyme that, by cleaving chemical bonds, breaks down nucleic acids into their constituent nucleotides. See also *Exonuclease*.

Nucleic acid: Large molecules, generally found in the cell's nucleus and/or cytoplasm, that are made up of nucleotide bases. The two kinds of nucleic acid are DNA and RNA.

Nucleotides: The building block of nucleic acids, each nucleotide is composed of sugar, phosphate, and one of free nitrogen bases (one base is for RNA). The sequence of the bases within the nucleic acid determines what proteins will be made.

Nucleus: The structure within eukaryotic cells that contains chromosomal DNA.

Oligonucleotide: A polymer consisting of a small number (about two to ten) of nucleotides.

Oncogene: Gene thought to be capable of producing cancer.

Oncogenic: Cancer causing.

Oncology: Study of tumours.

Operator gene: A region of the chromosome, adjacent to the operon, where a repressor protein binds to prevent transcription of the operon.

Operon: Sequence of genes responsible for synthesizing the enzymes needed for biosynthesis of a molecule. An operon is controlled by an operator gene and a repressor gene.

Opsonin: An antibody that renders bacteria and other antigenic material susceptible to destruction by phagocytes.

Organ culture: The maintenance or growth of organ primordia or the whole or part of an organ *in vitro* in such a way that it allows differentiation and preservation of the architecture and the cellular function also.

Paratope: The site on an antibody molecule that attaches to antigen. See also *Affinity labeling*.

Passage number: The number of times the cells in a culture have been subcultured.

Passage: The transfer or transplantation of cells from one culture vessel to another. This term is synonymous to 'subculture'.

Passive Immunity: Immunity acquired from receiving preformed antibodies.

Peptide: Two or more amino acids joined by a linkage called a peptide bond.

Phage: See *Bacteriophage*.

Phagocyte: A type of white blood cell that can ingest invading microorganisms and other foreign material. See also *Macrophage*.

Phagocytosis: The process in which particulate matter is ingested by a cell, involving engulfment of that matter by the cell's membrane.

Phenotype: Observable characteristics, resulting from interaction between an organism's genetic make-up and the environment. See also *Genotype*.

Plasmaphoresis: A technique used to separate useful factors from the blood.

Plasmid: A small circular form of DNA that carries certain form of genes and is capable of replicating independently in the host cell.

Polyclonal: Derived from different types of cells.

Polymerase: General term for enzymes that carry out the synthesis of nucleic acids.

Polypeptide: Long chain of amino acids joined to peptide bond.

Precipitin reaction: When antigen and antibody reacts together near their equivalence point, they often form cross-linked precipitates. If the reaction occurs in free solution the concentration of Ab-Ag complex can be determined by measuring increased turbidity with a nephelometer. If the reaction occurs in the supporting medium, such as agar gel, the reactants form precipitin arcs that can be used to identify antigens and antibodies in complex mixtures.

Primary culture: A culture started from cells, tissues, or organs taken directly from organisms. A primary culture may be regarded as such, until it is subcultured for the first time.

Probe: See *DNA probe*.

Prokaryote: An organism (e.g., bacterium, virus, blue-green algae) whose DNA is not enclosed within the nuclear membrane. See also *Eukaryote*.

Promoter: A DNA sequence that is located in front of a gene and controls gene expression. Promoters are required for binding of RNA polymerase to initiate transcription.

Prophage: Phage nucleic acid that is incorporated into the host's chromosomes but does not cause cell lysis.

Protein-A: A protein produced by the bacterium *Staphylococcus aureus* that specifically binds antibodies. It is useful in the purification of monoclonal antibodies.

Radioallergosorbent Test (RAST): Specific form of RIA for detecting antigen specific IgE, in which antigen is covalently coupled to cellulose discs. Antigen-specific IgE binding to the disc is detected using radiolabeled anti-IgE.

Radioimmunoassay (RIA): A technique for quantifying a substance by measuring the reactivity of radioactivity labeled forms of the substance with antibodies, and includes a variety of techniques that use Radiolabeled reagents to detect antigen or antibody. Antibody may be detected using plates sensitized with antigen. Test antibody is applied and this is detected by the addition of a radiolabeled ligand specific for that antibody. The amount of ligand bound to the plate is proportional to the amount of test antibody.

Radioimmunosorbant Test (RIST): A competitive RIA test used for the detection of IgE (the antigen), in which test IgE is competed with labeled IgE on plates sensitized with anti-IgE.

Recombinant DNA (rDNA): The DNA formed by combining segments of DNA from different types of organisms.

Recombinant DNA technology: See *Genetic engineering*.

Regulator gene: A gene that acts to control the protein synthesizing activity of other genes.

Replication: Reproduction or duplication (e.g., as in replication of an exact of a strand of DNA).

Replicon: A segment of DNA (e.g., chromosomes or plasmid) that can replicate independently.

Repressor: A protein that inhibits transcription of a gene by binding to an operator adjacent to a structural gene.

Restriction enzyme: An enzyme that breaks DNA in highly specific locations, creating gaps into which new genes can be inserted.

Retrovirus: An animal virus that contains the enzyme reverse transcriptase. This enzyme converts viral RNA into DNA that can combine with the DNA of the host cell to produce more viral particles.

Reverse transcription: Mechanism for RNA synthesis in which the RNA viruses use their RNA genome as a template for an RNA directed polymerase.

Ribonucleic acid (RNA): A molecule similar to DNA that functions primarily to decode the instructions for protein synthesis that are carried by genes. See also *Messenger RNA (mRNA); Transfer RNA (tRNA)*.

Ribosome: A cellular component containing protein and RNA that is involved in protein synthesis.

RNA polymerase: An enzyme that catalyses the formation of RNA on DNA templates.

Rocket elecrophoresis (Laurell): A modification of single radical immunodiffusion (SRID) in which antigens are quantitated by electrophores them through an antibody-containing gel, the pH of which is selected so that the antibodies are naturally charged and immobile. The antigen moves towards the anode, forming a rocket shaped precipitin arc where the height of the rocket is proportional to antigen concentration.

Sandwich immunoassays: Used to detect antibodies in systems where the test antibody acts as a bridge between solid phase unlabeled antigen and labeled antigen. The labeled antigen will only stick if specific antibody is present to bridge it to the solid phase.

Scale-up: Transition from small-scale production to production of large industrial quantities.

Secondary culture: A culture arising from the passage of a primary culture.

Selective medium: Nutrient material constituted such that it will support the growth of specific organisms while inhibiting the growth of others.

Single-cell proteins: Cell or protein extract from microorganisms grown in large quantities for use as protein supplement.

Southern analysis: Technique that uses DNA probes to detect the presence of specific DNA in restriction fragments separated by electrophoresis.

Splicing: The removal of introns and joining of exons to form a continuous coding sequence in RNA.

Stem cells: Formative cells blood cells capable of producing various types of differentiated cells.

Sterilize: Processes to make any milieu free from microorganisms.

Structural gene: A gene that codes for a protein, such as an enzyme.

Substrate: The substance used up during a reaction.

Suppressor gene: A gene that can reverse the effect of a mutation in other gene.

Suspension culture: A type of culture in which the cells multiply while suspended in the medium without becoming attached to an inert surface.

Svedberg unit (S): The unit in which the sedimentation coefficient of a particle is commonly expressed as S, when values are given in seconds, the basic unit is 10^{-13}.

T lymphocytes (T cells): White blood cells that are produced in the bone marrow but mature in the thymus. They are important in the body's defense against certain bacteria and fungi, help B-lymphocyte make antibodies, and help in the recognition and rejection of foreign tissue. T-lymphocytes may also be important in the body's defense against cancers.

Template: A molecule that serves as the pattern for synthesizing another molecule.

Thymus: A lymphoid organ in the lower neck, the proper functioning of which in early life is necessary for development of the immune system; the *in vivo* source of mature T cells.

Tissue culture: The maintenance or growth of tissues, *in vitro*, in a way that may allow differentiation and preservation of the architecture and conserves the functions also.

Toxin: Antigenic substance produced by microorganisms.

Toxoid: An inactivated antigen.

Transcription: Synthesis of messenger (or any other) RNA on a DNA template.

Transduction: Transfer of genetic material from one cell to another by means of virus or phage vector.

Transfection: Infection of a cell with nucleic acid from a virus, resulting in replication of the complete virus.

Transfer RNA (tRNA): RNA molecule that carries amino acids to sites on ribosomes where protein is synthesized.

Transformation: Change in genetic structure of an organism by incorporation of foreign DNA.

Transgenic organism: An organism formed by the insertion of foreign genetic material into the germ cell-lines of organisms. Recombinant DNA technique is commonly used to produce transgenic organisms.

Translation: Process by which the information on a messenger RNA molecule is used to direct the synthesis of a protein.

Transposon; A segment of DNA that can move around and be inserted at several sites in bacterial DNA or in a phage, thus, altering the host's DNA.

Tumour necrosis factor (TNFs): Rare protein of the immune system that appears to destroy some types of tumour cells without affecting healthy cells.

Vaccine: A preparation that contains an antigen consisting of whole disease causing organisms (killed or weakened), or parts of such organisms, used to confer immunity against the disease that the organisms cause. Vaccine preparation can be natural, synthetic, or derived by recombinant DNA technology.

Vector: The agent (e.g., plasmid or virus) used to carry new DNA into a cell.

Virion: An elementary viral particle consisting of genetic material and a protein covering.

Virus: A submicroscopic organisms that contains genetic information but can not produce itself. To replicate, it must invade another cell and use part of the cell's reproductive machinery.

Western blotting: A technique that uses antibodies to detect the presence of specific protein separated by antibodies.

Yeast: A general term for single-celled fungi that reproduce by budding. Many yeast can ferment carbohydrates.

Index

A

B

C

D

H

I

K

L

M

N

O

P

R

S

T

V

W

Y

3 1896 00116 1839

DATE DUE